COMPLETE REPERTORY

TO THE

HOMŒOPATHIC

MATERIA MEDICA.

LONDON :

W. DEWICK AND SONS, STEAM PRINTERS, 46, BARBICAN, CITY.

COMPLETE REPERTORY

TO THE

HOMŒOPATHIC

MATERIA MEDICA.

—o—

Second Edition.

—o—

REVISED, RE-ARRANGED, AND VERY MUCH ENLARGED.

DISEASES OF THE EYES.

———

BY E. W. BERRIDGE, M.D.,

Bachelor of Medicine and Bachelor of Surgery of the University of London;
Doctor of Medicine (by Examination) of the Homœopathic College of Pensylvania;
Formerly Resident Medical Officer to the Liverpool Homœopathic Dispensary.

Author of "Index to Cases of Poisoning in the Allopathic Journals;" "Pathogenetic Record," Contributions to the "American Journal of Homœopathic Materia Medica," "North American Journal of Homœopathy," "Hahnemannian Monthly," "Hering's Complete Materia Medica," "Monthly Homœopathic Review," "Gregg's Homœopathic Quarterly," "British Journal of Homœopathy," &c. &c.

—oo—

ἡ δέ Κρίσις χαλεπή.

—oo—

Entered at Stationer's Hall.

LONDON:

ALFRED HEATH, 114, EBURY STREET.

A

symp

can

each

Symp

Conco

sectio

C. Ge

and F

Aggra

these

peculia

ing, a

* F

impossil

with ea

ias beg

agethe

athica

temen

z give

khem

along

ay b

: the

iw th

' in

e,

PREFACE.

A PERFECT Repertory should contain a reference to *every* symptom of the Materia Medica under *every* rubric where it can possibly be looked for. To effect this, I have divided each chapter of this Repertory into two Sections: I.—The *Symptoms* themselves; and II.—Their *Conditions*, (including *Concomitants*).* Section I. is further divided into five sub-sections: A. Functional Symptoms; B. Anatomical Regions; C. General Character, Sequence, and Direction; D. Right Side; and E. Left Side: and Section II. into two subsections; A. Aggravations; and B. Ameliorations. All the symptoms in these sub-sections are arranged *alphabetically*, excepting the *peculiar symptoms*, which, not falling under any general heading, are placed last. All symptoms of a nearly identical

---

* Here we discover the great value of *Clinical Cases*. It is often difficult or impossible to decide from the provings *alone* what symptoms are really connected with each other; because, if the prover has repeated the dose after the medicine has begun to act on him, the symptoms produced by the different doses are mixed up together—a *rudis indigestaque moles:* whereas, if a group of symptoms is cured homœopathically, there can be no doubt of the necessary connection of its constituent elements. (Hence in a Materia Medica, such clinical symptoms should always be given in their integrity *as a group*, and not be merely scattered throughout the Schema under the various rubrics to which their constituent elements respectively belong.) In making use of such a clinical confirmation, however, we must not only be sure that it is a *cure* and not a *recovery*; but that the case has been cured by the *Homœopathic* and not by the *Allopathic* or *Antipathic* action of the medicine. For this reason, cases cured rapidly, permanently, and without perturbative action, by single doses of high potencies, without the use of auxiliaries of any kind, are the *most*, if not the *only*, reliable ones.

meaning are placed under the same rubric, according to the Table of Synonyms.

The *Conditions* including the *Concomitants*, are arranged in 23 groups as follows :—(1) Time, (2) Situation and External Influences, (3) Posture, (4) Touch, (5) Motion, (6) Head (including Mental Symptoms), (7) Eyes, (8) Ears, (9) Nose, (10) Face and Front of Neck, (11) Teeth, (12) Mouth, and Throat, (13) Abdomen (including Stomach, Anus, and all Functional Symptoms thereof, (14) Urinary Organs, (15) Sexual Organs, (16) Chest and Larynx, (17) Back and Nape of Neck, (18) Arms, (19) Legs, (20) Sleep, (21) Fever, (Chills, Heat, and Sweat), (22) Generalities (including Skin, Bones, Convulsions, Other Drugs, &c.)

The arrangement of the symptoms in Section II is in every respect exactly the same as that of Section I.

In the sub-section I. C. *Direction*, the symptoms are given in the chapter belonging to the organ in which they *commence*, thus " Shooting from Eyeball to Head " is given in the sub-section I. C. of the chapter on " Eyes," but not in that on " Head."

Sometimes in a complex group of symptoms one symptom *follows* another ; in this case if they are both in the *same* organ they are given in Section I., sub-section C. ; if in *different* organs, in Section II. Thus " Blindness followed by Heat in Eyes " would be given in I. C. under the rubric " *Symptoms Changing Character ;*" but " Blindness followed by Heat in Head," would be given in II under rubric " *Before Head Symptoms*," and also in the Head Chapter under " *After Eye Symptoms.*"

As our Materia Medica is still incomplete, we are often obliged to select the remedy to a certain extent *by Analogy* ;

hence we require a Collective view of the medicines acting on any organ which agree as to *Specific Character, Anatomical Regions, General Character, Sequence, Direction, Sides,* and *Conditions* (including *Concomitants*).

In order to give Collectives according to *Specific Character,* the following plan has been adopted :—Under every rubric in I. A., and in the *principal* subdivision of I. B., are placed all the medicines from all the other subdivisions which agree in that particular point ; and also all the varieties of that symptom which are given separately ; *enclosed in brackets.* Thus under "Shooting in Eyeball" are placed *bracketed* the medicines possessing any *variety* of Shooting which may be given separately, or Shooting in *right* or *left* eye separately, or Shooting in any *subregion* of eye (*e.g.* Orbit), or Shooting in any *direction* in eye, or Shooting *to or from eye from or to any other organ.* When a symptom refers necessarily to one subregion *only* (*e.g.* Closing of Eyelids), this collective is given there. In I. A. and I. B., the medicines not bracketed affect both sides *simultaneously ;* if either is affected separately, it is given in I. D. or I. E.

Collectives of medicines agreeing with regard to *Anatomical Regions,* the chief divisions of the *Functional Symptoms, General Character, Sequence, Direction,* and *Sides,* are given under their respective rubrics, and in *these* collectives doubtful symptoms *only* are bracketed. In these collectives also, the principal one contains the less ; thus under the general rubric "Eye to Face" are given all the medicines which have any variety of the above, *e.g.* "Eye to Lower Jaw," to make the collective complete ; but, "Shooting from Eyeball to Lower Jaw" is given under the latter rubric only, and not under both. In the rubrics "Changing or Alternating in Character or Place in Eye," collectives as to the *varieties* of change of character or place are also given ; thus we have collectives of "Eyeball then Orbit," "Heat then Shooting," &c., &c.

In the Rubrics "Right then Left," "Above then Below," and the reverse, Clinical symptoms are marked with an *asterisk*, to facilitate the application of Hering's Law of *Inverse Directions.*

To make the *Conditions* as useful as possible, we require to show (1) the conditions belonging to any symptom in the *whole body*; (2) those belonging to the *organ generally*; (3) those belonging to each *Anatomical Region*; (4) those belonging to each *variety of symptom* in the organ irrespective of the subregion to which it belongs; and (5) those belonging to *each symptom* separately. Thus, under the Rubric "By Reading" we have (1) the medicines found under this condition which have reference to *any* part of the body (this will be given in the General Chapter which will resemble Bœnninghausen's *Taschenbuch*); (2) those belonging to the *entire organ* which is the subject of each chapter; (3) those belonging to each *Anatomical Region, e.g.* Orbit; (4) those belonging to each *variety of symptom* in whatever subregion of the organ it may be; and (5) those belonging to *each individual symptom.* I have accordingly divided this Repertory into 17 chapters; the list of which will be found above where the groups of the Conditions are referred to.

In the last—the General—Chapter, the arrangement is similar to that of the preceding ones. First is the arrangement according to *Specific Character*, the medicines to which belong any *variety of symptom*, (*e.g.* Shooting) in *any* part of the body being arranged under their respective rubrics (as in Bœnninghausen's *Taschenbuch*); next comes the arrangement according to *Tissues* (*e.g.* Glands, Skin, Bones, Entire Body, &c). which corresponds to the Anatomical Regions of the preceding chapters; followed by *General Character Sequence* and *Direction*, *Right Side*, and *Left Side*, just as before. In the *Conditions* of this chapter the same rule is observed; thus, under aggravation " By Warmth " we have (1) a collective of all the medicines having aggravation of *any symptom* by warmth; (2) those having aggravation of any particular *variety of symptom* (*e.g.* Shooting) in *any* part of the body; (3) those having aggravation of any *Tissue* (*e.g.* Bones); and (4) those having aggravation of *any variety of symptoms in each of these tissues.* In this chapter *only* doubtful symptoms are bracketed.

With regard to the abbreviations of the names of the medicines, I have adopted an uniform and scientific method of cyphering, as it is quite time that such absurd names as Hepar Sulphuris, Alcohöl Sulphuris, &c., be discarded for a more scientific nomenclature. The cyphers of the *elements* and *simple haloid salts* are the same as their *chemical symbols;* the —*ate* salts are cyphered by adding —*a*, and the —*ite* salts by adding —*i*, to the cyphers of the corresponding haloid salt. The —*ic* acids are cyphered by adding —*x*, the —*ous* acids adding —*ix*, and the *hydracids* by adding —*hx* to the cypher of the element or compound radical from which they are formed. Thus :

Na. = Sodium.	S. = Sulphur.
Na-s.=Sulphide of Sodium.	S-x. = Sulphuric acid.
Na-sa.=Sulphate of Sodium.	S-ix. = Sulphurous acid.
Na-si.=Sulphite of Sodium.	S-hx. = Sulphydric acid.

In the medicines derived from the Animal and Vegetable kingdoms, each genus is invariably expressed by a different cypher and by that only.

Hahnemann and Bœnninghausen insisted upon the necessity of having the medicines in a Repertory distinguished by *different types* to show their relative value, but hitherto such classification has been entirely arbitrary. The plan I propose is based entirely on the *provings*, not on the clinical experience of any one individual, and shows the relative frequency with which any symptom has been produced, compared with every other symptom of the Materia Medica.

This plan, however, cannot be satisfactorily carried out till we have a complete Materia Medica arranged like that of C. Hering, but I give it here for future adoption if thought useful. It is this—count the number of distinct *Pathogenetic* symptoms of each medicine obtained from *different* provers irrespective of their conditions or concomitants; those symptoms being considered distinct which are given as such in this Repertory. Thus if " Dilated Pupils " has been produced by a medicine on 20 *different* provers, it is counted as *twenty* symptoms; but if 20 times in the *same* prover, only as *one*, even though the conditions and concomitants should vary each time. Then if the total number of *provers* upon whom a symptom of any medicine has occured amounts to 1-25th of the total number of symptoms of the medicine obtained as stated above, the medicine producing that symptom is placed in the first rank, *Italic Capitals*; if from 1-50th to 1-25th, in the second rank, *Plain Capitals;* if from 1-75th to 1-50, in the third rank, *Italics;* if below 1-75rd in the fourth rank, *Roman Letters.* Clinical symptoms never rise above the fourth rank, and all *doubtful* symptoms are bracketed. The names of medicines enclosed in brackets for reference (as in the collectives of Specific Character) are invariably in *Roman letters.* In the *Conditions* the same rule is observed, as also in the Collectives of *Anatomical Regions, General Character, Sequence, Direction, Right Side,* and *Left Side;* the rank of the medicine being decided according to the number of *provers* whose symptoms refer to each respective rubric.

C. Hering's Materia Medica, which is the most complete in arrangement and execution of any yet published, has been used so far as it has extended (*i. e.* up to *Formica*) as the basis of this Repertory, but I have added some additional symptoms from later provings. I have also added many valuable symptoms from cases of poisoning, reported in the Allopathic Journals, which will in due time appear in the "Pathogenetic Record," now being published as an appendix to the British Journal of Homœopathy.

In order to illustrate the use of this Repertory, I give the two following cases from my own practice :*

CASE I.—Aug. 9, 1871. At 2 P.M., a child put its finger into its mother's left eye, scratching the upper part of eyeball ; smarting in the eye followed, with heat, redness, and hot lachrymation; cannot open the eye from pain. Cold water applications relieve the pains and watering ; the light of day increases the watering.

* As the selection of the remedy by means of the Repertory and Materia Medica is the *only* sure and scientific way of prescribing, it may not be inopportune to warn the public against the use of those very imperfect and deceptive works published under the names of "Domestic Homœopathy," &c. &c. In the first place, the plan of many of these works is entirely erroneous, the medicines being arranged *under the names of diseases,* and followed by their symptoms, instead of being arranged under *the symptoms,* as in the Repertory. Secondly, these works are often written by men possessed of very little knowledge of Homœopathy, who wish to gain notoriety by continually thrusting themselves upon the notice of the public by *popular* books, tracts, pamphlets, journals, &c.—a sort of "Homœopathy made Easy,"—the chief feature of which consists in the glorification of the author, and the vilification of Hahnemann and his *true* followers. Thirdly, they almost all encourage the public in that *curse* of homœopathy, the alternation of medicines ; a method which is not only subversive of all *scientific* practice, but is, moreover, entirely opposed to the teachings of the inspired Hahnemann *from first to last,*—the apparent exceptions to this statement resting merely on perverted translations and mutilated quotations of his original works. To those who wish to practice Homœopathy scientifically, I can confidently recommend Simmons' Repertory on Cough, and Bell's Repertory on Diarrhœa and Dysentery, as most excellent. Fenton Cameron's pamphlet on "Imperfect Digestion, with an Appendix for those who desire to know the difference between True and Delusive Homœopathy," will best explain to the public the science of Homœopathy, and enable them to distinguish between its *true* practitioners and *pretenders,* of which latter class there are, unfortunately, many in the present day.

Diagnosis of the Remedy.

(As the symptoms arose from a mechanical cause, I did not consider the locality (*left* eye) as a characteristic of the case).

Page 290. **Relief from Cold.—Heat.** alo. amm-cl. (thu).
       „   **Lachrymation.** al-o.
       „   **Smarting.** al-o. n-x.

Page 293. **Relief from Washing.—Heat.** al-o. amm-cl. asr. k-na. (thu)
       „   **Lachrymation.** al-o. asr. mg-ca.
       „   **Smarting.** al-o. na-ca.

Page 175. **Worse from Natural Light.—Lachrymation.** al-o. bry. dig. dl-s. dt. eug. grp. k-bicra. kre. lyc. mg-cl. qu-sa. s-x. (str-i). vr-s. zn.

Thus *Alumina* alone corresponds to all these symptoms, and it will be found to have also Redness of eyes (page 16), Difficult opening of Eyelids (page 47) and Hot Lachrymation (page 24). Accordingly at 7 p.m., the symptoms having lasted five hours, I gave a single dose of *Alumina* C. M. (Finckè). In *fifteen minutes* all the symptoms were gone, except a little feeling of stiffness.

CASE II.—November 6th. Three weeks ago, when blowing her nose, she felt as if something broke in the right eye, which watered much. Since then, at times, when blowing nose, has had a feeling as if a tight skin came half way down over right eye, preventing the sight of that eye ; removed by rubbing. After it has gone, feeling as if something were pricking the eye ; eye waters. On the last two occasions this sensation came on without blowing the nose.

Diagnosis of the Remedy.

Page 209. **By Blowing Nose. Sight Impaired.** k-o.
       „   **Pellicle.** k-o.

As *Kali Oxidum (Causticum)* was the only medicine which possessed these most characteristic symptoms, and, moreover, corresponded to the remaining symptoms as a reference to the Repertory will show, I gave one dose of *Causticum* 6 m. (Jenichen).

Dec. 11. Reports that the symptoms ceased at once and did not return.

With these prefatory remarks, I give this work—the labour of many years—to the Homœopathic body, only asking that it may be *used*; and if others find it of as much service in the relief of suffering humanity as I have done, I shall feel amply repaid for all my trouble. Let me however, state here, that if we wish to obtain the *maximum* amount of benefit from Homœopathy, we can only do so by faithfully following the three great rules of the Master:—(1) The careful selection of the SIMILIMUM ; not an *imperfectly homœopathic* remedy, or *allopathic palliative :* (2) the SINGLE REMEDY; all *mixing* of medicines, or *a priori alternation* or change of medicines *without* a corresponding alternation or change of the symptoms of the patient, being opposed to this law; and (3) the MINIMUM DOSE, which experience has shown to be a dose of one of the *highest potencies*, (repeated at such intervals as the case may require, till an improvement or medicinal aggravation sets in, and then allowed to act uninterruptedly so long as the patient improves, *without repetition of the dose or change of medicine*), PROVIDED ALWAYS *that the medicine be* PERFECTLY HOMŒOPATHIC *to the case.*

The volumes on the *Head* (including the Mental Group) and alsó on the *Ears* are being prepared, and will· be published as soon as completed ; whether I publish any more on the same plan, depends upon the encouragement I receive from the profession ; I hope however, that others may be induced to take up the work, for to arrange the whole Materia Medica Repertorially, would alone occupy the lifetime of any one individual. I have spared no pains to make this work as accurate‴ and complete as possible, both in execution and arrangement. To this end, I have examined all the English, French, and German Repertories which I could obtain, in order to combine all their excellences, at the same time excluding their defects. I have also endeavoured to extract the symptoms from the most reliable, and where possible the original, sources, thereby avoiding the many clerical and printer's errors which have crept into our Materia Medica. I cannot hope however to have avoided all these, and I shall feel grateful to any one who will point out any omission or error in this work, as it is my intention at the end of the third volume, (on the *Ears*) to print an Appendix, giving a list of the *errata* and *addenda* to all three volumes, thus bringing the entire work down to the date of the latest portion of it.

4, HIGHBURY NEW PARK,

LONDON, N.

April, 1873.

SYNONYMS.

—o—

In this Table I have arranged under one rubric all the varieties of expression which *in practice* I have found to be synonymous. Hair-splitting distinction should be avoided in a Repertory, (though in the Materia Medica the *ipsissima verba* of the provers should be given), as different provers will often describe the same symptoms by different terms: conversely moreover, symptoms *verbally* the same may *actually* be different, according to their locality ; thus *Pressing Out* in the *Head Generally* is equivalent to *Bursting ;* in the *Forehead* to *Pressing Forwards ;* in the *Occiput* to *Pressing Backwards ;* in the *Vertex* to *Pressing Upwards,* &c. : all such symptoms I have arranged under their *real* not *verbal* rubrics.

Boring. Digging, Rooting.

Broken. Crushed, Demolished.

Bursting. Breaking, Expanding, Fulness, Pressing Asunder or Centrifugally, Torn Asunder, as if all would Come Out.

Coldness. Cool, Frozen, Icy, Subjective Coldness ; (Objective Coldness is given separately as a variety.)

Contractive. Compressive, Constrictive, Grasping, Pinching, Pressing Centripetally, Screwed together, Squeezing.

Convulsions. Contortion, Distortion, Spasms, Twitches.

Crampy. Griping, Spasmodic.

Cutting. Acute, Sharp.

Drawing. Dragging, Pulling.

Heat. Burning, as if Burnt, Scalding, Warm, Subjective heat. (Objective Heat is given as a variety separately).

Itching. Irritation, Tickling.

Numbness. Deadness, Insensibility, Torpidity.

Paralysis. Weakness, Weariness.

Pressing. Aching, Forcing, Pushing.

Scraping. Grating, as if Rubbed.

Screwing. Twisting.

Shooting. Darting, Knife-thrusts, Lancinating, Penetrating, Piercing, Pricking, Sticking, Stitching, Stinging.

Smarting. Abscess-like, Biting, Corrosive, Eroding, Festering-like, Raw, Sore, Ulcerative.

Sprained. Dislocated.

Tensive. Stretching, Tight.

Throbbing. Beating, Blows, Hammering, Jerking, Pulsating, Shocks, Twitching.

Undefined. Dull, Congestive, Neuralgic, Rheumatic, and all other vaguely described pains.

LIST OF MEDICINES.

———o———

a.   acetyl
a-x.   aceticum acidum
ac-s.   actæa spicata
aca.   acacia catechu
acan.   acanthus mollis
ach.   achillea millefolium
acl.   acalypha indica
aco.   aconitinum
acon.   aconitum napellus
acon-c.   ,,   cammarum
acon-f.   ,,   ferox
acon-l.   ,,   lycoctonum
ada   adamas
adi.   adianthum aureum
ægl.   ægle marmelos
ægo.   ægopodium podagraria
æsc.   æsculus hippocastanum
æsc-g.   ,,   glabra
æth.   æthusa cynapium
ag.   argentum metallicum
ag-cl.   ,,   chloridum
ag-cy.   ,,   cyanidum
ag-i.   ,,   iodidum
ag-na.   ,,   nitricum
ag-o.   ,,   oxidum
ag-pa.   ,,   phosphoricum
aga.   agaricus muscarius
aga-b.   ,,   bulbosus
aga-c.   ,,   campanulatus
aga-ca.   ,,   cacumenatus
aga-cm   ,,   campestris
aga-e.   ,,   emeticus
aga-g.   ,,   glutinosus
aga-p.   ,,   procerus
aga-pi.   ,,   piperitidis
aga-v.   ,,   verrucosus
agr.   agrostema githago
agv.   agave americana
ail.   ailanthus glandulosa
aju.   ajuga reptans
al.   aluminium metallicum
al-cl.   ,,   chloridum
al-o.   ,,   oxidum(alumina)
ali.   alisma plantago
all.   allyl.

46 allyl. allylia
47 alli.   allium cepa
48 alli-p.   ,,   porrum
49 alli-s.   ,,   sativum
50 alm.   alumen. (potash-alum)
51 aln.   alnus rubra
52 aln-s.   ,,   serratula
53 alo.   aloes
54 alp.   alpinia galanga
55 als.   alstonia scholaris
56 alsi.   alsine media
57 alt.   aletris farinosa
58 alth.   althæa
59 am.   amyl
60 am-a.   ,,   aceticum
61 am-alc.   ,,   alcohol
62 am-gly.   ,,   glycol.
63 am-na-alc. ,, sodium alcohol
64 am-ni.   ,,   nitrosum
65 am-o.   ,,   ether
66 am-zn.   ,,   zinc
67 amar.   amaranthus communis
68 amb.   ambra grisea
69 amm-a. ammonium aceticum
70 amm-br.   ,,   bromidum
71 amm-bz.   ,,   benzoicum
72 amm-ca.   ,,   carbonicum
73 amm-cl.   ,,   chloridum
74 amm-ct.   ,,   citricum
75 amm-i.   ,,   iodidum
76 amm-pa.   ,,   phosphoricum
77 amm-s.   ,,   sulphuratum
78 amm-sc.   ,,   succinicum
79 amm-t.   ,,   tartaricum
80 ammon. ammonia
81 amn-c. anamirta citrina
82 amo.   amomum cardamomum
83 amp.   ampelopsis quinquefolium
84 amph.   amphisbæna vermicularis
85 amy.   amygdalæ amaræ
86 amyl   amylia
87 amyl-sa. ,, sulphurica
88 amylen. amylene
89 amyr.   amyris gileadensis
90 ana.   anagyris fœtida

91	anac.	anacardium occidentale
92	anacy.	anacyclus officinarum
93	anacy-p.	„ pyrethrum
94	anag.	anagellis arvensis
95	anan.	anantherum muricatum
96	and.	andira inermis
97	ane.	anemone nemorose
98	anem.	anemorrhena asphodeloïdes
99	aneth.	anethum graveolens
100	ang.	angelica archangelica
101	ani.	anisodus luridus
102	ank.	anthrokokali
103	anm.	anamirta cocculus (cocculus indicus)
104	anth.	anthemis nobilis
105	anthr.	anthroxanthum odoratum
106	anthra.	anthracite
107	antiar.	antiaria toxicaria
108	ap.	apium graveolens
109	aph.	aphis chenopodium glaucum
110	apo.	apocynum cannabinum
111	apo-a.	„ androsemifolium
112	aps.	apis mellifica
113	aqui.	aquilegia vulgaris
114	ara.	aranea domestica
115	ara-d.	„ diadema
116	ara-s.	„ scinensia
117	arc.	arctium lappa
118	arct.	arctostophylos uva ursi
119	are.	areca catechu
120	arch.	archangelica officinalis
121	arg.	argemone mexicana
122	argas.	argas persicus
123	ari.	aristolochia milhomens
124	ari-c.	„ clematitis
125	ari-s.	„ serpentaria
126	arl.	aralia racemosa
127	arma.	armadillo vulgaris
128	arn.	arnica montana
129	art.	artemisia vulgaris
130	art-a.	„ absinthium
131	art-v.	„ vahliana (cina)
132	artan.	artanthe elongata
133	arum.	arum maculatum
134	arum-t.	„ triphyllum
135	arun.	arundo donax
136	arun-m.	„ mauritanica
137	as.	arsenicum metallicum
138	as-h.	arsenicum hydrogenisatum
139	as-i.	„ iodidum
140	as-o.	„ oxidum (album)
141	as-s.	„ sulphuratum
142	as-ters.	„ tersulphuratum
143	asag.	asagræa officinalis

144	asc.	asclepias tuberosa
145	asc-c.	„ currasavica
146	asc-g.	asclepias gigantea
147	asc-i.	„ incarnata
148	asc-s.	„ syriaca
149	asc-v.	„ vincetoxicum
150	ask.	askalabotes lævigatus
151	asp.	asparagus officinalis
152	asper.	asperula adorata
153	aspid.	aspidium filix mas
154	asr.	asarum europæum
155	asr-c.	„ canadense
156	ast.	astacus fluviatilis
157	ath.	athamanta oreoselinum
158	atp.	atropa belladonna
159	atp-m.	„ mandragora
160	atr.	atriplex
161	atrac.	atractylis gummifera
162	atrop.	atropinum
163	atrop-sa.	„ sulphuricum
164	au.	aurum metallicum
165	au-cl.	„ chloridum
166	au-f.	„ fulminans
167	au-na-cl.	„ et natrum chloridum
168	au-o.	„ oxidum
169	aza.	azalea procumbens
170	b.	boron
171	b-x.	boracicum acidum
172	ba-a.	baryta acetica
173	ba-ca.	„ carbonica
174	ba-cl.	„ chlorida
175	ba-i.	„ iodida
176	bal.	ballota lanata
177	bals.	balsamodendron myrrha
178	bap.	baptisia tinctoria
179	bar.	baryosma tongo
180	be.	beryllium
181	ber.	berberis vulgaris
182	bgn.	bignonia
183	bi.	bismuthum metallicum
184	bi-cl.	„ chloridum
185	bi-na.	„ subnitricum
186	bi-v.	„ valerianicum
187	bid.	bidens parviflora
188	bll.	bellis perennis
189	blt.	blatta americana
190	bnz.	benzine
191	boa.	boa crotaloides
192	bol.	boletus suaveolens
193	bol-l.	„ laricis
194	bol-s.	„ satanas
195	bom.	bombus
196	bothr.	bothrops lanceolatus
197	br.	brominum
198	br-x.	bromicum acidum
199	bra.	brayera anthelmintica
200	brf.	bromoformum

brg. borago officinalis
brom. bromal
brs. brassica napus
bru. brucea antidysenterica
bruc. brucia
bruc-na. „ nitrica
bry. bryonia alba
bry-d. „ dioica
btl. betula alba
btn. betonia
bu. butyl (tetryl)
buf. bufo rana
buf-s. „ sahytiensis
bung. bungarus lineatus
but. butea frondosa
bux. buxus sempervirens
bz. benzoyl
bz-x. benzoicum acidum
c-bicl. carbo bichloridum
c-bis. „ bisulphuratum
c-h. „ hydrogenisatum
c-o. „ oxidum
c-tetracl. „ tetrachloridum
c-x. „ acidum
ca-a. „ calcarea acetica
ca-asa. „ arsenica
ca-ca. „ carbonica
ca-cl. „ chlorida
ca-f. „ fluorida
ca-i. „ iodida
ca-o. „ oxida (caustica)
ca-pa. „ phosphorica
ca-s. „ sulphurata(hepar)
cac. cactus grandiflorus
cal. calla æthiopica
calth. caltha palustris
can. cannabis sativa
can-i. „ indica
cap. capsicum annuum
cap-j. „ jamaicum
car. carica alba
car-p. „ papaya
carum. carum carui
cary. caryophyllus aromaticus
cast. castoreum
castor. castor equorum
cau. caullophyllum thalictroides
cb-a. carbo animalis
cb-v. „ vegetabilis
cbz-x. carbazoticum acidum
cch. colchicum autumnale
ccn. coccionella septem-punctata
ccs. coccus cacti
cd. cadmium metallicum
cd-ca. „ carbonicum
cd-cl. „ chloridum

257 cd-i. cadmium iodidum
258 cd-sa. „ sulphuricum
259 ce. cerium metallicum
260 ce-ox. „ oxalicum
261 cer. cerastes
262 cetr. cetraria islandica
263 chæ. chærophyllum temulum
264 chd. chelidonium majus
265 che. chelone glabra
266 chi. china officinalis
267 chio. chiococca racemosa (cainca)
268 chlor. chloral
269 chm. chimaphila umbellata
270 chp. chenopodium vulvaria (atriplex olida)
271 chp-a. „ anthelminticum
272 chp-am. „ ambrosioides
273 chp-b. „ botrys
274 chv. chavica roxburghii
275 chv-b. „ betel
276 cic. cicuta virosa
277 cic-m. „ maculata
278 cic-t. „ tenuifolia
279 cich. cichorium intybus
280 cis. cistus canadensis
281 cit-c. citrullus colocynthis
282 citr. citrus limomum
283 cl. chlorinum
284 cl-hx. chlorhydricum (muriaticum) acidum
285 clb coluber berus
286 cld. caladium seguinum
287 cle. clematis erecta
288 clf. chloroformum
289 cll. collinsonia canadensis
290 clm. calamus aromaticus
291 clotho. clotho arietans
292 cln. calendula officinalis
293 clt. callotropis procera
294 clt-g. „ gigantea
295 clv. claviceps purpurea(secale)
296 cmc. comocladia dentata
297 cmf. cimicifuga racemosa
298 cmx. cimex lectularius
299 cn. cinchoninum
300 cn-cl. „ chloridum
301 cn-sa. „ sulphuricum
302 cnm. cinnamonium zeylandicum
303 cnn. canna angustifolia
304 cnv. convolvulus arvensis
305 cnv-d. „ duartinus
306 cnv-s. „ scammoniæ
307 co. cobaltum metallicum
308 coc. cocculus palmatus
309 cochl. cochlearia armoracia
310 cod. codeinum

311	cof.	coffea arabica
312	con.	conium maculatum
313	conv.	convallaria majalis
314	cop.	copaifera multijuga
315	cor.	corallia rubra
316	cori.	coriaria myrtifolia
317	cori-r.	„ ruscifolia
318	corian.	coriandrum sativum
319	cory.	corydalis formosa
320	cos.	costus dulcis
321	cot.	cotyledon umbilicus
322	cp.	capryl.
323	cpo.	caproyl
324	cph.	cephaelis ipecacuanha
325	cr.	chromicum metallicum
326	cr-o.	„ oxidum
327	cr-x.	„ acidum
328	cra.	cratægus
329	crb-x.	carbolicum acidum
330	crd.	carduus benedictus
331	crd-m.	„ marianus
332	crn.	cornus cincinata
333	crn-f.	„ florida
334	crn-s.	„ sericea
335	cro.	crocus sativus
336	crot.	croton tiglium
337	crot-c.	„ eluteria
338	crp.	carapa touloucoma
339	crs.	cerasus virginiana
340	crt.	crotalus horridus
341	crt-c.	„ cascavella
342	crt-co.	„ confluentus
343	crt-d.	„ durissus
344	crv.	cervus braziliensis
345	cs.	cæsium metallicum
346	csm.	cissampelos pareira
347	css.	cassia lanceolata
348	css-f.	„ fistula
349	ct-x.	citricum acidum
350	cth.	cantharis vesicatoria
351	ctn.	cetonia aurata
352	ctr.	citrallus chinensis
353	cu.	cuprum metallicum
354	cu-a.	„ aceticum
355	cu-asi.	„ arsenicum
356	cu-ca.	„ carbonicum
357	cu-sa.	„ sulphuricum
358	cub.	cubebæ
359	cuc.	cucurbita pepo
360	cum.	cuminum cyminum
361	cund.	cundurango
362	cup.	cupressus sempervirens
363	cus.	cuscuta europæa
364	cy.	cyanogen
365	cy-hx.	cyanhydricum acidum
366	cyc.	cyclamen europæum
367	cyn.	cynanchum argel
368	cynob.	cynobatus
369	cynog.	cynoglossum officinale
370	cyp.	cypripedium pubescens
371	cyper.	cyperus rotundus
372	cypr.	cyprinus barbus
373	cyt.	cytisus laburnum
374	cyt-s.	„ scoparius
375	delph.	delphinus amazonicus
376	di.	didymium metallicum
377	dic.	dictamnus albus
378	dichr.	dichroa febrifuga
379	dig.	digitalis purpurea
380	dig-l.	„ lutea
381	dim.	dimorephanthus edulis
382	dio.	dioscorea villosa
383	dios.	diosma fœtida
384	dios-c.	„ crenata
385	dl-s.	delphinium staphysagria
386	dlp.	delphininum
387	dol.	dolichos pruriens
388	dor.	doryphora decemlineata
389	dph.	daphne mezereum
390	dph-i.	„ indica
391	dph-l.	„ laureola
392	dps.	dipsacus sylvestris
393	dpt.	dipterix odorata
394	dra.	dracontium fœtidum
395	dra-p.	„ polyphyllum
396	drm.	dorema ammoniacum
397	dro.	drosera rotundifolia
398	dry.	dryobalanops camphora
399	dt.	datura stramonium
400	dt-a.	„ alba
401	dt-ar.	„ arborea
402	dt-f.	„ ferox
403	dt-fa.	„ fastuosa
404	dt-m.	„ metel
405	dt-s.	„ sanguinea
406	dt-t.	„ tatula
407	eb.	erbium metallicum
408	ecb.	ecbalium officinarum
409	ech.	echites suberecta
410	elæ.	elæagnus angustifolia
411	elaps.	elaps corallinus
412	ele.	eleis guineensis
413	elet.	elettaria cardamomum
414	elp.	elaphrium elemiferum
415	elt.	elater noctulicus
416	epg.	epigæa repens
417	equi.	equisetum arvense
418	erc.	erica vulgaris
419	erech.	erechthites hieraci- folius
420	erig.	erigonon canadense
421	ero.	erodium cicutarium
422	eru.	eruca
423	erv.	ervum ervilia
424	ery.	erythroxylon coca
425	eryn.	eryngium aquaticum

426 erys. erysimum officinale
427 eryth. erythræa chilensis (canchalagua)
428 erythr. erythrophlæum judiciale
429 et-fr. ethyl formiatum (formic ether)
430 et-o. ethyl oxidum (ether)
431 eug. eugenia iambos
432 eug-p. „ pimenta
433 eup. eupion
434 eupat. eupatorium perfoliatum
435 eupat-a. „ aromaticum
436 eupat-c. „ cannabinum
437 eupat-p. „ purpureum
438 euph. euphorbia officinarum
439 euph-a. „ amydaloides
440 euph-c. :, corollata
441 euph-cy. „ cyparissias
442 euph-e. „ esula
443 euph-h. „ helioscopia
444 euph-i. „ ipecacuanha
445 euph-l. „ lathyris
446 euph-p. „ peplus
447 euph-s. „ splendens
448 euph-v. „ villosa
449 euphr. euphrasia officinalis
450 evo. evonymus europæus
451 evo-a. „ atropurpureus
452 exo. exogonium purga (jalappa)
453 f-hx. fluorhydricum acidum
454 fag. fagus
455 fe. ferrum metallicum
456 fe-a. „ aceticum
457 fe-asi. „ arseniosum
458 fe-ca. „ carbonicum
459 fe-cl. „ chloridum
460 fe-cy. „ cyanidum
461 fe-i. „ iodidum
462 fe-l. „ lacticum
463 fe mgs. „ magneticum
464 fe-pa. „ phosphoricum
465 fe-s. „ sulphuratum
466 fe-sa. „ sulphuricum
467 fe-t. „ tartaricum
468 fel. fel tauri
469 fel-v. „ vulpis
470 fer. ferula officinalis
471 fer-g. „ glauca (bounafa)
472 fig. fuligo
473 fmr. fumaria officinalis
474 fœn. fœniculum vulgare
475 fœn-d. „ dulce
476 fr-x. formicum acidum
477 frg. fragraria vesca

478 frm. formica rufa
479 frm-o. „ omnivora
480 frm-s. „ subsericea
481 frn. franciscea uniflora
482 frs. frasera carolinensis
483 frx. fraxinus
484 fu-v. fucus vesiculosus
485 ga-x. gallicum acidum
486 gad. gadus morrhuæ
487 gal. galium aparine
488 gale. galeopsis ochroleuca
489 gau. gaultheria procumbens
490 gel. gelseminum sempervirens
491 gettys. gettysburg
492 geum. geum rivale
493 geum-u. „ urbane
494 gl. glucinum
495 glan. glanderinum
496 glb. galbanum officinale
497 glech. glechoma hederaceum
498 glo. glonoinum
499 glp. galipea cusparia. (augustura)
500 gn-c. gentiana cruciata
501 gn-l. „ lutea
502 gna. gnaphalium polycephalum
503 gna-a. „ arenarium
504 gna-m. „ margaritaceum
505 gns. genista tinctoria
506 grc. garcinia morella (gamboge)
507 grc-c. „ elliptica
508 gri. grindelia robusta
509 grn. geranium maculatum
510 grn-d. „ dissectum
511 grn-o. „ odoratum
512 grn-r. „ robertianum
513 grp. graphites
514 grt. gratiola officinalis
515 grs. gossypium herbaceum
516 gua. guano
517 guar. guarea trichilioides
518 gui. guiacum officinale
519 gym. gymnocladus canadensis
520 gyn. gynocardia odorata
521 hæm. hæmatoxylon campechianum .
522 ham. hamamelis virginica
523 hdm. hedeoma pulegioides
524 hed. hedysarum ildefonsianum
525 hel. helianthus
526 heli. helianthemum vulgare
527 helo. heloella esculenta
528 hem. hemisdesmus indicus
529 hg. mercurius (hydrargyrum) metallicus

530	hg-a.	mercurius aceticus
531	hg-am-cl.	„ ammonio-chloridus
532	hg-bibr.	„ bibromidus
533	hg-bicl.	„ bichloridus
534	hg-bini.	„ biniodidus
535	hg-br.	„ bromidus
536	hg-cla.	„ chloratus
537	hg-cl.	„ chloridus
538	hg-cy.	„ cyanidus
539	hg-i.	„ iodidus
540	hg-me.	„ methidus (mercuric methide)
541	hy-o.	„ oxidus
542	hg-pa.	„ phosphoricus
543	hg-s.	„ sulphuratus (cinnabar)
544	hg-sa.	„ sulphuricus
545	hier.	hieraceum pilosella
546	hier-u.	„ umbellatum
547	hll.	helleborus niger
548	hll-f.	„ fœtidus
549	hlm.	helminthocortos officinarum
550	hln.	helonias dioica
551	hln-e.	„ erythrosperma
552	hlt.	heliotropum peruvianum
553	hlx.	helix pomatia
554	hom.	homeria collinea
555	hpm.	hippomane mancinella
556	hpp.	hippomanes
557	hpt.	hepatica triloba
558	hrc.	heracleum spondylium
559	hrn.	herniaria glabra
560	hum.	humulus lupulus
561	hur.	hura braziliensis
562	hur-c.	„ crepitans
563	hyd.	hydrocotyle asiatica
564	hydr.	hydrastis canadensis
565	hydro.	hydrophobinum
566	hydrus.	hydrus colubrinus
567	hyo.	hyoscyamus niger
568	hyo-a.	„ albus
569	hyo-s.	„ scopolia
570	hyp.	hypericum perfoliatum
571	hyp-p.	„ pulcrum
572	hypoph.	hypophyllum sanguineum
573	i.	iodinum
574	if	iodoform
575	ilex.	ilex aquifolium
576	ilex-p.	„ paraguaensis
577	ill.	illicium anisatum
578	imp.	imperatoria ostruthinum
579	in.	indium metallicum
580	ind.	indigo
581	inu.	inula helenium
582	ipo.	ipomœa jalappa

583	ir.	iridium metallicum
584	irs.	iris versicolor
585	irs-f.	„ fœtidissimus
586	irs-g.	„ germanicus
587	irs-ps.	„ pseudacoras
588	irs-t.	„ tricolor
589	itu.	itu resina
590	jan.	janipha manihot
591	jat.	jatropha curcas
592	jat-m.	„ multifida
593	jat-u.	„ urens
594	jcr.	jacaranda caroba
595	jnc.	juncus effusus
596	jnc-p.	„ pilosus
597	jnp.	juniperus communis
598	jnp-s.	„ sabina
599	jnp-v.	„ virginiana
600	jug.	juglans regia
601	jug-c.	„ cinerea
602	jus.	justicia adhatoda
603	k-a.	kali aceticum
604	k-asa.	„ arsenicum
605	k-asi.	„ arseniosum
606	k-bica	„ bicarbonicum
607	k-bicra.	„ bichromicum
608	k-br.	„ bromidum
609	k-ca.	„ carbonicum
610	k-cl.	„ chloridum
611	k cla.	„ chloricum
612	k-cra.	„ chromicum
613	k-cy.	„ cyanidum
614	k-ct.	„ citricum
615	k-fcy.	„ ferrocyanidum
616	k-i.	„ iodidum
617	k-mna.	„ manganicum
618	k-na.	„ nitricum
619	k-o.	„ oxidum (causticum)
620	k-ox.	„ oxalicum
621	k-permna.	„ permanganicum
622	k-sa.	„ sulphuricum
623	k-scy.	„ sulphocyanidum
624	k-sia.	„ silicatum
625	k-t.	„ tartaricum
626	kao.	kaolin
627	kd.	kakodyl
628	kd-o.	„ oxidum
629	kis.	kissengen
630	klm.	kalmia latifolia
631	kre.	kreasotum
632	kreu.	kreutznach
633	krm.	krameria triandra (ratanhia)
634	l-x.	lacticum acidum
635	la.	lanthanium metallicum
636	lac.	lac vaccinum
637	lac-b.	„ „ butyrum
638	lac-bu.	„ „ butyraceum
639	lac-c.	„ caninnm

751	na-asa.	natrum arsenicum
752	na-asi.	„ arseniosum
753	na-ba.	„ biboracicum
	(borax)	
754	na-br.	„ bromidum
755	na-ca.	„ carbonicum
756	na-cl.	„ chloridum
757	na-hpa.	„ hypophosphoricum
758	na-i.	„ iodidum
759	na-na.	„ nitricum
760	na-o.	„ oxidum
761	na-pa.	„ phosphoricum
762	na-sa.	„ sulphuricum
763	na-sc.	„ succinicum
764	na-si.	„ sulphurosum
765	naj.	naja tripudians
766	naph.	napthalinum
767	narc.	narcissus pseudo-narcissus
768	narth.	narthex asafœtida
769	nb.	niobium metallicum
770	nbl.	nabulus serpentaria
771	nct.	nectandra rodiæi
772	nct-p.	„ puchury major
	(pichurim)	
773	ner.	nerium oleander
774	ner-a.	„ antidysentericum
775	ngl.	nigella sativa
776	ngl-d.	„ damascena
777	ni.	niccolum metallicum
778	ni-ca.	„ carbonicum
779	nic.	nicotiana tabacum
780	nitro-bnz.	nitro-benzine
781	no.	norium metallicum
782	nrc.	narcotinum
783	nrc-a.	„ aceticum
784	nrc-cl.	„ chloridum
785	nst.	nasturtium officinale
786	nst-a.	„ aquaticum
787	nuph.	nuphar lutea
788	nym.	nymphæa odorata
789	oci.	ocimum canum
790	œn.	œnanthyl
791	œna.	œnantha crocata
792	œna-a.	„ apifolia
793	œno.	œnothera biennis
794	oid.	oidium
795	ol-a.	oleum animale
796	ol-m.	„ morrhuæ
797	ol-t.	„ terebinthinæ
798	oni.	oniscus asellus
799	ono.	ononis arvensis
800	oph.	ophelia chiretta
801	opo.	opoponax chironicum
802	org.	orgianum majorana
803	ori.	origanum vulgare
804	oro.	orobanche virginiana
805	os.	osmium metallicum

806	os-bino.	osmium binoxidum
807	os-x.	„ acidum
808	ost.	ostrya virginica
809	ott.	ottonia anisum
810	ox-x.	oxalicum acidum
811	oxl.	oxalis acitosella
812	ozæ.	ozænin
813	p.	phosphorus
814	p-h.	„ hydrogenisatus
815	p-x.	phosphoricum acidum
816	pæo.	pæonia officinalis
817	pan.	panacea
818	pap.	papaya vulgaris
819	par.	paris quadrifolia
820	pass.	passerina chamædaphne
821	pau.	paullinia pinnata
822	pau-s.	„ sorbilis
823	pav.	pavia ohio
824	pb	plumbum metallicum
825	pb-a.	„ aceticum
826	pb-bini.	„ biniodium
827	pb-ca.	„ carbonicum
828	pb-cra.	„ chromicum
829	pb-i.	„ iodidum
830	pb-na.	„ nitricum
831	pc-x.	picricum acidum
832	pcr.	picræna excelsa
833	pd.	palladium metallicum
834	pe.	pelopium metallicum
835	ped.	pediculus capitis
836	pet.	petroleum
837	peu.	peucedaneum officinale
838	phen-h.	phenyl hydride
	(benzol)	
839	phenyl.	phenylia (aniline)
840	phenyl-sa.	phenylia sulphurica
841	phil.	philadelphus coronarius
842	phl.	phellandrium aquaticum
843	phlo.	phlomis esculenta
844	phs.	phaseolus angulatus
845	phy.	phytolacca decandra
846	phys.	physalis
847	physo.	physostigma venenosum
848	picro.	picrotoxin
849	pim.	pimpernella saxifraga
850	pim-a.	„ anisum
851	pin.	pinus sylvestris
852	pin-a.	„ abies
853	pip.	piper niger
854	pip-m.	„ methysticum
855	pist.	pistachia vera
856	plb.	plumbago littoralis
857	plb-e.	„ europæa
858	plc.	plectranthus fruticosus
859	plg.	polygonum hydropiper
860	plg-a.	„ amphibium
861	plg-m.	„ maritimum

862	plm.	polemonium cæruleum
863	pln.	plantago major
864	pln-l.	„ lanceolata
865	plp.	polyporus officinalis
866	pne.	punica granatum
867	pnx.	panex ginseng
868	pnx-q.	„ quinquefolium
869	pod.	podophyllum peltatum
870	pog.	pogostemon patchouli
871	pol.	polygala senega
872	pol-a.	„ amara
873	pop.	populus tremuloides
874	ppv.	papaver somniferum (opium)
875	ppv-d.	„ dubium
876	ppv-r.	„ rhœas
877	prd.	pardanthus chinensis
878	prf.	paraffin
879	prin.	prinos verticillatus
880	prm.	primula vera
881	prn.	prenanthus
882	pra.	persica vulgaris
883	prt.	portulaca
884	pru.	prunus domestica
885	pru-l.	„ laurocerasus
886	pru-m.	„ mahelep
887	pru-p.	„ padus
888	pru-sp.	„ spinoea
889	prun.	prunella vulgaris
890	psboa.	pseudoboa fasciata
891	psc.	piscidia erythrina
892	pso.	psoricum
893	psr.	psoralea bituminosa
894	pst.	pastinaca sativa
895	psy.	psycotria emetica
896	pt.	platinum metallicum
897	pt-cl.	„ chloridum
898	pt-i.	„ iodidum
899	pth.	pothos fœtidus
900	ptl.	ptelea trifoliata
901	ptm.	potamageton natans
902	ptn.	potentilla tormentilla
903	ptn-a.	„ aurea
904	ptn-r.	„ reptans
905	ptr.	pterocarpus marsupium
906	pts.	petroselinum sativum
907	ptv.	petiveria tetrandra
908	pul.	pulsatilla nigricans
909	pul-n.	„ nuttaliana
910	pulm.	pulmonaria vulgaris
911	pulmo.	pulmo vulpis
912	pup.	pupalia geniculata
913	qu.	quinia
914	qu-asa.	„ arsenica
915	qu-bicl.	„ bichlorida
916	qu-cy.	„ cyanida
917	qu-pa.	„ phosphorica
918	qu-sa.	„ sulphurica

919	quas.	quassia amara
920	raph.	raphanistrum arvense
921	rb.	rubidium metallicum
922	rbn.	robinia pseudo-acacia
923	rehm.	rhemannia chinensis
924	rh.	rhodium metallicum
925	rhe.	rheum palmatum
926	rhm.	rhamnus catharticus
927	rhm-f.	„ frangula
928	rho.	rhododendron chrysan-themum
929	ric.	ricinus communis
930	rmx.	rumex crispus
231	rmx-a.	„ acetosella
932	rmx-p.	„ patientia
933	rn-a.	ranunculus acris
934	rn-b.	„ bulbosus
935	rn-f.	„ flammula
936	rn-fi.	„ ficaria
937	rn-g.	„ glacialis
938	rn-r.	„ repens
939	rn-s.	„ sceleratus
940	rosa.	rosa canina
941	rosa-c.	„ centifolia
942	rs.	rhus toxicodendron
943	rs-g.	„ glabrum
944	rs-l.	„ laurina
945	rs-r.	„ radicans
946	rs-v.	„ veneneta
947	rs-vx.	„ vernix
948	rsm.	rosmarinus officinalis
949	rtt.	rottleria tinctoria
950	ru.	ruthenium metallicum
951	rubi.	rubia officinarum
952	rud.	rudbeckia hirta
953	rut.	ruta graveolens
954	s.	sulphur
955	s-h.	„ hydrogenisatum
956	s-i.	„ iodidum
957	s-o.	„ oxidum
958	s-x.	sulphuricum acidum
959	sa-a.	seccharum album
960	sa-l.	„ lactis
961	sa-mgs.	„ „ odo-magneticum
962	sang.	sanguinaria canadensis
963	sant.	santalum album
964	sas.	sassafras officinalis
965	sb.	antimonium metallicum (stibium)
966	sb-asa.	„ arsenicum
967	sb-asi.	„ arseniosum
968	sb-cl.	„ chloridum
969	sb-o.	„ oxidum
970	sb-s.	„ sesquisulphur-atum (crudum)
971	sb-t.	„ tartaricum (tartar emetic)

972	sbc-x.	sebacicum acidum
973	scol.	scolopendron heros
974	scor.	scorpio europæus
975	scp.	scoparia
976	scr.	scrofularia nodosa
977	scr-m.	„ marilandica
978	scu.	scutellaria laterifolia
979	se.	selenium metallicum
980	sed.	sedinha
981	sedum.	sedum acre
982	sedum-t.	„ telephium
983	sep.	sepia officinalis
984	si.	silicium metallicum
985	si-cl.	„ chloridum
986	si-x.	„ acidum (silica)
987	silph.	silphium laciniatum
988	sld.	solidago virgaurea
989	slm.	salamandra maculata
990	slv.	salvia officinalis
991	slx.	salix alba
992	slx-p.	„ purpurea
993	smb.	sambucus nigra
994	smb-e.	„ ebulus
995	smc.	semecarpus anacardium (anacardium orientale)
996	smi.	smilax officinalis (sarsaparilla)
997	smi-a.	„ aspera
998	smp.	sempervivum tectorum
999	smr.	simaruba cedron
1000	sn.	stannum metallicum
1001	sn-cl.	„ chloridum
1002	snc.	senecio aureus
1003	snc-o.	„ obovatus
1004	sng.	sanguisorba officinalis
1005	snp.	sinapis alba
10.6	snp-n.	„ nigra
1007	snt.	santoninum.
1008	so-a.	solanum arrabenta
1009	so-d.	„ dulcamara
1010	so-l.	„ lycopersicon
1011	so-m.	„ mammosum
1012	so-n.	„ nigrum.
1013	so-ps.	„ pseudo-capsicum
1014	so-t.	„ tuberosum
1015	so-t-æg	„ ægrotans
1016	so-v.	„ vesiculosum
1017	spar.	spartium scoparium
1018	spg.	spiggurus martini
1019	sph.	sophora japonica
1020	spi.	spigelia anthelmintica
1021	spi-m	„ marilandica
1022	spil.	spilanthes oleracea
1023	spir.	spiranthes autumnalis
1024	spo.	spongia tosta
1025	spo-f.	„ fluviatilis (badiaga)
1026	spr.	spiræa ulmaria
1027	sr.	strontiana metallica
1028	sr-ca.	„ carbonica
1029	sr-cl.	„ chlorida
1030	srb.	sorbus aucuparia
1031	srr.	sarracenia purpurea
1032	stach.	stachys betonica
1033	stach-r.	„ recta
1034	stc.	sticta pulmonaria
1035	ster.	sterculia acuminata
1036	stl.	stillingea sylvatica
1037	str.	strychnos nux vomica
1038	str-i.	„ ignatia
1039	str-t.	„ tieute
1040	str-tx.	„ toxifera.
1041	stry.	strychnia
1042	stryph.	stryphnodendron barbatinum
1043	styr.	styrax officinale
1044	styr-b.	„ benzoin
1045	sum.	sumbulus moschatus
1046	sxf.	saxifraga granulata
1047	syc.	sycosin
1048	sym.	symphytum officinale
1049	syph.	syphilin
1050	syr.	syringa vulgaris
1051	ta.	tantalum metallicum
1052	tam.	tamus communis
1053	tb.	terbium metallicum
1054	tcn.	ticunas
1055	te.	tellurium metalicum
1056	te-o.	„ oxidum
1057	te-x.	„ acidum
1058	tep.	teplitz
1059	tephr.	tephrosia apollinea
1060	teu.	teucrium marum verum
1061	teu-c.	„ creticum
1062	teu-ch.	„ chamædris
1063	teu-s.	„ scorodonia
1064	th.	thorium metallicum
1065	thasp	thaspium aureum
1066	the.	thea
1067	thl.	thlapsi bursa pastoris
1068	thr.	theridion curassivicum
1069	thu.	thuya occidentalis
1070	thv.	thevetia ruscifolia
1071	thv-n.	„ nereifolia
1072	thy.	thymus vulgaris
1073	thy-s.	„ serpyllum
1074	ti.	titanium metallicum
1075	til.	tilia europæa
1076	tl.	thallium metallicum
1077	tl-sa.	„ sulphuricum
1078	tn-x.	tannicum acidum
1079	tnc.	tanacetum vulgare
1080	tnc-b.	„ balsamita
1081	tng.	tanghinia venenifera
1082	tourn.	tournfortia argusina
1083	trach.	trachinus vipera

1084	trd.	tradescantia diuretica
1085	trf.	trifolium arvense
1086	trf-p.	„ pratense
1087	trf-r.	„ repens
1088	trg.	trigonocephalus lachesis
1089	trg-a.	„ atrox
1090	trg-c.	„ contortrix
1091	trg-j.	„ jararaca
1092	trg-p.	„ piscivorus
1093	tri.	triosteum perfoliatum
1094	trich.	trichosanthes dioica
1095	trl.	trillium repens
1096	trl-p.	„ pendulum
1097	trm.	trombidium muscæ domesticæ
1098	trn.	tarantula hispanica
1099	trx.	taraxacum dens leonis
1100	tss.	tussilago petasites
1101	tss-f.	„ farfara
1102	tt-x.	tartaricum acidum
1103	tub.	tuber cibarium
1104	tx-b.	taxus baccata
1105	tx-e.	„ erecta
1106	tyl.	tylophora asthmatica
1107	u.	uranium metallicum
1108	u-cl.	„ chloridum
1109	u-na.	„ nitricum
1110	u-o.	„ oxidum
1111	ulm.	ulmus campestris
1112	unc.	uncaria gambir
1113	upas.	upas antiar
1114	ure.	uredo caricis
1115	urea.	urea
1116	urea-na	„ nitrica
1117	urg.	urginea scilla
1118	urt.	urtica dioica
1119	urt-m.	„ marina
1120	urt-u.	„ urens
1121	ust.	ustilago madis
1122	v.	vanadium metallicum
1123	vac.	vaccininum
1124	val.	valeriana officinalis
1125	van.	vanilla planifolia
1126	var.	variolinum
1127	vbr.	viburnum prunifolium
1128	vbr-o.	viburnum odoratissimum
1129	vcc.	vaccinium myrtillus
1130	verb.	verbena officinalis
1131	verb-h.	„ hastata
1132	verb-j	„ jamaicensis
1133	verb-u.	„ urticæfolia
1134	vi-o.	viola odorata
1135	vi-t.	„ tricolor
1136	vin.	vinca minor
1137	vit.	vitis vinifera
1138	vnc.	vincetoxicum officinale
1139	vp-r.	vipera redi
1140	vp-t.	„ torva.
1141	vr-a.	veratrum album
1142	vr-s.	„ sabadilla
1143	vr-v.	„ viride
1144	vr-b.	verbascum thapsus
1145	vrn.	veronica officinalis
1146	vrn-b.	„ beccabunga
1147	vrt.	veratrinum
1148	vsc.	viscum album
1149	vsp.	vespa vulgaris
1150	vsp-c.	„ crabro
1151	vtx.	vitex agnus castus
1152	w.	tungsten metallicum
1153	wis.	wisbaden
1154	woo.	woorari
1155	xan.	xanthoxylon fraxineum
1156	xanth.	xanthium spinosum
1157	xyp.	xyphosura americana
1158	y.	yttrium metallicum
1159	ziz.	zizia aurea
1160	zn.	zincum metallicum
1161	zn-a.	„ aceticum
1162	zn-ca.	„ carbonicum
1163	zn-cl.	„ chloridum
1164	zn-cy.	„ cyanidum
1165	zn-fcy.	„ ferrocyanidum.
1166	zn-i.	„ iodidum
1167	zn-o.	„ oxidum
1168	zn-sa	„ sulphuricum
1169	zn-v.	„ valerianicum
1170	zng.	zingiber officinalis
1171	zr.	zirconium metallicum

EYES.

SECTION I. SYMPTOMS. A. FUNCTIONS.

OBJECTS, FALSE APPEARANCE OF.

ac-s. acon. æth. ag-na. aga. al-o. alm. am-ni. amm-ca.
amm-cl. anan. anm. arn. art-v. as-o. atp. au. ba-ca. ba-cl.
bap. ber. bry. buf. c-bis. ca-ca. ca-o. ca-s. can. can-i. cap. cb-a.
cb-v. chd. chi. chio. chlor. cic. cit-c. cl-hx. cle. clf. cmc. cmf.
co. con. cop. cph. crb-x. cro. cth. cu. cy-hx. cyc. dig. dl-s. dph.
dph-i. dro. dt. ele. ery. eug. euph. euph-c. euphr. f-hx. fe.
fe-mgs. frm. frm-s. gel. grp. grt. gua. hæm. hg. hg-bicl. hpp.
hyo. i. irs-f. jnc. jnp-s. k-bicr. k-ca. k-na. k-o. kre. lac-c.
lac-d. lau-c. lct. led. li-ca. lo-i. lpd. ly-b. lyc. men. mg-ca.
mg-cl. mgs. mgs-au. mn-ca. morph. mph. mrl. msc. mtr.
myris. n-x. na-ba. na-ca. na-cl. ner. ni-ca. nic. os. ox-x. p.
p-x. par. pb. pet. phy. physo. pnx. pod. pol. ppv. pru-l. pso.
pt. ptv. pul. rho. rn-b. rs. rs-r. rut. s. s-x. sb-t. sep. si-x. smc.
smi. sn. so-d. spi. spo. sr-ca. srr. str. str-i. tep. thr. thu. til.
trg. val. vi-o. vin. vr-a. vr-s. vr-v. vrb. vtx. wis. woo. zn.

BLACK, (dark). acon. al-o. amm-ca. amm-cl. anan.
anm. as-o. atp. au. ba-ca. ca-ca. ca-s. cap. cb-v. chi. cic. clv.
dl-s. dt. euphr. hg. k-ca. k-o. lyc. mg-ca. mn-ca. msc.
n-x. (na-cl). p. p-x. pet. physo. rut. s-x. sep. si-x. smc. str.
thu. val. vr-a.

BLUE, (lilac, purple, violet). ac-s. acon. atp. cph.
dt. hpp. i. kre. lyc. ni-ca. s. snt. sr-ca. trg. zn.

BRIGHT. al-o. amm-ca. anan. as-o. atp. au. ba-ca bry.
ca-ca. can. cb-a. cb-v. chd. chlor. cic. cit-c. clv. con. cro.
dig. dph. dro. euphr. grp. hyo. i. jnp-s. k-ca. k-o. lau-c. lyc.
men. mgs. mn-ca. na-ba. na-cl. ner. p-x. pol. ppv. pt. pul. rs.
sb-t. so-d. spi. sr-ca. str. str-i. trg. val. vi-o. vr-a. zn.

CLOSER together. myris.

CONFUSED (indistinct). ag-na. anan. anm. atp. au. bry.
c-bis. ca-ca. can. chd. chi. chio. cic. cl-hx. cle. co. con. crb-x.

A

cund. dl-s. dro. dt. ele. ery. eug. euphr. f-hx. frm-s. gel. grp. hæm. hyo. i. irs-f. (k-bicr). k-ca. k-o. lct. led. lyc. mph. mrl. n-x. na-ca. na-cl. na-sa. os. p. phy. pnx. pod. pol. ppv. pt. rs-r. si-x. til. trg. vi-o. woo.

Outlines. chi. k-bicr. p. pod.

DISTORTED. atp. hyo.

FAR, too. (atp). can-i. cb-a. chlor. cic. dt. gel. hg-bicl. myris. na-cl. ox-x. p. s. smc. sn. srr. thr.

GREEN. art-v. chi. clf. dig. dt. hg. lac-c. mg-cl. nic. p. rut. s. sep. snt. sr-ca. tep. vr-v. zn.

GREY. anan. dt. n-x. p. sep. si-x. str.

INVERTED. atp. eug. gel. glo. gua. k-ca. ly-b.

LARGE, too. æth. anan. atp. ber. can-i. dig. dl-s. dt. euph. hyo. k-o. mll. myris. na-cl. ni-ca. os. ox-x. p. physo. ppv. pru-l. vrb.

LOW down. can-i. dl-s.

MOVING. acon. ag-na. aga. al-o. amm-ca. anan. anm. arn. atp. au. ba-ca. ba-cl. bap. ber. bi-na. bry. ca-ca. ca-o. ca-s. can. can-i. cb-a. chd. cic. cl-hx. con. crb-x. cy-hx. dl-s. dro. dt. ery. eug. euph. euph-c. euphr. fe. frm. grt. gua. hg. hll. hyo. i. jnc. jnp-s. k-bicr. k-ca. k-o. kre. lac-d. lct. lpd. ly-b. lyc. men. mg-ca. mgs. mrl. msc. myris. na-cl. ner. nic. p. p-x. par. pet. pnx. pol. ppv. pru-l. pso. pul. rho. rn-b. rs. rs-r. rut. s. s-x. se. sep. si-x. smc. spi. spo. str. str-i. tep. thu. til. urg. val. vin. vr-a. vr-s. vtx. wis. woo. zn.

Backwards. atp.

Backwards and Forwards. atp. cic. crb-x. frm. p. tep.

Circularly. acon. ag-na. al-o. amm-ca. anm. arn. atp. au. ba-ca. ba-cl. ber. bi-na. bry. ca-ca. ca-o. ca-s. can. can-i. cb-a. chd. cic. cl-hx. con. cy-hx. dl-s. dro. ery. euph. euph-c. fe. grt. gua. hg. hll. jnc. k-bicr. k-ca. k-o. kre. lct. lpd. ly-b. lyc. mg-ca. mrl. msc. na-cl. ner. nic. p. p-x. par. ppv. pru-l. pso. pul. rho. rn-b. rs. rs-r. rut. s. s-x. se. sep. si-x. smc. spi. str. tep. thu. urg. val. vin. vr-a. vr-s. vtx. zn.

Slowly. cy-hx.

Slowly, then Quickly. msc.

Semicircle, in a. dl-s.

From Below Upwards. gua.

Jumping. men.

Sideways. cic. grt. lac-d.

To Right. lac-d.

To Left. grt.

Swaying. ner. str-i.

Undulating. atp.

Vertically. arn. con. dt. hyo. lpd. p-x. si-x. spo.

Downwards. arn. dt. lpd. p-x.

Up and Down. con. si-x. spo.

Vibrating. acon. atp. ca-ca. cic. dro. dt. eug. euphr. hg. hyo. i. jnp-s. k-o. lyc. men. msc. p. pet. pol. s-x. smc. str-i. tep. thu. til. wis. zn.

On the Surface. atp.

In all directions. lac-d.

MULTIPLIED. æth. aga. (alm). amm-ca. atp. au. ba-ca. bry. ca-ca. chd. cic. cle. clv. cmf. con. cy-hx. cyc. dig. dph. dt. ery. eug. euph. gel. grp. hg. hg-bicr. hyo. i. (k-bicr.) k-ca. k-i. kis. led. lyc. mgs-au. mtr. n-x. na-cl. ner. ni-ca. nic. pb. pet. physo. pnx. pol. pul. s. sb-t. spo. srr. thr: vr-a. vr-v.

Antero-Posteriorly. euph.

Horizontally. dt. n-x. ner. pol. sbt.

Vertically. atp. dt. (k-bicr). pol.

The Left image Highest. dt.

The Right image Highest. pol.

The two images alternately Approach and Recede from each other. con.

The Left image seen with Right eye. na-cl.

NEAR, **too.** (atp). cic. dt. (k-ca). ly-b. morph. physo. (pol). srr.

OBLIQUE. atp. buf. dt. myris.

PART VISIBLE. au. ca-ca. can. chio. cl-hx. cro. dl-s. dt. i. k-ca. k-o. lac-c. li-ca. lo-i. lyc. mtr. na-cl. p. pb. rs-r. sep. spi. ti. vr-v.

Centre Visible. pb. dt. mtr.

Circumference Visible. cro.

Horizontal. au. chio.

Lower part Visible. au.

Upper part Visible. au. chio.

Vertical. au. ca-ca. cl-hx. i. k-o. li-ca. lyc. na-cl. pb.

Left side Visible. i. li-ca. lyc.

Right side Visible. ca-ca.

Beginning and End Visible. k-o. pb.

RED. anan. atp. ca-s. can. chlor. cmc. con. cph. cro. dig. dt. hyo. lac-c. mg-cl. myris. rut. s. smi. smr. snt. spi. sr-ca: trg. vr-s. vr-v.

SMALL. cb-v. (chd). chlor. dt. glo. hg-bicl. hyo. pet. ppv. pt. thu.

STRANGE. ba-cl. ca-a. can-i. cic. cro. dl-s. dt. glo. hyo. na-cl. ppv. pt. rs-r. vr-a.

STRIPED, amm-ca. amm-cl. atp. con. i. k-ca. mgs. mtr. na-cl. p. pul. sep.

VARIEGATED. ag-na. atp. ba-ca. cic. con. dig. dt. euph. fe-mgs. k-ca. k-na. k-o. lac-c. ni-ca. p. p-x. s. sn.

WHITE, (pale). aga. al-o. amm-ca. atp. can. chd. chi. (cop). cro. dig. dl-s. dro. ery. grt. k-ca. k-o. p-x. pb. pet. pul. (rn-b). rs. rut. s. si-x. srr.

WIDE apart, cb-a.

YELLOW (orange). al-o. am-ni. amm-cl. art-v. as-o. atp. clf. cth. dig hyo. k-bicr. k-ca. lac-c. mn-ca. nic. p-x. ptv. s. sep. si-x. snt. sr-ca. tep. zn.

OBJECTS, IMAGINARY.

ac-s. ach. acon. æsc. ag. ag-na. aga. al-o. alo. am-ni. amm-ca. amm-cl. amb. anan. anm. aps. art-v. arum-t. as-o. asc. atp. au. ba-ca. ber. bi-na. br. bry. buf. c-bis. ca-ca. ca-pa. ca-s. cac. can. can-i. cast. cb-a. cb-v. chd. chi. chio. cit-c. cl-hx. cle. clv. cmc. cmf. co. cof. con. cop. cph. crd. cro. crot. crt-c. cth. cu. cu-asi. cund. cy-hx. cyc. dig. dl-s. dph. drm. dro. dt. elaps. ery. evo. eug. eupat-p. euph. euphr. f-hx. frm. frm-s. gel. glo. glp. gn-c. grp. hæm. hg. hg-i. hur. hydr. hyo. i. itu. jat. jnp-s. k-ca. k-cla. k-na. k-o. klm. kre. krm. lac-c. lau-c. lch. lct. led. lpd. ly-b. lyc. men. mg-ca. mg-cl. mgs. mgs-ar. mgs-au. mim. mn-ca. morph. msc. mtr. myris. n-x. na-ba. na-ca. na-cl. na-sa. narth. ner. nic. ol-a. ol-t. p. p-x. par. pb. pet. phy. physo. pim. pnx. pol. ppv. pru-l. pso. pt. ptv. pul. qu-sa. rho. rmx. rn-b. rs. rs-r. rut. s. s-x. sang. sb-t. scr-m. sep. si-x. smb. smc. smi. so-d. so-n. spi. spo. sr-ca. srr. str. str-i. sum. tep. thr. thu. til. trg. trn. tx-b. urg. val. vi-o. vi-t. vin. vr-a. vr-s. vr-v. vrb. woo. zn. zng.

BLACK. ac-s. acon. ag-na. aga. al-o. amm-ca. amm-cl. anan. anm. asc. atp. au. ba-ca. buf. ca-ca. ca-pa. ca-s. can. cb-a. cb-v. chd. chi. clv. cmf. co. cof. con. cop. cu-asi. (cund). dig. dl-s. dt. elaps. ery. evo. glo. hg. hg-i. hyo. itu. jat. k-ca. k-o. klm. lau-c. lct. lyc. mg-ca. mn-ca. msc. (myris). n-x. na-ca. na-cl. narth. nic. ol-a. ol-t. p. p-x. pb. pet. pnx. ppv. pso. pul. qu-sa. rs. rut. s. sb-t. scr-m. sep. si-x. so-d. spi. sr-ca. str. tep. thr. thu. trg. val. vr-a. woo. zn.

Centre, atp. thu.

BLUE. as-o. can-i. clv. (cph). crt-c. (cund). dt. elaps. fe-mgs. k-ca. pso. sr-ca. trg. zn.

BRIGHT (fiery). acon. æsc. ag-na. al-o. alo. amm-ca. anan. as-o. atp. atrop. au. ba-ca. br. bry. ca-ca. ca-pa. ca-s.

can. cast. cb-v. chd. chi. cit-c. cl-hx. cle. clf. clv. co. con. cph. cro. cu. cu-asi. cyc. dig. dl-s. dph. dro. dt. elaps. ery. eug. euphr. f-hx. fe-mgs. gel. glo. grp. hg. hur. hydr. hyo. i. jat. k-ca. k-cla. k-o. klm. lau-c. led. lyc. men. mgs. mgs-ar. mn-ca. mtr. n-x. na-ba. na-ca. na-cl. na-sa. narth. ner. nic. ol-a. p. p-x. par. pet. pol. ppv. pru-l. pt. pul. qu-sa. s. sang. sb-t. sep. si-x. smc. smi. so-d. spi. spo. sr-ca. str. str-i. thr. thu. til. trg. tx-b. val. vi-o. vin. vr-a. woo. zn. zng.

Border. atp. thu. ˙

BROWN. (aga). na-cl.

BUBBLE **Bursting.** pul.

CIRCLES. am-ni. anan. bry. ca-pa. cac. can. cb-v. cit-c. cph. dig. elaps. f-hx. fe-mgs. i. k-ca. k-na. lch. mn-ca. na-ca. p. pso. pul. (s). sep. str-i. thu. tx-b. woo. zn.

Black. elaps. mn-ca. (s).

Blue. fe-mgs. zn.

Bright. anan. bry. ca-ca. can. cit-c. (cph). fe-mgs. pul. thu. tx-b. woo.

  On Inner Edge. cb-v. k-ca.

  At Side of Visual Ray. can. ˎ

Green. zn.

Grey. lch.

Increasing in Size. k-ca.

Moving Circularly. k-ca. tx-b.

Rays with. (cit-c). k-ca.

Red. cac. elaps. fe-mgs.

Side of Visual Ray at. can.

Sparks. mn-ca.

Variegated. (cph). k-na. p. sep. zn.

Vibrations Bright. dig.

White. can. k-ca.

Yellow. am-ni. k-ca. mn-ca. zn.

Zigzags. fe-mgs. sep. str-i.

COBWEB. aga. k-ca. k-o. mgs-ar. mrl. n-x. trn.

CORPSES. **(Skeletons).** as-o. atp. ca-s. can-i. crt-c. cth. hur. na-ca. ppv. smc. str.

  CROSS **Bright.** dt.

  High up. dt.

CRYSTALS **with Black tips.** (cund).

CURLS. (cund). i. k-ca.

CYPHERS. p. p-x. s.

Increasing in Size. p. s.

ELLIPSE, **Bright with Dark Centre.** thu.

FAR **off.** dt.

FEATHERS. (al-o). ca-ca. kre. lyc. mg-ca. na-ca. na-cl. phy. pol. spi.

FIGURES of Living Objects. æth. ag-na. aga. amb. anm. as-o. atp. br. bry. ca-ca. ca-pa. ca-s. can-i. cch. chi. clv. cmf. cof. con. (cu). dig. drm. dt. hg. hyo. k-o. lac-c. lau-c. mg-ca. mg-cl. mg-sa. mgs-au. myris. na-ca. nic. p. p-x. ppv. pru-l. ptv. pul. rhe. rs. s. sep. si-x. smb. str. trn. vr-a. zn.

Black. anm.

Moving with the Eye. anm.

High up. dt.

Moving. dt.

Moving from Right to Left. ca-pa.

Moving Downwards. dt.

Moving Upwards. dt.

Moving from Sides. dt.

Moving with the Eye. anm.

Side of Visual Ray at. dt. lac-c. myris.

FLAMES. atp. ba-ca. bry. ca-ca. ca-s. can. cph. dig. dt. ery. f-hx. hyo. k-ca. k-o. na-cl. p-x. ppv. pul. s. so-d. spi. spo. str. vi-o. vin. vr-a.

Moving. f-hx.

Red. f-hx. spi.

White Circle. can.

FLASHES **Bright.** ag-na. as-o. atp. atrop. br. clf. clv. cro. dl-s. dt. elaps. ery. f-hx. glo. i. k-ca. mgs. mgs-ar. mtr. na-ca. na-cl. ner. pul. sb-t. sep. si-x. spi. str. thr. thu trn. zn.

Moving Downwards. i.

Moving from Left to Right. elaps.

Side of Visual Ray at. thu.

GREEN. can-i. chi. dt. k-ca. k-o. lac-c. mg-cl. n-x. (na-sa). nic. p. rut. sep. sr-ca. vr-v. zn.

GREY. ag-na. ca-pa. chd. dt. elaps. lch. n-x. p. pnx. sep. si-x. str.

HALO. al-o. atp. ba-ca. ca-ca. chi. cic. cmc. con. cph. dig. dl-s. dt. euph. hyo. k-ca. k-na. k-o. mg-cl. mim. n-x. p. p-x. ptv. pul. rut. s. sep. smc. smi. sn. sr-ca. trg. vr-v. zn.

Black. k-o. p.

Blue. cph. sr-ca. trg.

Bright. ca-ca. trg.

Green. k-o. mg-cl. p. rut. sep. vr-v. zn.

Grey. dt. p. sep.

Red. atp. (cmc). cph. dt. ptv. rut. s. sr-ca. trg. vr-v.

Starlike. pul.

Variegated. atp. ba-ca. cic. con. hyo. k-na. k-o.
White. chi.
Yellow. hyo.
HIGH up. atp. dt. hg. mg-cl. rn-b.
HORNS Black. (cund).
INCREASING in Size. k-ca. p. s. so-d.
INCREASING and DECREASING in Size. lau-c.
LEAF. hg. (na-sa).
White. (na-sa).
LIGHT. al-o. chi. eug. k-cla. lau-c. p. qu-sa. val.
Red. chi.
Yellow. chi.
LOW down. cit-c. dt. hg. rs-r.
MIST (clouds). ach. acon. ag. ag-na. aga. al-o. amb.
amm-cl. anan. arum-t. atp. (au). bi-na. bry. c-bis. ca-ca.
ca-pa. cac. can. cast. cb-a. chd. chio. (cit-c). clv. con. cro.
crot. cth. cund. cy-hx. cyc. dig. dl-s. dt. (ery). frm-s. gel. glo.
glp. grp. grt. hæm. hg. hg-i. jnp-s. k-ca. k-o. klm. lac-d.
ly-b. (lyc). mg-ca. mg-cl. mrl. msc. myris. n-x. na-cl. (na-sa).
narth. ni-ca. ol-a. p. p-x. par. pb. pim. pln. pnx. pod. pru-l.
pt. pul. qu-sa. rmx. rn-b. rs-r. rut. s. sep. smi. so-n. spi. srr.
trg. trn. vi-t. vin. zn.
  Black. (ery). hg-i. ol-a. p.
    Moving. hg-i.
  Bright. k-ca. lyc.
  Grey. anan.
  High up. atp. mg-cl.
  Moving. atp. con. evo. hg-i. pod.
  Moving Upwards. jnp-s.
  Moving from Left to Right. atp.
  Red. (ery).
  White. atp. con.
    High up. atp.
    Moving. atp. con.
    Moving from Left to Right. atp.
  Yellow. k-ca.
MOVING. aga. amm-cl. anm. atp. au. buf. ca-ca. ca-s.
can. cb-v. chi. clv. co. cof. con. cop. (cund). dig. dl-s. dt.
ery. evo. f-hx. hg. hg-i. hyo. itu. k-ca. k-o. klm. lch. lct. lyc.
mg-ca. n-x. na-ca. na-cl. narth. ol-a. p. pb. pod. ppv. pul. rs.
rut. s. sb-t. sep. si-x. so-d. spi. thu. trg. zn.
MOVING with EYE. anm. ca-ca. dt. n-x. na-cl.
(qu-sa). s. thu.
MOVING CIRCULARLY. aps. ba-cl. k-ca. msc. tx-b.
urg. zn.

MOVING DOWNWARDS. dt.ery.i.k-ca.na-ba.p-x.thu.
MOVING UPWARDS. dt. jnp-s.
MOVING UP and DOWN. (ery). msc.
MOVING towards EACH OTHER. dig.
MOVING from SIDES. dt.
MOVING from RIGHT to LEFT. ca-pa. na-ba.
MOVING from LEFT to RIGHT. atp. elaps.
NEAR EYES. lyc. na-sa. s.
OBJECTS Previously Seen, (images retained long on retina). lac-c. nic.
PYRIFORM body. (cund).
Blue. (cund).
Red. (cund).
RAIN. au. k-ca. na-ca. na-cl. thu.
RAYS. atp. cit-c. i. k-ca. mtr. srr. trg.
RED. atp. cac. chi. (cmc). cot. (cph). (cund). dt. elaps. (ery). f-hx. fe-mgs. lac-c. ptv. rut. s. spi. sr-ca. trg. vr-v.
ROCKS. High up. mg-cl.
ROPE Across Sky. rn-b.
SEMICIRCLE. con. dt. vi-o.
Bright. dt. vi-o.
High up. dt.
High up. dt.
SERPENTINE bodies. ag-na. (cund). ery. str-i.
Black. (cund).
Moving. (cund).
Bright. ery.
Moving. (cund).
SHADOWS. ca-ca. pol. rut.
SIDE of VISUAL RAY at. can. cit-c. dt. grp. lac-c. mgs. myris. str. str-i. thu.
SPIRITS. as-o. atp. ca-s. can-i. cb-v. (cu). dt. hur. hyo. na-cl. ppv. pt. pul. s. sep. si-x. so-d. trg. trn.
Increasing in Size. so-d.
SPOTS (balls, points). ac-s. acon. ag-na. aga. al-o. amm-ca. amm-cl. anan. anm. as-o. asc. atp. au. ba-ca. bry. buf. ca-ca. ca-pa. ca-s. can. cb-a. cb-v. chd. chi. cit-c. clv. cmf. co. cof. con. cop. cot. cro. cu. cu-asi. cyc. dig. dl-s. dph. dt. elaps. ery. evo. glo. hg. hur. hyo. i. itu. jat. k-ca. k-o. klm. krm. lac-c. lau-c. lch. lct. lyc. mg-ca. mgs. mn-ca. msc. (myris). n-x. na-ca. na-cl. na-sa. narth. ner. nic. ol-a. ol-t. p. p-x. par. pb. pet. pnx. pol. ppv. pru-l. pso. pul. (qu-sa). rs. rut. s. sb-t. scr-m. sep. si-x. so-d. spi. sr-ca. srr. str. tep. thu. trg. val. vr-a. woo. zn.
Black. ac-s. acon. ag-na. aga. al-o. amm-ca. amm-cl.

anan. anm. asc. atp. au. ba-ca. buf. ca-ca. ca-pa. ca-s. can.
cb-v.·chd. chi. clv. cmf. co. cof. cop. cu-asi. dig. dl-s. dt.
elaps. ery. evo. glo. hg. hyo. itu. jat. k-ca. k-o. klm. lau-c.
lct. lyc. mg-ca. mn-ca. msc. (myris). n-x. na-ca. na-cl. narth.
nic. ol-t. p. pb. pet. pnx. ppv. pso. pul. (qu-sa). rs. rut. s.
sb-t. scr-m. sep. si-x. so-d. spi. sr-ca. str. tep. thu. val.
vr-a. woo. zn.

Bright. dl-s. thu.
With Bright Border. atp.
Low down. (cit-c). dt. hg.
Moving. aga. amm-cl. anm. atp. au. buf. ca-ca. ca-s.
can. cb-v. chi. clf. co. cof. con. cop. dig. dl-s. ery. hg. hyo.
itu. k-ca. k-o. klm. lct. lyc. mg-ca. n-x. na-ca. na-cl. narth.
ol-a. p. pb. ppv. pul. rs. rut. s. sb-t. sep. si-x. so-d. spi.
thu. zn.
Moving with Eye. ca-ca. dt. (qu-sa). (si-x).
Moving Downwards. thu.
Near Eyes. lyc. s.
Side of Visual Ray at. thu.
Symmetrical Lines in. cb-a.
Blue. as-o. clv. crt-c. dt. k-ca.
Moving. clv.
Bright (sparks). acon. ag-na. amm-ca. anan. as-o. atp.
au. ba-ca. bry. ca-ca. chd. cit-c. clv. con. cro. crt-c. cu.
cu-asi. cyc. dig. dph. dt. elaps. ery. glo. hg. hur. hyo. i.
jat. k-ca. k-o. lau-c. lyc. mgs. mn-ca. n-x. na-cl. na-sa.
narth. ner. nic. ol-a. p-x. par. pet. pol. ppv. pru-l. s. sb-t.
sep. (si-x) so-d. spi. sr-ca. srr. str. tep. thu. val. vr-a. zn.
Far off. dt.
High up. dt. hg.
Low down. (cit-c).
Moving. clv. con. ery.
Moving with Eye. na-cl. thu.
Moving Circularly. zn.
Moving Downwards. ery. p-x. thu.
Side of Visual Ray at. (cit-c). dt. thu.
Brown. (aga). na-cl.
Far off. dt.
Green. dt. k-ca. lac-c. n-x. sr-ca.
Low down. dt.
Moving. dt.
Moving with Eye. n-x.
Grey. ag-na. ca-pa. chd. lch. n-x. p. pnx. si-x str.
Moving. lch.
High up. dt. hg.

Low down. (cit-c). dt. hg.

Moving. aga. amm-cl. anm. atp. au. buf. ca-ca. ca-s. can. cb-v. chi. clv. co. cof. con. cop. dig. dl-s. dt. ery. hg. hyo. itu. k-ca. k-o. klm. lch. lct. lyc. mg-ca. n-x. na-ca. na-cl. narth. ol-a. p. pb. ppv. pul. rs. rut. s. sb-t. sep. si-x. so-d. spi. thu. trg. zn.

Moving with Eye. ca-ca. dt. n-x. na-cl. (qu-sa). (s). thu.

Moving Circularly. zn.

Moving Downwards. ery. k-ca. thu.

Near Eyes. lyc. s.

Red. atp. cot. elaps. lac-c.

Side of Visual Ray at. (cit-c). dt. thu.

Symmetrical Lines in. cb-a.

White. al-o. amm-ca as-o. elaps. ery. k-ca. krm. p-x. pnx. s. sr-ca. thu. trg.

Moving. thu. trg.

Moving Downwards. k-ca. p-x.

Yellow. aga. amm-cl. cb-a. cot. lac-c. lch. na-sa.

Symmetrical Lines in. cb-a.

SQUARES. elaps. hydr.

Red. elaps.

White. elaps.

STARS. al-o. amm-ca. atp. (ca-ca). cast. cro. hyo. k-ca. k-o. mgs. mgs-ar. na-ca. (na-sa). p. physo. pso. pul. trn.

Blue. pso.

Bright. al-o. amm-ca. atp. (ca-ca). cast. cro. k-ca. (na-sa). p.

Moving with Eye. ca-ca.

Near Eye. (na-sa).

Green. (na-sa).

Near Eye. (na-sa).

Halo. pul.

High up. atp.

Moving with Eye. ca-ca.

Near Eye. (na-sa).

Shooting. mgs. mgs-ar.

Variegated. physo.

White. al-o. amm-ca. atp. k-ca. k-o. na-ca.

High up. atp.

Yellow. (na-sa).

Near Eye. (na-sa).

STRIPES, (bars, columns). con. crd. dig. dl-s. dt. elaps. hydr. i. na-ca. na-cl. nic. p-x. s. thu. zn.

Black. p-x. s. zn.
  Moving. s.
  Upwards to Left. zn.
Blue. dt.
  Moving with Eye. dt.
  Vertical. dt.
Bright. dig. dl-s. dt. na-ca. na-cl. nic.
  High up. dt.
  Moving towards Each Other. dig.
  Upwards to Right. dt.
  Vertical. dl-s. dt.
Green. dt.
  Moving with Eye. dt.
  Vertical. dt.
High up. dt.
Moving. s.
  Moving with Eye. dt.
Moving towards Each Other. dig.
Red. elaps.
  Transverse. elaps.
Transverse. elaps.
Upwards to Left. zn.
Upwards to Right. dt.
Variegated. con.
Vertical. dl-s. dt.
SYMMETRICAL LINES **in.** cb-a.
THREADS (**hairs**). al-o. cb-a. con. (cund). elaps. (ery).
k-ca. pln. pol. spi. trg.
  Moving. con. (ery). trg.
  Moving Up and Down. (ery.).
White. elaps.
TRANSVERSE. elaps. rn-b.
UPWARDS to LEFT. zn.
UPWARDS to RIGHT. dt.
VARIEGATED. atp. au. ba-ca. cic. con. (cph). cund.
dig. ery. k-ca. k-na. k-o. p. physo. sep. zn.
VEIL. (**net**). ach. acon. ag. aga. al-o. amb. amm-cl.
arn. art-v. arum-t. as-o. atp. au. ba-ca. ber. bi-na. bry.
buf. c-bis. ca-ca. ca-pa. ca-s. can. cast. cb-a. chd. chi.
chio. clv. con. cro. crot. cth. cu. cy-hx. cyc. dig. dl-s. dro.
dt. elaps. euph. euphr. gel. glp. gn-c. grp. hæm. hg. hg-i.
hyo. i. jnp-s. k-bicr. k-ca. k-o. klm. kre. krm. lct. lpd.
ly-b. lyc. mg-ca. mg-cl. mgs-ar. mgs-au. morph. mrl. msc.
n-x. na-ba. na-ca. na-cl. narth. ni-ca. nic. ol-a. p. p-x.

par. pb. pet. pim. pln. pnx. pol. ppv. pru-l. pt. pul. qu-sa.
rho. rn-b. rs. rs-r. rut. s. sb-t. scr-m. sep. si-x. smc. smi.
so-d. spi. srr. thr. thu. til. trg. trn. vi-t. vin. vrb. woo. zn.

Black. (p). s.

Blue. (elaps).

Crooked. (na-cl).

Grey. elaps. p. si-x.

Watery. cb-a.

White. dl-s. elaps. lpd. srr.

Yellow. k-bicr.

VERTICAL. dl-s. dt.

VIBRATIONS, (flickering). acon. æsc. aga. al-o. alo.
amm-ca. aps. as-o. atp. ca-ca. ca-s. cb-v. chd. chi. cic. cit-c.
cl-hx. cle. clv. co. con. cro. cu. dig. dl-s. dph. dro. dt. ery.
euphr. f-hx. frm. gel. grp. hg. hur. hydr. hyo. i. jnp-s. k-ca.
k-o. klm. led. lyc. men. mgs. mtr. na-ba. na-cl. ner. nic.
p. p-x. par. pet. pol. pru-l. pt. pul. rs-r. s. s-x. sang. sb-t.
sep. si-x. smc. smi. sr-ca. str. str-i. sum. thr. thu. til. trg.
vi-o. vin. vr-a. vr-s. zn. zng.

Black. dl-s. thr. trg.

Bright. acon. æsc. al-o. alo. amm-ca. as-o. atp.
ca-ca. ca-s. cb-v. chd. chi. cit-c. cl-hx. cle. clv. co. con.
cro. dig. dl-s. dph. dro. (dt). euphr. f-hx. gel. grp. hg. hur.
hydr. hyo. i. k-ca. k-o. klm. led. lyc. men. mgs. mtr. na-ba.
na-cl. ner. nic. p. p-x. pet. pol. pt. pul. s. sang. sb-t. sep.
smc. sr-ca. str. str-i. thr. thu. til. trg. vin. vr-a. zng.

Circle of. dig.

Red. f-hx.

Side of Visual Ray at. grp. mgs. str.

Variegated. dig. k-ca.

White. sep.

Yellow. hydr.

VISIONS. acon. al-o. art-v. atp. ca-ca. can. can-i. cb-a.
cb-v. dt. hg. k-o. led. na-ca. p. p-x. ppv. pul. rs. smb. str.
thu. trn.

Beautiful. can. can-i. ppv.

Horrible. atp. ca-ca. cb-a. cb-v. dt. k-o. p. ppv. pul.
smb. trn.

Ludicrous. atp. can-i.

WATER. ca-s. hg. sb-t.

WAVES. ca-ca. hur. k-o. na-ba. (p). rs-v. sr-ca.

Concentric. (p).

Green. sr-ca.

Irregular Lines. rs-r.

Light of. ca-ca. hur. k-o. na-ba.
Moving Downwards. na-ba.
Moving from Right to Left. na-ba.
WHITE. al-o. amm-ca. as-o. atp. can. chi. con. dl-s. elaps. ery. k-ca. k-o. krm. lpd. na-ca. (na-sa). p-x. pnx. rn-b. s. sep. sr-ca. srr. str-i. thu. trg.
YELLOW. aga. amm-cl. cb-a. chi. cot. hydr. k-ca. lac-c. lch. mn-ca. na-sa. nic. zn.
ZIGZAGS. can. con. f-hx. fe-mgs. grp. hur. na-cl. p. rs-r. sep. str-i. trg. vi-o.
Bright. f-hx. na-cl. p. str-i.
Circle of. fe-mgs. sep. str-i.
Low down. rs-r.
Red. f-hx.
Side of Visual Ray at. str-i.
Variegated. sep.
White. str-i.
Side of Visual Ray at. str-i.

PHOTOMANIA (DESIRE FOR LIGHT).

acon. amm-cl. atp. ca-a. ca-ca. dt. gel. rut.
ARTIFICIAL **Light.** dt.
NATURAL **Light.** dt.

PHOTOPHOBIA (AVERSION TO LIGHT), SEE CONDITIONS—LIGHT.

SIGHT DAZZLED.

acon. as-o. ba-ca. buf. ca-ca. cb-a. chd. cic. con. crt-c. dig. dro. dt. euph. euphr. grp. hg. hyo. k-ca. k-o. lau-c. lyc. mn-ca. mrl. n-x. na-ca. na-cl. ner. p. p-x. pol. s. sa-l. sep. si-x. str. str-i. val.

SIGHT IMPAIRED. (DIMNESS. BLINDNESS).

ach. acon. æsc-g. ag. ag-na. aga. aga-c. al-o. alm. alo. amb. amm-ca. amm-cl. anan. anm. aps. arn. art-v. arum-t. as-o. asc. asr. ast. atp. au. ba-ca. bi-na. br. bru. bry. buf. c-bis. ca-a. ca-ca. ca-pa. ca-s. cac. can. cap. cast. cau. cb-a. cb-v. ccs. cd-sa. chd. chi. chio. cic. cit-c. cl hx. cle. clv. cmf. co. cochl. cof. con. cop. cot. cph. crb-x. crd. cro. crot.

crt. cth. cu. cund. cy-hx. cyc. dig. dl-s. dol. dph. drm. dro.
dt. elaps. ery. eug. eupat. eupat-p. euph. euph-c. euphr.
evo. f-hx. fe. fe-mgs. frm. frm-s. gel. glo. glp. gn-c. gn-l.
grp. grt. gui. hæm. hdm. hg. hg-bi. hg-i. hg-s. hur. hyo.
i. jnp-s. k-bicr. k-ca. k-i. k-na. k-o. klm. kre. krm. lac-d.
lac-f. lam. lau-c. lch. lct. led. lol. lpd. ly-b. lyc. men.
mg-ca. mg-cl. mgs. mgs-ar. mgs-au. mim. mll. mn-ca.
morph-a. mrl. msc. mtr. myris. n-x. na-ba. na-ca. na-cl.
na-sa. narth. ner. ni-ca. nic. ol-a. ol-t. os. p. p-x. par. pb.
pet. phl. phy. physo. pim. pln. pnc. pnx. pol. ppv. pru-l.
pso. pt. ptv. pul. qu-sa. rhe. rho. rmx. rn-b. rs. rs-r. rs-v.
rut. s. s-x. sa-a. sang. sb-s. sb-t. scr-m. se. sep. si-x. smc.
smi. smr. sn. so-d. so-n. spi. spo. sr-ca. srr. str. str-i. stry.
sum. thr. thu. til. trg. trn. trx. urg. val. vi-o. vi-t. vin.
vp-r. vr-a. vr-s. vr-v. vrb. woo. zn. zng.

TRANSIENT. acon. ag. ag-na. aga. al-o. amb. arn.
art-v. as-o. asr. atp. au. br. bry. ca-ca. ca-s. cac. can. cap.
cb-a. chd. chi. cic. cl-hx. cle. cochl. con. cop. cro. crt.
cyc. dig. dl-s. dph. dro. ery. euphr. fe. gn-l. grp. grt. gui.
hg. hyo. i. jnp-s. k-ca. k-na. k-o. lau-c. led. lyc. men.
mg-ca. mg-cl. mgs-au. mn-ca. msc. mtr. myris. n-x. na-ba.
na-cl. narth. ner. nic. p. pb. pet. pol. ppv. pru-l. pt. pul.
qu-sa. rn-b. rut. s. sang. sb-t. sep. si-x. smc. so-d. spi. str.
sum. thu. til. trg. urg. vi-t. vp-r. vr-a. vr-s. zn.

MYOPIA and PRESBYOPIA.

See Conditions—Looking at Distant & Near Objects.

B. ANATOMICAL REGIONS.

EYEBALL (including Conjunctiva Bulbi).

ach. acon. æsc. æth. ag. ag-na. aga. al-o alli. alm. alo.
amb. amm-ca. amm-cl. anag. anan. anth. aph. apo. aps.
ara. arn. art-v. arum. arum-t. as. as-h. as-i. as-o. asc. asp.
asr. ast. atp. au. ba-a. ba-ca. ba-cl. bap. bar. ber. bi-na.
blt. br. bru. bry. buf. buf-s. bz-x. c-bis. ca-a. ca-ca. ca-i.
ca-o. ca-pa. ca-s. cac. can. can-i. cap. cast. cau. cb-a. cb-v.
cbz-x. cch. ccs. cd-sa. chd. chi. chio. chlor. clv. cmf. cop.
cori. cot. cr-o. crot. cu. cu-a. cu-ca. cu-sa. cund. cy. cy-hx.
cyc. dig. dl-s. dph. dph-i. drm. dro. dt. elaps. erig. ery.
eryn. et-fr. eug. eupat. eupat-p. euph. euphr. evo. f-hx.
fe. fe-mgs. frm. frm-o. frm-s. gel. glo. glp. gn-c. gn-l. grn.
grc. grp. grt. gui. gym. hæm. hed. hg. hg-bi. hg-bicl. hg-cl.

hg-cy. hg-s. hll. hpm. hrc. hum. hur. hydr. hyo. hyp. i.
ind. irs. jat. jnp-s. jug. k-bicr. k-ca. k-cla. k-i. k-na. k-o.
klm. kre. krm. lac-ac. lac-c. lac-d. lac-f. lam. lau-c. lch.
lct. led. li-ca. lo-c. lo-cœ. lo-i. lpd. lpt. ly-b. lyc. men.
menth. mg-ca. mg-cl. mg-sa. mgs. mgs-ar. mgs-au. mitch.
mn-ca. morph-a. mph. mrl. msc. mtr. mur. myr. myris.
n-x. na-ca. na-cl. na-sa. narth. ner. ni-ca. nic. ol-a. os.
ox-x. p. p-x. pæo. pan. par. pau. pb. pb-a. pd. ped. pet.
phl. phy. physo. pim. plb. pnc. pnx. pol. ppv. pru-l. pso.
pt. ptv. pul. pul-n. qu-cy. qu-sa. rhe. rho. rmx. rn-b.
rn-s. rph. rs. rs-r. rs-v. rut. s. s-x. sa-a. sa-l. sang. sb-s.
sb-t. scr-m. sep. si-x. smb. smc. smi. sn. snp-n. so-d. so-n.
so-o. so-t. spi. spi-m. spo. spo-f. sr-ca. srr. stach. stc. str.
str-i. sum. teu. thr. thu. til. trg. tri. trn. trx. urg. urt.
urt-m. val. vi-o. vi-t. vp-t. vr-a. vr-s. vrb. vsp. vtx. woo.
xan. ziz. zn. zn-s. zng.

APPEARANCE, EXPRESSION, **Anxious.** acon.
alo. arn. as-o.

Astonished. glo. lau-c.

Bright, &c. ach. acon. æth. ag-na. (alm). alo. arn. as-o.
atp. bap. bry. clv. cmf. (con). cori. crot. cth. cu. cy-hx. dt.
eupat. hg-bicl. hyo. jat. jnp-s. k-ca. k-o. lch. (lyc). mgs.
morph-a. msc. mtr. na-cl. pb. pet. ppv. pul. sep. so-n. spi.
str. trg. trn. val. vp-t. vr-a.

Dim, &c. acon. æth. (alm). anan. arn. as-o. asc. asr.
ast. atp. ber. br. bru. bry. buf. c-bis. ca-s. cb-a. (cch). chd. chi.
cle. clv. cmc. cmf. con. (cph). crn. crt-c. cu. cu-asi. cyc. dig.
dph-i. dt. elaps. ery. eryn. eug. fe. gel. glo. gym. hg.
hg-bicl. hg-s. hyo. jnp-s. (k-bicr). k-ca. k-i. kre. lau-c. lch. ly-b.
lyc. mn-ca. mrl. msc. mtr. n-x. narth. p. p-x. pb. phy.
pol. ppv. qu-sa. rs-v. s. sang. sb-t. sep. sn. spi. spo. trg.
urg. val. vr-a. zn. zn-s.

Glassy. anm. atp. bry. cmc. (con). cro. dt. elaps. glo.
p-x. ppv. s. sep. sn. spi.

Impudent. (dt).

Spiteful. (dt).

Staring. ach. acon. æth. al-o. amm-ca. amy. anm.
arn. art-v. as-o. asr. atp. ba-cl. bru. bry. c-bis. ca-s. can.
cast. chi. cic. cl-hx. cle. clv. con. cro. crot. crt-c. cth. cu.
cu-a. cu-sa. cy. cy-hx. dig. dol. dph. dt. ery. eupat-p. glo.
glp. gui. hg. hg-bicl. hll. hyo. k-ca. lau-c. lch. lyc. mgs.
mgs-ar. mrl. msc. mtr. myris. nic. p-x. pb. pol. ppv. pru-l.
rs. rut. s. sb-t. sep. spi. spi-m. (spo). str. str-i. urg. vr-a.
zn.

Downwards. dt. ery.

Sideways. (dt).

Strange. æth.

Suspicious. dt.

Transparent. (acon).

Upward-looking. jat. .

Velvety. (con).

Wild. (alm). as-o. atp. clv. cu. cu-ca. dt. glo. hyo. lau-c. pb. ppv. spi-m. vp-t.

BORING. alli. aps. ber. bi-na. (br). (ca-a). ca-ca. (ca-o). (ca-s). cch. (cis). (cof). (con). (cu-asi). (elaps). (euph-a). (frm). hg. (i). k-ca. (lo-cœ). (myris). na-cl. nic. (ol-a). p. (ptv). pul. s. spi. (srr). thu. woo.

BROKEN **as if.** (lch). si-x.

BRUISED. acon. (alm). anm. (as-o). ca-pa. ca-s. (chlor). (cu). gel. (glo). (lch). (ly-b). lyc. (mg-cl). (na-cl). (pln). (pol). (pt). (ptv). (rs). s. sb-t. (smi). (str). urt. vr-a. vtx.

BURSTING. acon. al-o. aps. asr. (au). bap. bi-na. (buf-s). ca-s. can-i. (ccs). cot. dl-s. frm-s. (gel). grn. grp. gui. hyo. k-o. lac-ac. (lau-c). (mg-ca). (morph). (morph-a). myris. n-x. na-ca. (na-cl). (na-sa). par. pb. pol. pru. sb-t. spi. stach. srr. thu. woo.

COLDNESS. acon. (æsc). ag-na. al-o. amm-ca. asr. ber. (br). buf. ca-ca. ca-pa. chd. (chlor). con. cro. (dt). et-fr. f-hx. grp. hg-s. (hur). k-ca. k-o. lch. (li-ca). lyc. mgs-ar. mgs-au. narth. (ni-ca). (nic). p-x. par. pim. pnx. pol. pt. rs-r. s. sa-l. (sep). spo. thu. (trn). urg.

Burning. et-fr.

COLOR **Dark. (blue, brown, &c.).** (acon). (aga). (anm). (aps). (arn). (art-v). (as-h). (as-o). atp. (au). (ba-ca). (ber). (bi-na). (buf). (c-bis). (ca-ca). (ca-s). (can). (cch). (chd). (chi). (clv). (cn-sa). (con). (cph). (crn). (cu). (cyc). (dig). (dl-s). (dph). (dro). (dt). (ery). euphr. (fe). (glo). (grp). (gui). (hæm). (hg). (hg-bicl). (hg-s). (hll). (hpm). (hur). (hyo). (irs). (jat). (jnp-s). k-bicr. (k-ca). (k-o). (lyc). (mg-ca). (mrl). (mtr). (myris). (n-x). (na-ca). (ner). (p). (p-x). pb. (pod). (ppv). (pul). (rs). (rs-v). rut. (s). (s-x). (sa-l). (sb-t). (sep). (si-x). (smc). (smi). sn. (so-d). (spi). (spo-f). (sr-ca). (str). (str-i). (trg). (trn). (trx). (tx-b). vr-a. (vr-s). (woo). (zn).

Green. (cch) (myris). (p). (pb). (rs). (vr-a).

Red. acon. æth. (ag). ag-na. aga. al-o alli. (alm). alo. amb. amm-ca. amm-cl. anan. apo. aps. arn (as). as-o. asr. ast. atp. atrop. au. ba-ca. (ba-cl). bap. ber. bi-na.

br. bru. bry. buf. (c-bis). (ca-a). ca-ca. (ca-o). ca-pa.
ca-s. can. can-i. cap. (cb-a). (cb-v). (cch). ccs. chd.
chi. (chio). chlor. cit-c. cl-hx. cld. cle. cln. cmc. cmf.
(cnv-d). cof. con. cop. cor. (cot). cph. crot. cth. cu.
cu-a. cu-asi. cu-ca. cy-hx. dig. dl-s. dph-i. dt. elaps. (ery).
(eryn). (eug). (eupat). (eupat-p). euph. euphr. fe. frm. gel.
glo. glp. gn-l. grc. grp. grt. hæm. hg. (hg-a). hg-bi. hg-bicl.
hg-s. (hll). hur. (hydr). hyo. i. (ind). irs. k-bicr. (k-br).
k-ca. k-cla. k-i. (k-na). k-o. klm. kre. krm. (lac-f). lau-c.
(lch). lct. led. lpd. ly-b. lyc. mg-ca. mg-cl. (mgs). (mgs-ar).
mim. morph-a. mph. (mrl). mtr. myr. myris. n-x. (na-ba).
na-ca. na-cl. na-sa. ner. ni-ca. nic. ol-a. p. (p-x). (par).
(pau). pb. (pb-a). ped. pet. (phy). (plb). pnc. (pod). pol.
ppr. (pru-l.) pso. ptv. pul. qu-cy. qu-sa. rho. rn-b. rn-s.
rph. rs. rs-r. rs-v. rut. s. s-x. sa-a. sb-s. sb-t. scr-m. sep.
si-x. (smi). smr. sn. so-d. so-o. so-t. spi. spo. spo-f. sr-ca.
srr. str. str-i. teu. thu. trg. trn. trx. (u-na). (val). vi-o. (vin).
vp-t. vr-a. vr-s. woo. ziz. zn.

White. (acon). (ag-na). (atp). (buf). (ca-i). (cub). (frm).
(hg-bicl). (k-bicr). (pb). (s).

Yellow. acon. æsc. aga. amb. (anan). anm. as-h. as-o. atp.
(blt). bry. ca-s. cbz-x. chd. chi. cle. clv. con. crn. crt. (crt-c).
cth. cu-sa. (dig). (eupat). (eupat-p). fe. gel. hg-cl. i. k-bicr.
mg-cl. mtr. myr. (n-x). p. p-x. pb. (pnc). ppv. pul. rs. s.
sb-s. sep. (spi). str. str-i. trg. vp-r. vr-a. woo.

CONGESTION see COLOR **Red.**

CONTRACTIVE. acon. ag. aga. (amph). (anan). (ber).
bi-na. (bry). (chd). (chi). (crn). cro. (crot). crt-c. (dl-s). elaps.
(eug). (euph). (euphr). evo. grt. hæm. (hll). jnp-s. k-ca.
k-na. krm. lac-d. (lch). lpd. (lpt). ly-b. lyc. mgs-au. (myris).
n-x. na-ba. na-ca. (ner). p-x. pb. physo. (ppv.) pru-l. (pt).
(rho). rs. sep. (si-x). (sn). (so-d). (so-t). (spi). (str). (trg).
(urg). vi-t. vr-a. (vrb). woo.

Band, like a. lac-d.
Cord, like a. (amph). pru-l.
Horizontally. lac-d.
Vertically. (lch).
CRACKING (**snapping**). con.
CRAMPY. (aga). amb. (arn). (au). buf. can. (chd).
(cit-c). (crot). (eug). glp. (hll). (k-cla). (mn-ca). (msc).
na-ca. (narth). (p-x). (pt.) (vi-o).
CREEPING. (ach). (aga). (art-v). (as-o). (asr). atp.
(ber). chi. (cop). cro. crot. frm-o. (k-bicr). mgs-ar. na-sa. ol-a.
(par). (phl). (pol). (pt). (rn-b). sep. spi. str.

CUTTING. (alli). amm-ca. aps. (atp). au. ca-ca. (ca-s). (chi). cit-c. (cl-hx). (cr-o). (crd). crt-c. cth. (cund). (dl-s). (dro). hg. (hg-s). (i). (k-i). (na-ba). ol-a. pet. pul. (pul-n). rs. s. sep. (spi). (srr). stry. (thu). trg. (vi-t). vr-a. (zn). (zng).

DISCHARGE. ach. (acon.) æth. ag-na. aga. al-o. (alm). amm-ca. amm-cl. anan. anm. aps. art-v. arum-t. as-o. as-ters. asc. atp. ba-ca. ba-cl. ber. bi-na. br. bry. buf. c-bis. ca-a. ca-ca. ca-s. cast. cb-a. cb-v. cch. ccs. chd. chi. cic. cl-hx. cn-sa. cof. con. cph. cro. dig. dl-s. dro. (dt). erig. ery. eryn. (eupat). euph. euphr. fe. glp. grc. grp. grt. gui. hg. hll. hydr. hyo. i. k-bicr. k-ca. k-i. k-na. k-o. kre. (lac-ac). lch. lct. led. lpt. ly-b. lyc. men. mg-ca. mg-cl. mgs. mgs-ar. mgs-au. mn-ca. mrl. mtr. n-x. na-ba. na-ca. na-cl. na-sa. ni-ca. ol-a. ox-x. p. p-x. par. pb. pet. phy. pol. pru-l. pt. pul. pul-n. rhe. rho. rs. rs-r. rut. s. s-x. sb-s. sep. si-x. smi. sn. spi. spo. str. str-i. thu. trx. vi-t. (u-na). vr-a. vr-s. ziz. zn.

Corrosive. lyc. na-cl. s. (u-na).

Fetid. led.

Foam. ber.

Hard (æth.) ag-na. aga. al-o. (as-ters). atp. ba-ca. (bi-na). ca-ca. ca-s. chd. chi. cn-sa. (cof). con. (cph). (dig.) (dl-s). dro. (euph.) (euphr). fe. grp. gui. (hll). k-ca. (k-na). k-o. (kre). led. lyc. mtr. n-x. na-ca. ox-x. p-x. par. (pol). rhe. rho. rs. s. (sb-s). si-x. spi. (str). thu. trx. (vr-s).

Mucus. ach. æth. ag-na. aga. al-o. amm-ca. amm-cl. anan. anm. aps. art-v. arum-t. as-o. asc. atp. ba-ca. ba-cl. bry. c-bis. ca-a. ca-ca. ca-s. cb-a. cb-v. ccs. chd. cic. cl-hx. cn-sa. con. cro. dig. dro. erig. ery. eryn. euph. euphr. fe. glp. grc. grp. grt. hg. hydr. i. k-bicr. k-ca. k-i. k-na. k-o. kre. lct. led. lpt. ly-b. lyc. men. mg-ca. mg-cl. mgs. mgs-ar. mgs-au. mn-ca. mrl. mtr. n-x. na-ba. na-ca. na-cl. ni-ca. ol-a. ox-x. p. p-x. par. phy. pol. pru-l. pt. pul. pul-n. rho. rs. rs-r. s. s-x. sb-s. sep. si-x. sn. spi. str. str-i. thu. trx. vr-a. ziz. zn.

Pus. ag-na. al-o. (alm). amm-ca. art-v. as-o. atp. br. bry. (buf). ca-ca. ca-s. cb-v. chd. cro. dl-s. (dt). (eryn). euph. euphr. glp. grp. grt. k-ca. k-i. k-o. led. lyc. mg-ca. mn-ca. (mrl). (mtr). n-x. na-cl. na-sa. p. par. pb. pru-l. pt. pul. rhe. rho. rs. rut. s. s-x. sep. si-x. sn. (spi). spo. str. str-i. thu. trx. (u-na). (zn).

Tenacious (glutinous). (eupat). (lac-c).

Thick. hydr.

Thin (watery). mrl. na-cl. (pet). s. str.

White. ber. hydr. lch. (rs.)

Yellow. aga. (ca-ca). hg. k-bicr. n-x. rs. str. ziz.

DRAWING. acon. aga. (alli). (alo). (arn.) art-v. as-o. asr. (ast). atp. (bar). (ber). buf. ca-s. can. (cb-v). cch. (ccs). chd. (chio). (cic). cit-c. (cl-hx). con. (cor). cro. (crt-c). (cth). (dph). (dro.) (f-hx). (grp). (grt). (hg-s). (hll). (jcr). (k-i). k-o. klm. kre. (li-ca). (lo-cœ). lo-i. (ly-b). mgs. (mgs-ar). (mn-ca). myris. n-x. (na-ba). (narth). (nic). ol-a. p. (p-x). (par). pb. (pod). pol. (pru-l). pt. pul. (rhe). rho. (rs). (rut). (s). se. (si-x). (sn). (spo). sr-ca. (str). thu. (trg). (trx). tx-b. (val). vr-s. zng.

DRYNESS. acon. ag-na. aga. al-o. (anm). (arn). art-v. as-o. asr. atp. atrop-sa. ba-ca. bar. ber. bry. ca-ca. (cb-v). chi. cit-c. cle. (cln). co. cor. (cph). (cr-o). cro. crt. (cyc). dl-s. dph. (dph-i). drm. elaps. euph. euphr. gel. (glp). grc. (grp). grt. hg-bicl. (hpm). k-bicr. k-ca. k-o. kre. lch. li-ca. lyc. mg-ca. mg-cl. (mgs). (mgs-ar). (mgs-au). mn-ca. mrl. mtr. myris. (n-x). na-ca. na-cl. na-sa. narth. ni-ca. ol-a. p. pæo. pol. (pet). phl. ppv. pru-l. pul. qu-sa. rho. rs. s. (sa-l). si-x. (smi). spi. srr. str. (str-i). thu. trg. vr-a. zn.

Appearance of. kre.

ERUPTIONS. ach. (æth). ag-na. (al-o). (alm). (alo). amb. amm-cl. (anan). (aps). arn. as-o. (asc). atp. (au). ba-ca. (br). (bry). (buf). (c-bis). (ca-a). ca-ca. (ca-i). ca-pa. (ca-s). can. cap. cb-a. (cch). chd. (chio). (chlor). chm. cit-c. (cle). (co). (con). (cro). crot. (cth). (cub). (dig). dl-s. (elaps). (ery). (eryn). (euph). euphr. f-hx. (fe). (fe-pa). (frm). grp. (gui). hg. (hg-bicl). (hg-s). (hll). hydr. (i). jug-c. k-bicr. (k-ca). k-i. (k-o). kre. krm. lau-c. (lch). (led). lyc. (men). (mgs-ar). (mgs-au). (mrl). (msc). mtr. (myris). (n-x). (na-ba). na-ca. (na-cl). (na-sa). (ner). p. (p-x). (par). pet. phy. (pol). pul. (rho). (rn-s). (rs). rut. s. sb-s. sb-t. (se). sep. si-x. (smi). sn. (so-o). (spi). (spo). (srr). (str). (str-i). (te). thu. trg. (trm). (trn). (trx). (tx-b). (u-na). (val). (vtx). woo. (ziz). zn.

Abscess. (ca-ca). (ca-s). (hg.) (na-ca). (pul). (si-x).

Blisters. (arn). (ca-s). euphr. (k-bicr). (na-sa). sb-t. (thu). woo.

Boils. (bry). (ca-pa). (i). (na-cl). (p).

Cancer. as-o. atp. ca-ca. cb-a. hydr. p. sep. si-x. thu. trg.

Dry. (kre). (tx-b).

Encysted Tumors. (ca-ca). (thu).

Erythema Circumscripta. (ery).

Fistula. (alm). ca-ca. chd. dl-s. f-hx. grp. pet. pul. rut. s. si-x. sn. trg.

Fungus. as-o. can. cb-a. p. sep. thu.

Hæmatodes. atp. ca-ca. lyc. sep. si-x.

Medullaris. atp.

Granulations (roughness). ag-na. (aps). (as-o). (eryn). (k-bicr.) phy. sb-t.

 Hard. sb-t.

 White. sb-t.

Feeling of. elaps. (k-bicr). myris. (trn).

Hard. (au). (bry). (ca-ca). (dl-s). (gui). (lch). (rn-s). sb-t. (thu).

Herpes. (bry). (ery). (kre). (rs). (sep). (trn). (tx-b). (woo).

 Dry. (kre). (tx-b).

 Red areola with. (tx-b).

Hot. (c-bis). (smi). (sn). (woo).

Itching. (c-bis) (ca-ca) (na-cl). (se). (smi).

Moist. (ca-ca). sb-s.

Pimples. ach. (al-o). (asc). (au). ba-ca. (bry). (ca-s). (dl-s). (gui). (hg-s). (hur). (k-ca). (lyc). (msc). (n-x). (na-cl). (pet). (rho). (rn-s). (rs). (s). (smi). (sn). (thu). (trg). (trn). (trx).

 Hard. (gui). (rn-s).

 Hot. (sn).

 Pressing. (sn).

 Smarting. (gui).

 Undefined pain. (asc).

Pterygium. ag-na. as-o. can. chd. chm. euphr. (frm). krm. myris. pul. rut. spi. (trm). zn.

 Pustules. (æth). (al-o). (alo). atp. (c-bis). (ca-s). (chd). (chio). (con). (cro). (cth). hg. jug-c. k-bicr. (lyc). (na-cl). (p). (pet). (pol). (rs). (s). (se). (sep). (thu).

 Hot. (c-bis).

 Itching. (c-bis).

 Red areola with. k-bicr.

 Soft. (bry).

 White. (k-bicr).

Red areola. k-bicr. (tx-b).

Rhagades (cracks). (anan). (grp). (zn).   •

Scabs. (buf). (co). (con). (f-hx). (grp). (hg). (lyc). (sb-t). (sep). (spo). (srr). (te).

 Undefined pain. (spo).

 Yellow. (spo).

Scales, (scurf). (kre). (pul).

Shooting. (smi).

Smarting. (gui). (s).
Smooth. (au).
Soft. (bry).
Spongy. (alm).
Stye. (Al-o). (amb). (aps). (as-o). (au). (ca-ca).
(ca-s). (cch). (cit-c). (con). (cth). (cub). (dig). (dl-s).
(elaps). (fe). (fe-pa). (grp). (hg). (k-o). (lyc). (men).
(mgs-au). (na-cl). (p). (p-x). (pol). (pul). (rs). (s). (sep).
(sn). (so-o). (thu). (trg). (u-na). (val). (ziz).
    Smarting. (s).
Tubercles (warts). (alm). (au). (bry). (ca-ca). (dl-s).
(hg-s). (k-i). (k-o). (lch). (n-x). (rn-s). (sb-s). (sb-t). (srr).
(thu).
    Smooth. (au).
    Spongy. (alm).
    Undefined pain. (bry). (sb-s).
    White. (sb-s).
Ulcers. amb. (anan). arn. (as-o). atp. (buf). (ca-a).
ca-ca. (ca-i). ca-pa. (ca-s). cap. (cch). cit-c. (cle). (con).
(cro). crot. dl-s. (euph). (euphr). (frm). (hg). (hg-bicl).
(k-i). (led). (lyc). (mrl). mtr. (na-ba). na-ca. (na-cl). p.
(pul). (rs). (rut). s. (sb-s). si-x. (spi). (str). (str-i). trg.
(woo). (zn).
    Undefined pain. (asc). (bry). (hg-s). (sb-s). (sn).
(spo). (thu).
Urticaria. (chlor). (f-hx). (smi).
    Hot. (smi).
    Itching. (smi).
    Shooting. (smi).
Vesicles. amm-cl. (arn). atp. ba-ca. (br). cth. euphr.
(lch). (mgs-ar). (pol). (rs). s. (se). srr.
    White. (k-bicr). (sb-s). sb-t.
    Yellow. (spo).
FALSE SENSATIONS. ag-na. (aga). (al-o). alli. amb.
(amm-cl). (amph). anm. apo. aps. arn. art-v. as-o. asc. atp.
au. ba-ca. (bar). ber. bru. bry. buf. ca-ca. ca-o. ca-pa. ca-s.
cap. (cau). (cb-a). cb-v. ccs. chd. chi. cis. (co). con. cor. cro.
(crt-c). dig. (dl-s). drm. (dt). et-fr. euph. euphr. f-hx. fe.
frm. frm-s. gel. (grp). grt. hæm. hg. hg-s. hur. hyo. i.
k-bicr. k-ca. (k-i). k-na. k-o. kre. lac-d. lch. li-ca. (lo-cœ).
ly-b. lyc. (men). mg-cl. (mg-sa). mgs. mgs-ar. mgs-au.
mph. msc. n-x. na-ba. na-ca. na-cl. (na-sa). narth. ner.
ni-ca. (nic). ol-a. ox-x. p. p-x. pb. ped. pet. phy. pol.
ppv. pt. ptv. pul. rhe. rho. rn-b. rs. rs-r. s. (s-x). sang. sb-t.

(se). (sep). si-x. smc. smi. (sn). spi. sr-ca. srr. (str-i).
(te). teu. thu. trg. trn. trx. urg. urt. vi-t. zn. (zng).

Cutting. hg. k-bicr.

Fixed. k-i.

Hair. ccs. (k-na). mgs-au. na-ca. (nic). pul. rn-b. sang.
(te). (trn).

Hard. ner.

Lime. rs-r.

Mucus (grease). aps. ca-ca. (euph). pul.

Pellicle (film). cro. k-o. ol-a. (s). scr-m.

Sand (dust, foreign body). ag-na. (aga). (al-o). (alli).
amb. (amm-cl). (amph). anm. apo. aps. arn. art-v. as-o.
asc. atp. au. ba-ca. (bar). ber. bru. bry. buf. ca-ca. ca-o.
ca-pa. ca-s. cap. (cau). (cb-a). cb-v. ccs. chd. chi. (co).
con. cor. cro. (crt-c). dig. (dl-s). drm. (dt). euph. euphr.
(f-hx). fe. frm. frm-s. gel. (grp). grt. hæm. hg. hg-s. hur.
hyo. i. k-bicr. k-ca. k-i. k-na. k-o. kre. lch. li-ca. lo-cœ.
ly-b. (lyc). (men). mg-cl. (mg-sa). (mgs). mgs-ar. (mgs-au).
mph. msc. n-x. na-ba. (na-ca). na-cl. (na-sa). narth. ner.
ni-ca. (nic). ol-a. ox-x. p. p-x. ped. pet. phy. plb. pol.
ppv. pt. ptv. pul. rhe. rho. rn-b. rs. (rs-r). s. (s-x). (sang).
sb-t. (se). (sep). si-x. smc. smi. (sn). spi. sr-ca. srr. (str-i).
teu. thu. trg. trn. trx. urt. vi-t. zn. (zng).

Smoke. (alli). (chi). sang.

Snow-flakes. et-fr.

Splinter (thorn). ca-o. s. trn.

Stones, surrounded by. k-na. lac-d.

Water. ber. buf. (dt). (ni-ca). (trn). urg.

Wind. ag-na. (asr). cro. f-hx. hg-s. mgs-ar. narth.
(sep). thu.

GNAWING. (hyo). (k-i). (kre). ox-x. (pt). rn-s. s. (str-i).
vtx.

HÆMORRHAGE. arn. atp. ca-ca. cb-v. crt. elaps.
(ery). euphr. (grp). mtr. (pb). rut. str.

HARD. (acon). (bry). (cit-c). (dl-s). (n-x). (rn-s). (rs).
(spi). (spo-f).

HEAT, (burning). ach. acon. (æsc). æth. ag-na. aga.
al-o. alli. (alm). amb. amm-ca. amm-cl. anan. aph. apo.
aps. ara. arn. (art-v). as. as-i. as-o. asr. ast. atp. au. ba-ca.
bap. bar. ber. bi-na. br. bru. bry. (buf). bz-x. c-bis. (ca-a).
ca-ca. ca-o. (ca-pa). ca-s. can. can-i. cap. cast. cb-a. cb-v.
(cch). (ccs). chd. chi. chio. (chlor). cic. cit-c. cl-hx. cld.
cle. (cmf). co. con. cor. crb-x. cro. crot. crt. cth. cu. cy-hx.
cyc. dig. dl-s. dph. drm. (dro). dt. elaps. ery. eryn. et-fr.

eug. euphr. f-hx. fe. frm-s. (gel). glo. glp. grc. grp. gym.
hg. (hg-a). (hg-bi). hg-bicl. (hg-s). hll. hpm. (hur). hydr.
(ind). (irs). (itu). jnp-s. jug. k-bicr. k-ca. k-i. k-na. k-o.
(klm). kre. krm. lau-c. lch. lct. led. li-ca. lo-c. (lo-cœ).
lo-i. lpd. ly-b. lyc. (men). mg-ca. mg-cl. mg-sa. mgs. mgs-ar.
(mgs-au). mn-ça. mph. mrl. mtr. mur. myris. n-x. na-ba.
na-ca. na-cl. na-sa. narth. (ner). ni-ca. nic. ol-a. os. p. p-x.
pæo. par. pb. pb-a. pet. phl. phy. pim. plb. (pnc). (pnx).
pol. ppv. pru-l. pso. pt. ptv. pul. (pul-n). (rhe). rho.
(rn-b). (rn-s). rs. rs-r. rs-v. rut. s. s-x. (sang). sb-t. sep.
si-x. (smi). sn. so-d. so-t. spi. spo. (spo-f). sr-ca. srr. (stc).
str. str-i. stry. (te). (thr). thu. til. trg. trn. trx. (tx-b).
(urg). val. vi-o. (vin). vp-t. vr-a. vr-s. vrb. vtx. woo. ziz.
zn. zng.

Cold. et-fr.

HEAVINESS. (acon). æsc. al-o. anan. aps. arum-t.
as. as-o. asc. ast. atp. (atrop). (ber). br. (c-bis). (ca-ca). (ca-o).
(cac). cb-v. (chd). chi. (cit-c). (cl-hx). cmc. cmf. (con).
cph. (cr-o). crb-x. crn. cro. crot (crt-c). (dig). (dl-s). (dph-i).
ery. (euph). euphr. fe. (gel). glo. (glp). hæm. hg-s. hll. hpm.
hur. itu. k-bicr. k-ca. k-o. (lac-c). (lac-f). lch. (lpd). lyc.
mitch. mrl. (mtr). myr. na-ba. (na-ca). (na-sa). (nuph). (ol-m).
p. (p-x). pan. pb. (pd). (physo). (pnx). pod. (ppv). (pru-l).
ptv. (pul-n). (rs). rs-r. s. sep. (si-x). so-t. (spi). (spo). stach.
(str). str-i. stry. (thr). thu. (trn). (vi-o). (vr-a). (vr-v).

INFLAMED. See COLOR Red.

ITCHING. ach. acon. (æth). (ag). (ag-na). aga. al-o.
alli. (alm). amb. amm-ca. amm-cl. anan. (anm). aps. (arn).
art-v. arum. as-o. asc. atp. (au). ba-ca. (bar). ber. (br). bru.
(bry). buf. buf-s. (by-x). (c-bis). ca-a. ca-ca. (can-i). cb-a.
cb-v. chd. (chi). (chio). (chlor). (cit-c). cl-hx. (cle). con. cot.
(cr-o). crd. cro. (crot). (crt). (crt-c). cth. cu. cyc. (dl-s). dph.
dro. (dt). (elaps). eug. (euph). (euphr). (f-hx). fe. (frm).
frm-s. (glo). (glp). grc. grp. (grt). hg. (hg-a). hg-bicl. hg-s.
(hll). (hur). (hyo). (i). (ind). (jat). (jnc). k-bicr. k-ca. (k-i).
k-na. k-o. klm. kre. (krm). lam. (lau-c). (lch). (led). (lo-cœ).
(lo-i). lpd. ly-b. lyc. mg-ca. mg-cl. mgs. mgs-ar. mgs-au. mim.
mn-ca. mrl. msc. n-x. na-ba. na-ca. na-cl. (na-sa). narth. ner.
ni-ca. (nic). (ol-a). p. p-x. pæo. (par). (pb). (pb-a). pd. (ped).
pet. phl. (phy). (pnc). (pnx). (ppv). (pru). pru-l. pt. pul. rho.
rn-b. (rs). rs-r. (rut). s. (s-x). sb-s. (sb-t). (se). sep. si-x. (smi).
smr. (sn). (spi). (spo). (sr-ca). srr. str. str-i. stry. (te). (til).
trg. trn. tx-b. urg. vi-t. (vin). (vsp). (vr-a). (vr-v.) vtx. zn.

Desire to rub the eyes. aga. con. cot. cro. gym. k-bicr. k-o. urg.

LACHRYMATION. ach. acon. ag-na. aga. al-o. alli. (alm). alo. amb. amm-ca. amm-cl. (amph). anan. anth. aps. arn. art-v. arum-t. as-i. as-o. asr. ast. atp. au. ba-ca. bap. bar. ber. blt. br. bru. bry. buf. c-bis. ca-ca. (ca-i). ca-o. ca-pa. ca-s. cap. cast. cau. cb-a. cb-v. cch. cd-sa. chd. chi. cit-c. cl-hx. cle. clv. cmc. cmf. co. cof. con. cor. cph. cr-o. (crb-x). cro. crot. crt. crt-c. cth. cu. cu-asi. dig. dl-s. dph. dph-i. dt. (ery). eug. eupat. eupat-p. euph. euphr. f-hx. fe. fe-mgs. frm. gel. glp. grc. grp. grt. gym. hg. hg-bi. hg-s. hll. hrc. hydr. (hyo). i. irs. jnp-s. k-bicr. k-ca. k-i. k-na. k-o. kre. lac-d. (lac-f). lau-c. lch. led. lo-c. (lo-cœ). lpd. lpt. ly-b. lyc. men. mg-ca. mg-cl. mg-sa. mgs. mgs-ar. mgs-au. mitch. mrl. msc. myris. n-x. na-ba. na-ca. na-cl. na-sa. ner. ni-ca nic. ol-a. os. p. p-x. par. pau. pb. pb-a. (ped). pet. phl. phy. physo. plb. pnx. pol. ppv. pru-l. pt. ptv. pul. pul-n. qu-cy. qu-sa. rhe. rho. rn-b. rn-s. rs. (rs-r). rs-v. (rut). s. s-x. (sa-l). (sang). sb-t. se. sep. si-x. smc. smi. sn. snc. (snp). so-n. so-t. spi. spo. sr-ca. srr. str. str-i. stry. te. teu. thu. trg. trn. trx. tx-b. (u-na). urg. val. vi-o. vr-a. vr-s. vr-v. vtx. woo. xan. ziz. zn.

Cold. (trg).

Excoriating. as-o. led. pul. (u-na).

Greasy. s.

Hot (acrid). acon. al-o. arn. as-o. atp. au. bry. (ca-ca). (ca-i). cb-v. cd-sa. cit-c. con. cph. dig. dl-s. eug. euphr. glp. (grc). grp. hg. jnp-s. (k-na). k-o. kre. led. lyc. mgs. n-x. na-cl. (na-sa). p. p-x. pb. pb-a. pul. rs. s. sep. spi. str. str-i. teu. zn.

Salt. atp. kre. rs.

Thick. trn.

Appearance of. ca-ca. cro. hyo. kre. na-cl. ppv. sa-l. sep. so-n. teu. trg. vr-a.

Feeling of. arum-t. as-i. ba-ca. chi. cor. cro. (hg-s). hyo. kre. mitch. mrl. myris. n-x. na-cl. ner. ped. pt. s. sep. si-x. smr. sn. spi. teu.

LOOSE, feel. alli. cb-a. spi.

MOTION in. acon. ber. cb-a. cis. (dt). eug. (ly-b). mgs. (pt). (rs).

Bubbling. ber.

Jumping like something. (dt).

Passing round, like something. cis. (rs).

Pendulum, like. mgs.

Rolling. eug.
Undulation. acon. (pt).
Whirling. (ly-b).
MOVEMENTS. ach. acon. æsc. æth. ag-na. aga. al-o.
(alm). amb. amm-cl. amph. amy. anan. anm. aps. ara. arn.
art-v. arum-t. as-o. asr. ast. atp. ba-ca. bar. ber. br. bry. buf.
(c-bis). ca-ca. (ca-i). ca-pa. cb-a. cb-v. cbz-x. cch. ccs. chd.
chi. cic. cit-c. cl-hx. clv. con. (cop). cori. cph. crd. cro. crot.
crt. crt-c. cth. cu. cub. cy-hx. cyc. dig. dl-s. dph. dt. (ery).
eryn. eug. f-hx. (frm). gel. glo. glp. grp. grt. hg. hg-bicl. hll.
hur. hyo. (hyp). i. ind. jat. jnp-s. k-bicr. k-ca. k-cla. k-i. k-o.
kre. krm. (lac-ac). (lac-d). (lac-f). lau-c. lch. lyc. men. mg-ca.
mg-cl. mgs. mgs-ar. mn-ca. mrl. msc. mtr. n-x. na-ca. na-cl.
narth. ni-ca. nic. ol-a. p. p-x. par. pb. pet. phl. phy. pnc. pnx.
pol. ppv. pru-l. pt. pul. qu-sa. rhe. rho. rs. rs-r. rut. s. s-x.
(sa-l). sb-s. se. sep. si-x. smc. (smi). sn. so-d. so-t. spi.
(spi-m). (spo). sr-ca. str. str-i. thu. trg. trn. urg. vi-o. vr-a.
vrb. woo. zn.

Convulsions (rolling, quivering, twitching). ach.
acon. (æsc). æth. ag-na. aga. al-o. alo. (amb). amm-cl. (amph).
amy. anan. anm. (aps). arn. (art-v). (arum-t). as-o. (asr).
(ast). atp. au. (ba-ca). (bar). (ber). bry. buf. (c-bis). ca-ca.
ca-pa. cb-a. (cb-v). cbz-x. (cch). (ccs). (chd). chi. cic. (cit-c).
(cl-hx). clv. con. cori. (cph). (crd). (cro). crot. (crt). (crt-c).
cth. cu. (cub). cy-hx. cyc. dig. dl-s. (dph). dt. eryn. eug.
(f-hx). (frm). gel. glo. glp. (grp). (grt). hg. hg-bicl. hll.
(hur). hyo. i. (ind). (jat). (jnp-s). (k-bicr). (k-ca). (k-cla). k-i.
(k-o). (kre). (krm). (lac-ac). (lac-d). (lac-f). lau-c. (lch).
(lyc). men. (mg-ca). (mg-cl). (mgs). mgs-ar. mn-ca. mrl.
msc. mtr. (n-x). (na-ca). na-cl. (narth). ni-ca. (ol-a). (p).
p-x. par. pb. pet. (phl). (phy). (pnc). pnx. (pol). ppv.
pru-l. pt. pul. qu-sa (rhe). (rho). (rs). rs-r. (rut). s. (s-x).
(sa-l). (sb-s). (se). (sep). si-x. smc. (smi). sn. (so-d). (so-t).
spi. sr-ca. (str). str-i. (thu). trg. (trn). (urg). (vi-o). vr-a.
vr-s. (vrb). (woo). (zn).
    Feeling of. ara. ca-ca. (can). clv. (dt). glo. (lch).
(ol-a). pet. rs-r. trn.
    Squinting. acon. æth. al-o. (alm). aps. (art-v). as-o. atp.
ca-ca. ca-pa. clv. cu. cub. cyc. dig. dt. eryn. gel. hll. hyo.
k-i. men. pb. pul. rs. s. s-x. spi. (spi-m).
    Feeling of. ca-ca. men. pod. pul.
    Downwards. æth. (cb-a). (chd). (elaps). (grp). (ind).
(k-o). (phy). (ppv). (sep). (spi). (urg).
    Feeling of. (can). (ol-a).

Upwards. ach. acon. aga. amy. anan. arn. as-o. buf. cic. cu. cub. glo. hll. jat. lau-c. (lch). msc. (na-cl). nic. pb. ppv. spi. vr-a.

Inwards. (alm). (art-v). (ca-ca). (cyc). (hyo). pb.

Outwards. (cph). (cro). glo. lau-c. (mtr). (rhe). (rut). s-x. vr-a.

Feeling of. arn.

To the left. buf. dig.

From side to side. cu.

As if turned round. (chi).

As if taken out, squeezed, and put back. trg.

NUMB. (acon). (as-h). hg-s. (mrl). (naj). (narth). (pb). (ppv). pt. trg.

PARALYSIS. (acon). (ag-na). (aga). al-o. (amb). (amm-ca). amph. (anan). (anm). aps. arn. art-v. as-o. asr. ath. atp. atrop. au. ba-ca. ba-cl. (bap). (br). bru. bry. ca-ca. (ca-s). can. (cap). cb-a. (cb-v). (chd). chi. (chlor). cle. con. cro. (cu). cy-hx. cyc. (dro). (dt). (elaps). (eug). (euph). (fe). (gel). glp. grp. (hg). hg-btcl. (hll). hur. (hyo). i. ind. (k-ca). k-i. k-o. (li-ca). (lpd). ly-b. lyc. (men). (mg-ca). (mg-cl). mg-sa. mrl. (mtr). (myris). n-x. (na-ba). na-ca. (na-cl). (nic). (p). p-x. (pæo). pb. ped. (pet). (physo). (pnx). pol. ppv. pru-l. (ptv). (pul). rhe. (rs). (rs-v). (s-x). (sa-l). sb-t. (sep). (si-x). sn. (so-d). spi. srr. (str). stry. (thu). trg. (trn). urg. val. (vi-t). vr-a. vr-s. (zn).

PECKING. (pet).

PRESSING. ach. acon. æth. ag-na. aga. (al-o). (alo). amb. (amm-ca). (amm-cl). (amph). anag. anan. anm. aps. (arn). art-v. (arum-t). as-o. (asr). (ast). (ath). atp. atrop. atrop-sa. au. ba-a. ba-ca. bap. (ber). bi-na. br. bry. buf. c-bis. (ca-a). ca-ca. (ca-o). ca-s. (can). (can-i). cap. (cau). cb-a. (cb-v). (cch). (ccs). chd. chi. (chio). (cic). (cit-c). cl-hx. (cld). (cle). clv. cmc. cmf. cn-sa. co. cof. con. cop. (cor). cph. (crd). cro. crot. (crt). crt-c. cth. cu. cyc. dig. dl-s. dph. (drm). dro. dt. elaps. erig. ery. (eryn). evo. (euph.) euphr. (f-hx). fe. (fe-mgs). (frm-s). (gel). glo. glp. gn-c. gn-l. grp. grt. (gui). gym. hæm. hg. (hg-bi). hg-bicl. (hg-i). hg-s. (hll). hur. (hydr). (hyo). i. ind. itu. (jcr). (jnp-s). k-bicr. k-ca. k-cla. (k-i). k-na. k-o. (klm). kre. krm. lac-c. (lac-f). lam. lau-c. lch. lct. led. lo-i. lpt. (ly-b). lyc. men. menth. mg-ca. mg-cl. mg-sa. (mgs-ar). mgs-au. mn-ca. (morph-a). mph. mrl. (msc). mtr. myr. (myris). n-x. (na-ba). na-ca. na-cl. na-sa. narth. ner. ni-ca. nic. nuph. ol-a. (ox-x). p. p-x. (pan). par. pb. (pd). pet. (phl). phy. pnx. pol. (ppv). pru-l. pso.

pt. ptv. pul. pul-n. (qu-sa). rhe. rho. rn-b. rn-s. rs. (rs-r).
rs-v. rut. s. s-x. sang. (sb-s). sb-t. (scu). se. sep. si-x. smb.
smc. smi. sn. snp-n. so-d. (spi). spo. sr-ca. str. str-i. stry.
sum. (te). (teu). (thr). thu. trg. (trx). (urt). val. vr-a. vr-s.
(vr-v). xan. (zn). (zng).

Like a Plug, &c. (asr). chi. (hll). n-x. (na-sa). smc.

As if pressed about in all directions. atrop.

PROJECTING. acon. æth. (alm). alo. amy. anan. anm.
(aps). arn. as-o. atp. au. br. bru. ca-pa. ca-s. cap. (cch.) chi. cic.
cl. con. cth. cu. cy-hx. dl-s. dro. dt. glo. glp. gui. gym. hg.
hg-bicl. hyo. (k-bicr). mgs-ar. morph-a. mrl. msc. myris. na-ba.
pb. ppv. pru-l. rs. (s). (si-x). sn. spi. spo. str. urg. vp-r. vp-t. vr-a.

Feeling. atp. (cmc). glo. gui. rs. scu.

SCRAPING. (chd). (k-bicr). (p). (pb). (pru-l). pul. s.
(si-x). sn.

SENSITIVE. **See** CONDITIONS—TOUCH, &c.

SHOOTING. ach. acon. (æsc). (æth). (ag). aga. al-o.
alli. (alo). amm-ca. amph. (anag). anan. (anm). aps. arn. as-o.
atp. (au). ba-ca. (bar). ber. (blt). (br). bry. buf. c-bis. ca-a.
ca-ca. (ca-o). ca-s. cap. cb-a. cb-v. (chd). (chi). (chio). (cic).
(cis). cit-c. cl-hx. (cld). (cle). clv. (cmc). co. con. (cot). cph.
(crd). cro. crot. (crt). (cth). (cub). cyc. dl-s. (dph). drm.
(dro). (dt). (ecb). elaps. (eug). euphr. (f-hx). fe. (frm-s).
(gel). glo. (glp). (grp). (grt). (gym). hed. hg. (hg-bi). hg-bicl.
hg-cy. (hg-s). hll. hpm. hur. (hyp). (i). (ind). (irs-f). (itu).
(jnp-s). (k-bicr). k-ca. k-cla. (k-i). k-o. klm. (krm). (lac-f).
lau-c. (li-ca). lpd. ly-b. lyc. men. mg-ca. mg-cl. (mgs).
mgs-ar. mgs-au. (mn-ca). mph. mrl. mtr. (myris). (n-x).
na-ba. na-ca. na-cl. na-sa. narth. (ner). (ni-ca). (nic). ol-a.
p. p-x. (pæo). (pan). par. pau. pb. pet. phl. (phy). pnx. pru-l.
(pso). (ptv). pul. (rho). (rn-s). rs. rs-v. s. (s-x). sa-l. (sang).
sb-s. (sb-t). se. sep. si-x. smi. (sn). (snc). snp-n. so-t. (spi).
spo. sr-ca. srr. str. (str-i). stry. thu. trg. trn. (trx). (tx-b).
(u-na). (urg). (val). (vi-t). (vr-a). (vr-v). vtx. woo. (ziz).
(zn). (zng).

Cold. s. sa-l.

Hot. aps. (as-o). (con). (rho). (trg).

SMALL (**contracted**). (can-i). (crot). hg-s. (na-ba). (pb).
(rho). (woo).

Feeling. al-o. cro. grt. (gui). hg-bicl. (kre). (lac-d).
mrl. (par). (trg).

SMARTING. acon. æsc. æth. ag-na. aga. al-o. alli. amb.
amm-ca. anan. aps. arn. art-v. arum-t. as-o. (asc). asp. asr.
atp. (au). (ba-ca). bap. (bar). ber. br. bry. buf-s. (c-bis). ca-ca.

ca-s. (cac). cap. cast. cb-a. cb-v. cch. ccs. (chd). chi. (cl-hx).
cld. cle. (cln). cit-c. cmc. cmf. cmx. co. con. cor. cot. cr-o. crn.
cro. crot. cth. (cu). (cu-asi). dig. dl-s. dph. dro. dt. erig. eryn.
eug. eupat. euph. euphr. fe. fe-mgs. (frm). gel. glo. glp.
(gn-l). grp. (grt). (gui). gym. hg. (hg-i). hg-s. hll. (hur).
hydr. (hyo). i. (jat). k-bicr. k-ca. k-i. k-na. k-o. klm. kre. (krm).
(ind). (lac-ac). (lac-f). lau-c. lct. (led). li-ca. lo-c. lo-cœ. (lo-i).
lpt. lyc. mg-ca. mg-cl. mg-sa. mgs. (mgs-ar). mgs-au. mn-ca.
mrl. msc. (mtr). n-x. (na-ba). na-ca. na-cl. ner. ni-ca. nic.
ol-a. ox-x. p. p-x. pæo. par. (pb). ped. pet. phl. phy. (pim).
(pln). (pnc). (pnx). pod. pol. pru-l. pso. (pt). (ptv). pul.
(pul-n). rhe. (rho). rmx. rn-b. rn-s. rs. rs-r. rs-v. rut. s. s-x.
sa-l. sang. (sb-s). (sb-t). se. sep. si-x. smc. smr. sn. snp-n.
so-t. spi. sr-ca. srr. stc. str. (str-i). stry. (te). teu. thu. trg.
trn. trx. (u-na). (urt). val. (vi-t). (vr-a). (vr-v). vtx. woo.
ziz. (zn).

SOFTNESS. (rs). (thu).
Feeling of. (na-sa).
STICKY feeling. elaps.
STIFFNESS. acon. (al-o). anm. as-o. atp. ber. (ca-ca). ca-s.
chi. (chlor). cic. clv. eryn. (hg-s). hyo. k-o. klm. (krm). (men).
mgs. mgs-ar. mrl. mtr. p. p-x. pol. pru-l. (rs). s. (spi). str-i.
stry. trg. vr-a.
STRAINED. dph. s.
SUNKEN. (æth). ag-na. amb. anan. anm. as-h. as-o. ber.
buf. c-bis. ca-ca. chi. cic. cit-c. clv. cn-sa. crn. crt. cu. cu-a.
cyc. dl-s. dro. dt. ery. fe. glo. hg. hg-cy. hyo. i. irs. k-bicr. k-ca.
lau-c. lyc. mgs-ar. morph-a. n-x. ner. ox-x. p. p-x. pb. phy.
pnc. pod. ppv. pru-l. pul. qu-sa. rph. rs. s. smc. sn. spi. spo.
str. teu. til. trg. urg. vp-t. vr-a.
Feeling. amb. hg-s. lac-f. teu.
SWEAT. (ca-pa).
SWELLING. (acon). æth. (ag). ag-na. (aga). (al-o). alli.
(alm). (amb). anan. anm. (aps). arn. (arum-t). (as). as-o.
(asr). atp. au. ba-ca. (ba-cl). br. bru. bry. buf. (ca-ca). ca-pa.
ca-s. (can-i). cap. (cb-v). (cch). (cd-cl). chd. (chio). (chlor).
(cit-c). (cl-hx). (cln). (clv). (cmc). (cmf). cn-sa. cochl. (con).
cro. (crot). (cu). (cyc). (dig). dt. (elaps). (ele). (ery). (eryn).
(eupat-p). (euph). euphr. (fe). (fe-mgs). (gel). (glo). (grp).
gui. (hg). hg-bi. hg-bicl. hg-s. (hll). hum. hur. (hyo). (i).
k-bicr. (k-br). (k-ca). k-i. (k-o). (kre). (lch). (lct). led. (lyc).
mg-ca. (mg-cl). (mgs-au). (mn-ca). (morph-a). (msc). mtr.
myris. n-x. na-ca. (na-cl). (ner). ol-m. ni-ca. (p). (p-x). pb. (pet).
(phy). (physo). (pln). (pol). ppv. (pru-l). (pso). ptv. pul. rhe.

(rho). (rn-b). (rph). rs. (rs-r). rs-v. (rut). s. (sa-a). sb-t. sep.
si-x. (smi). (sn). (spi). (spi-m). (spo). (srr). str. (str-i). (te).
(teu). (thu). til. (trg). (u-na). (urg). (urt). urt-m. (urt-u).
(val). (vp-r). (vsp). woo. (zn).

Air-like. (p).

Bag-like. (k-ca).

Blue. (phy).

Chemosis. acon. aps. (atp). cd-cl. euphr. k-bicr. k-br.
k-i. physo. (vsp).

Hard. (acon). (thu).

Œdematous. (aps). (arn). (as-o). (chio). (crot). (hur).
(i). (k-bicr). (k-i). mg-ca. (pb). (phy). (rph). (rs). (rs-r).
rs-v. (sa-a). (te). (u-na). (urt). urt-m. (urt-u).

Red. (acon). (aps). (ner). rs. (sep). (te). (thu). (vsp).

Watery. (pul).

Feeling of, (feel large). acon. (al-o). (aps). asr. bap.
(ber). bi-na. (buf-s). ca-s. can-i. cch. (ccs). (chd). (cit-c). cld.
(cmc). cmf. con. cph. crd. cro. (cyc). dph. (dt). gel. grp. gui.
(hg-s). hyo. k-o. lch. men. mg-ca. (morph). (morph-a). mrl.
myris. n-x. na-ca. na-cl. ni-ca. p-x. par. pb. phy. pol. ppv.
pru-l. (rs). (rs-r). (sa-l). sb-t. sep. spi. srr. thu. trg. trx. (val).
(vi-o). (vr-v).

Veins swelled. acon. (alm). amb. (atp). (ca-s). dt.
(ery). (mg-ca). (pru-l). sa-a. spi.

TEARING. (acon). (ag-na). (aga). al-o. (alli). (amb).
amm-cl. (anm). arn. as-o. asr. atp. (au). (au-cl). ba-ca. (bar).
ber. (bi-na). bry. (ca-a). ca-ca. (ca-o). (can). (cast). (cb-v).
cch. ccs. chd. (chi). cit-c. (cl-hx). (cle). (con). cph. cro.
cth. (dl-s). dph. (dro). (euph). grt. (hg-bicl). (hyo). (hyp).
(i). (jnp-s). (k-ca). (k-i). (k-na). k-o. (krm). led. ly-b. lyc.
(men). mg-ca. (mg-cl). mg-sa. mgs. (mrl). na-ba. na-ca. na-sa.
(ni-ca). (ol-a). p. (p-x). par. (pb). (phl). (pnc). (pru). (pru-l).
pul. (rs). rut. s. (s-x). sb-t. sep. (si-x). smc. (spi). (spo). str.
(str-i). (teu). (thu). (trg). urg. (val). vr-a. zn.

TENSIVE. (ach). (acon). æth. al-o. (amm-ca). aps. (as-o).
au. ba-a. ba-ca. (bar). ca-ca. (con). cro. (cth). (dl-s). (dro). dt.
glp. (grt). (hg-s). (hll). hyp. i. jnp-s. k-ca. (k-o). lau-c. lct.
led. (ly-b). (lyc). (men). mrl. (myris). n-x. (na-ba). na-ca.
na-cl. narth. (ner). ni-ca. (nic). ox-x. p. (par). (phl). pol. pt.
pul. s. (s-x). (sb-t). sep. si-x. (sn). spi. (spo). stach. str. (thu).
trg. vi-t. (zn).

Like a Thread Stretched. (par). (s). (trg).

Laterally. (s).

THROBBING. aga. (amm-cl). aps. arn. as-o. asr. (atp).

(ba-a). (ba-ca). ber. (br). bry. (buf). bz-x. (c-bis). ca-ca. (cch). (ccs). (chd). (chi). (cl-hx). (cph). (cr-o). (cro)'. crot. (cth). (dig). dl-s. (euphr). (glo). hur. hyo. (i). (k-ca). (k-o). klm. (lau-c). (li-ca). (men). (mg-ca). (mgs). mgs-ar. mgs-au. mn-ca. mtr. (myris). (n-x). na-cl. (na-sa). ni-ca. p. (par). (pb). (pet). pol. (pru-l). rhe. (rho). (rs). (rs-r). (s). (s-x). (sep). sn. (so-t). (sr-ca). srr. (stry). (thr). thu. (trg). trn. (woo). (zn).

Single Throbs. cr-o.

TINGLING. aga. (art-v). (cro). crot. (drm). (ly-b). (par). (pol). spi.

UNDEFINED **Pain.** acon. (æth). ag-na. aga. al-o. (alli). alo. (amm-ca). (amm-cl). amph. anan. (anm). aps. arn. art-v. (arum-t). as. as-o. asc. ast. atp. atrop. atrop-sa. au. ba-ca. bap. (ber). bry. buf. bz-x. ca-ca. (ca-o). ca-pa. ca-s. cap. (cast). cau. cb-a. cb-v. cch. (ccs). chd. chi. (chio). cic. cit-c. (cl-hx). cld. cle. cmc. cmf. cn-sa. co. (cof). con. cph. crb-x. crn. cro. crot. (crt-c). (crv). cth. (cu). (cu-asi). cund. (delph). dig. dl-s. dph. dph-i. (drm). (dro). dt. (elaps). erig. ery. eryn. (eupat). euphr. (f-hx). fe. (fe-mgs). frm. (gel). gn-l. (grc). grp. gui. (gym). hg. hg-bi. (hg-i). (hg-s). hll. hpm. (hur). (hydr). hyo. hyp. i. (irs). (irs-f). (jan). (jcr). jnp-s. jug. k-bicr. k-ca. (k-cla). k-i. (k-na). k-o. klm. kre. lac-ac. lac-c. lac-d. (lau-c). led. li-ca. (lo-c). lo-i. lpd. (lpt). (ly-b). lyc. (mg-ca). mg-cl. (mg-sa). mgs-ar. mll. mn-ca. mph. mrl. (msc). mtr. myr. n-x. na-ba. na-ca. na-cl. narth. ner. (ni-ca). nic. (nuph). (ol-a). (ox-x). p. p-x. (pau). pb. (pd). pet. (phy). (pnx). pod. pol. ppv. (pru-l). (pso). pt. pul. pul-n. (qu-sa). rho. rn-b. rn-s. rs. (rs-r). rut. s. (s-x). (sa-a). (sang). (sb-s). (sb-t). (scu). (se). sep. si-x. smc. smi. sn. snp-n. (so-o). spi. spo-f. srr. str. str-i. stry. thu. trg. tri. trn. (trx). (urt). val. vr-a. vr-s. (vsp). (vtx). (woo). (xan). (ziz). zn. (zng).

WRINKLED. ag-na. br. (chio). (dt). (zn).

Feeling. anan.

EYEBALL SUPERIORLY.

acon. aga. alli. amm-cl. anan. as-o. ast. br. ca-ca. ca-o. cac. cb-a. cb-v. ccs. chd. cmf. co. cot. crt-c. dl-s. drm. hg. hll. i. lo-cœ. lo-i. mrl. ox-x. p-x. phy. pim. pru-l. s. sep. si-x. sn. snc. spi. sr-ca. str-i. thu. vi-t.

BORING. s.

BRUISED. s.

BURSTING. acon.
COLOR Red. str-i.
CONTRACTIVE. chd.
CUTTING. hg.
DRAWING. pru-l.
DRYNESS. s.
FALSE SENSATIONS, Hair. ccs.
Sand. aga. anan. ca-ca. ca-o. ccs. co. sn. str-i. vi-t.
Smoke. alli.
HEAT. p-x. pim. spi.
ITCHING. aga.
PRESSING. aga. cb-a. cb-v. chd. drm. lo-i. mrl. ox-x.
phy. sep. spi.
SHOOTING. cb-a. hll. p-x.
SMARTING. cac. spi.
TEARING. amm-cl.
TINGLING. aga. drm.
UNDEFINED. (acon). as-o. cmf. crt-c.

EYEBALL INFERIORLY.

aga. aps. chi. glp. jnp-s. men. p-x. pol. s. se. sep. spi.
str. zn.
COLOR, Yellow. str.
DRYNESS. s.
FALSE SENSATIONS, Sand. se. smc. (spi.)
Smoke. chi.
HEAT. glp.
PRESSING. p-x. pol. spi.
SMARTING. spi.
TENSIVE. jnp-s.

EYEBALL EXTERNALLY.

ca-a. ca-pa. cyc. dt. i. k-bicr. p-x. ptv. pul. rn-b. rs. smi.
sn. spi. spo. trx. vr-a. vtx. woo.
BRUISED. vtx.
COLOR, Red. ca-a. ca-pa. pul. smi.
ERUPTIONS, Blisters. woo.
HEAT. trx.
PRESSING. rn-b.
SHOOTING. cyc. trx.
SWELLING. ptv.

EYEBALL INTERNALLY.

acon. ag-na. art-v. ber. ca-ca. ca-pa. ery. eug. glp. hæm.
jnp.-s. k-bicr. k-o. li-ca. mtr. p-x. pru-l. pul. rs. rs-v. rut.
s. str-i. thr. thu. trm. trx. woo. zn.
BORING. s.
BRUISED. s.
COLOR, **Red**. acon. ag-na. ca-pa. eug. hæm. p-x.
pru-l. pul. rs-r. rs-v. zn.
Yellow. p-x.
DRYNESS. art-v. ber.
ERUPTIONS, **Blisters**. woo.
Pterygium. trm. zn.
Pustules. k-bicr.
FALSE SENSATIONS, **Pellicle**. k-o.
HEAT. glp. thr.
ITCHING. str-i.
PRESSING. ber.
SWELLING. ag-na.
TENSIVE. jnp-s.

EYEBALL ANTERIORLY.

acon. s-x. sb-s.
HEAT. s-x.
PRESSING. acon. s-x.
SHOOTING. acon. sb-s.

EYEBALL POSTERIORLY.

anth. asc. atp. au. bi-na. ca-pa. can. cau. co. f-hx. glo. led.
menth. mrl. p. p-x. pd. s. sep. spi. spo-f. srr. thr. thu. urg.
BORING. thu.
COLDNESS. ca-pa.
HEAVINESS. thr.
ITCHING. sep.
PRESSING. anth. au. can. cau. f-hx. led. menth. mrl
p-x. s. thr.
SHOOTING. p.
SMARTING. srr.
TEARING. bi-na. urg.
UNDEFINED. atrop. co. sep. spi.

EYEBALL INTERIORLY.

acon. al-o. alli. anag. art-v. as-o. asr. atp. ba-a. ba-ca. cch. chd. cis. cmf. dt. glo. hg. k-ca. lac-ac. lac-f. li-ca. men. mrl. pol. rn-b. spi. trn. vr-s.

BORING. cch.
BURSTING. acon.
DRAWING. cch.
DRYNESS. asr.
HEAT. hg.
PRESSING. anag. art-v. atp. ba-a. ba-ca. cmf. dt. hg. men. mrl. rn-b.
SHOOTING. k-ca.
SMARTING. al-o. spi.
TEARING. asr.
THROBBING. asr. trn.
UNDEFINED. as-o. cmf. li-ca.

EYEBALL CIRCUMFERENCE.

æsc. crt-c. gel. spo.
CUTTING. crt-c.
PRESSING. spo.

EYEBALL ROUND CORNEA.

ag-na. as-o. ba-ca. ca-s. hg-s. k-bicr. na-ca. pul. s. thu.
COLOR **Red.** ag-na. as-o. (ca-s). hg-s. k-bicr. pul. s.
ERUPTIONS **Blisters.** (ca-s).
Pimples. ba-ca.
Ulcers. na-ca.
Vesicles. s.

EYEBALL, CENTRE OF.

k-bicr. krm. lac-ac. lac-f. rs.
FALSE SENSATIONS, **Pellicle.** krm.
HEAT. krm.
SMARTING. lac-ac.

c

SCLEROTIC.

acon. anan. aps. as-o. atp. blt. ca-s. clv. cmc. con. dt. elaps. eupat. hg. hur. i. k-bicr. led. pau. pnc. rs. so-t. srr. str.

COLOR **Dark**. pb.

Red. aps. as-o. atp. ca-s. cmc. dt. elaps. eupat. hg. hur. i. led. pau. rs. so-t. srr. str.

Yellow. acon. anan. as-o. blt. clv. con. eupat. i. k-bicr. pnc.

SWELLING. atp. k-bicr. led.

Veins of. atp.

CORNEA.

acon. æth. ag-na. (alm). amm-ca. amm-cl. aps. art-v. atp. au. ba-ca. bry. buf. ca-ca. (ca-i). ca-pa. ca-s. can. cap. cch. chd. chi. con. cph. crot. cu, dig. dt. euph. euphr. fe. (frm). glp. grp. hg. hg-bicl. hyo. k-bicr. k-i. k-o. kre. lac-ac. ly-b. lyc. mg-ca. n-x. na-ca. na-cl. nic. p. pb. pb-a. physo. pol. ppv. pul. rs. rut. s. sa-a. sb-t. sep. si-x. smi. sn. so-d. spi. spo. str. thu. trg. trx. urg. val. vr-a. zng.

APPEARANCE, **Bright**. con.

Glassy. con.

ARCUS SENILIS. ca-ca.

COLOR. **Dark**. aps. crot. euph. euphr. glp. k-bicr. n-x. spi.

Red. (alm). amm-ca. au. can. nic. pb. pb-a. s. thu.

White. ag-na. (ca-i). (frm). hg-bicl. (k-bicr). pb. s.

ERUPTIONS, **Abscess**. ca-ca. ca-s. hg. si-x. ,

Pimples. rs.

Pustules. æth. ca-s. hg. k-bicr. (p). sep.

Ulcers. (aps). as-o. atp. buf. ca-ca. (ca-i). ca-pa. ca-s. con. crot. euphr. (frm). hg. na-ca. rut. s. sa-a. si-x. trg.

Vesicles. rs.

OPACITY (**specks**). æth. ag-na. (alm). aps. art-v. as-o. atp. au. ca-ca. ca-s. can. cap. cch. chd. chi. con. crot. (cu). euphr. (frm). glp. (k-bicr). k-i. k-o. lyc. mg-ca. n-x. pb. physo. pol. pul. (rs). rut. s. sa-a. sep. si-x. str. trx. zng.

PROJECTING. (alm.) aps. cch. (k-bicr). k-i. s. si-x.

SMARTING. lac-ac.

SUNKEN. æth.

CHAMBERS OF EYE.

as-o. (atp). ca-s. crot. hg-bicl. pb. s.
DISCHARGE, **Pus.** as-o. (atp). ca-s. crot. hg-bicl.
pb. s.

IRIS.

acon. æth. ag. ag-na. aga. aga-p. (alm). amy. anan. anm.
aps. arn. art-v. as-o. ast. atp. au. ba-a. br. buf. c-bis. ca-a. ca-ca
ca-s. can. cap. cb-a. cch. chd. chi. chlor. cic. cl-hx. cle. clf.
cln. clv. con. cop. cph. cro. crt. cth. cu. cu-a. cub. cy. cy-hx.
cyc. cyt. dig. dl-s. dph. dph-i. dt. ery. euph. fe. gel. glo. glp.
grp. gui. hæm. hg. hg-bicl. hg-cy. hg-s. hll. hyo. hyp. i. jat.
jnp-s. k-br. k-i. k-o. kre. lam. lau-c. lch. lct. led. lol. lyc. men.
mgs. mgs-ar. mgs-au. mn-ca. morph. morph-a. mrl. msc. mtr.
myris. n-x. na-ca. narth. ner. nic. ol-t. p. p-x. par. pb. ped.
pet. phy. physo. pnc. pnx. pol. ppv. pru-l. qu-sa. rhe. rho.
rn-b. rph. (rs). rut. s. sang. sb-t. scu. si-x. smb. smc. smi.
smr. sn. so-d. so-n. spi. spi-m. sr-ca. srr. str. str-i. thu. trg.
trx. tx-b. urg. val. vi-o. vi-t. vr-a. vrb. vtx. woo. zn.
APPEARANCE **Dim.** cch. cph. (k-bicr).
COLOR **Discolored.** as-o. atp. cle. hg. hg-bicl. na-cl.
ol-t. rs. s. zn.
Green. rs.
Red. s.
ERUPTIONS, **Tubercles.** hg-s.
PROLAPSUS. (alm).
PUPILS **Contracted.** acon. ag. ag-na. aga. aga-p.
amy. anan. anm. arn. art-v. as-o. ast. atp. au. c-bis. ca-a.
ca-ca. can. cap. cch. chd. chi. chlor. cic. cl-hx. con. cop. cph.
(crb-x). cro. crot. cth. cu. cu-a. cub. dig. dl-s. dph. dph-i.
dro. dt. glo. glp. hæm. hg-bicl. hg-cy. hll. hyo. jat. jnp-s. k-o.
lam. lau-c. led. men. mgs-ar. mn-ca. morph. morph-a. msc.
mtr. myris. na-ca. ner. nic. p. p-x. pb. phy. physo. pnc.
pnx. pol. ppv. pru-l. pul. qu-sa. rhe. (rho). rs. rut. s. sb-t.
sep. si-x. smb. smc. sn. srr. str. str-i. thu. trx. urg. vi-o. vi-t.
vr-a. woo. zn.
Dilated. acon. æth. ag-na. aga. aga-p. (alm). anan. anm.
aps. arn. art-v. as-o. atp. au. br. buf. c-bis. ca-a. ca-ca. ca-s.
can. cap. cb-a. chi. chlor. cic. cl-hx. cln. clv. con. cph. cro.

crt. cth. cu. cub. cy. cy-hx. cyc. cyt. dig. dl-s. dph. dro. dt
ery. euph. gel. glo. glp. gui. hg. hg-bicl. hg-cy. hyo. hyp. i.
jnp-s. k-bicr. k-br. k-i. k-o. kre. lam. lau-c. lch. lct. led. lol.
lyc. men. mgs. mgs-ar. mgs-au. mn-ca. morph. morph-a. mrl.
msc. mtr. myris. n-x. na-ca. narth. ner. nic. p. (p-x). par. pb.
ped. physo. pnc. pnx. ppv. pru-l. pul. qu-sa. rhe. rho. rph. rs.
sang. scu. smb. smc. smi. smr. sn. so-d. so-n. spi. spi-m. sr-ca.
str. str-i. thu. trg. trx. tx-b. urg. val. vr-a. vrb. vtx. woo. zn.

Insensible.   acon. æth. ag-na. amy. arn. atp. ba-ca. buf.
chi. chlor. cph. (crb-x). cu. cy-hx. dig. dt. fe. hg-bicl.
hyo. k-bicr. lyc. mgs-ar. mtr. myris. n-x. pb. pnc. pol. ppv.
pru-l. rn-b. (rs). spi. trg.

Irregular.   ba-a. ca-ca. grp. hg-bicl. n-x. (nic). (rs). s.
si-x. trg.

Mobile.   anan. atp. buf. cph. mtr. pb. ppv. s. str-i.

LENS.

acon. aga. alli. amm-ca. amm-cl. anm. arn. art-v. as-o. atp.
au. ba-ca. bry. buf. ca-ca. ca-pa. ca-s. can. cap. cch. chd. chi.
clv. con. cro. cub. dig. dl-s. dt. euph. euphr. glp. gui. hg. hyo.
k-o. kre. ly-b. lyc. men. mg-ca. mn-ca. n-x. na-ca. na-cl. p.
pb. pol. ppv. pul. rs. rut. s. sa-a. sang. sb-t. sep. si-x. smi. sn.
so-d. spi. srr. str. str-i. te. trx. val. vr-a.

CATARACT.   acon. aga. alli. amm-ca. amm-cl. anm. arn.
art-v. as-o. atp. au. ba-ca. bry. buf. ca-ca. ca-pa. ca-s. can. cap.
cch. chd. chi. clv. con. cro. cub. dig. dl-s. dt. euph. euphr. glp.
gui. hg. hyo. k-o. kre. ly-b. lyc. mg-ca. mn-ca. n-x. na-ca. na-cl.
p. pb. pol. ppv. pul. rs. rut. s. sa-a. sang. sb-t. sep. si-x. smc.
smi. sn. so-d. spi. srr. (str). str-i. te. trx. val. vr-a.

Reticulated.   k-o. pb.

COLOR, **Black.**   anm. atp. ca-ca. can. chi. clv. (con).
dig. gui. hg. hyo. n-x. p. pb. pul. rs. rut. s. sb-t. si-x. so-d.
spi. (str).

Green.   cch. p. pul.

Grey.   ba-ca. can. chd. con. euphr. hyo. k-o. mg-ca. n-x.
ppv. pul. rut. s.

Red.   buf.

White.   atp. buf. cub.

SWELLING.   cch.

FUNDUS.

atp. p.
COLOR **Green.** p.
Red. atp.

ORBIT.

acon. æth. aga. al-o. alm. alo. amm-cl. anan. anm. aps.
arn. art-v. as-o. asc. atp. au. ba-a. ba-ca. bar. ber. bi-na. bry.
buf. c-bis. ca-a. .ca-ca. ca-o. ca-s. cac. cch. chd. chi. chio.
cit-c. cl-hx. con. crn. crot. crt. crt-c. cu. cu-asi. cy-hx. dig.
dl-s. dph. elaps. euph-a. f-hx. frm. frm-s. gel. glo. glp. hg.
hg-i. hg-s. hll. hur. hyo. i. jan. itu. k-ca. k-i. k-o. kd-o. lau-c.
lct. led. li-ca. lo-cœ. ly-b. lyc. men. mg-ca. mg-cl. mg-sa.
mgs. mn-ca. morph. morph-a. mrl. msc. myris. n-x. na-ca.
na-cl. na-sa. narth. ner. nic. nuph. ol-a. os. ox-x. p. p-x. pæo.
par. pau. pb. pet. phy. pol. pru-l. pt. ptv. pul. qu-sa. rho.
rs. rut. s. s-x. sb-s. se. sep. si-x. smc. smi. smr. sn. snp-n.
so-d. spi. spo. sr-ca. srr. str-i. thu. trg. trn. u-na. val. vr-a.
vr-v. vrb. ziz. zn. zng.

BORING.   ca-ca. ca-s. cch. ol-a. srr.
BRUISED.   crt. cu. pol. rs.
BURSTING.   buf. buf-s. gel. morph. morph-a. pb.
COLDNESS.   sep.
CONTRACTIVE.   spi. vrb.
CRAMPY.   aga.
CUTTING.   chi. srr.
DRAWING.   cch. mn-ca. s. sn. val.
EMPTINESS, **Feeling of.**   s. sep.
FALSE SENSATIONS, **Wind.**   sep.
GNAWING.   hyo.
HEAT.   men. nic. s. trn.
HEAVINESS.   crot. crt-c. glo. hur. nuph.
ITCHING.   buf-s. p.
MOTION IN, **Whirling.**   ly-b.
PRESSING.   acon. al-o. alo. anm. arn. as-o. atp. au. ba-ca.
c-bis. ccs. chd. chi. chio. cit-c. con. crt. cy-hx. dph. frm-s. gel.
glp. hll. hur. hyo. k-ca. k-o. lct. led. ly-b. msc. narth. ner.
nic. p. p-x. pæo. par. pb. pol. pru-l. qu-sa. rho. rut. s. sb-s.
sep. si-x. smc. sn. spi. sr-ca. str-i. trg. val. vr-a.
SHOOTING.   acon. æth. au. ca-ca. glo. k-o. lau-c. ly-b.
p-x. rho. rs. sb-s. val. ziz.

SMALL **Feeling.** par. trg.
SMARTING. (chd). glo. pt. si-x.
TEARING. acon. al-o. atp. au. bi-na. ca-ca. cl-hx. con. dph. mg-ca. mrl. p. phl. s-x. sep. smc. spi.
TENSIVE. men, pt. spi. thu.
THROBBING. amm-cl. ba-ca. ca-ca. dig. mgs. sn. trn.
TINGLING. ly-b.
UNDEFINED. alo., anan. atp. chd. chi. con. crt-c. gel. hg. i. jan. (ly-b). na-ca. nuph. ox-x. p. pb. pru-l. pul. se. spi. trg.

ORBIT CIRCUMFERENCE.

anm. aps. arn. ca-ca. cch. cl-hx. crn. li-ca. ly-b. mrl. na-cl. na-sa. narth. p. p-x. phl. phy. rho. rs. s. so-d. str-i. val. zng.
BRUISED. rs.
BURSTING. na-sa.
CONTRACTIVE. crn. so-d.
DRAWING. s. val. zng.
HEAVINESS. crn.
ITCHING. p.
PRESSING. anm. arn. mrl. str-i.
SHOOTING. p-x.
TEARING. ca-ca. cch. cl-hx. mrl.
UNDEFINED. anm. aps. (ly-b). p. phy.

ORBIT SUPERIORLY.

acon. al-o. alo. amm-cl. ba-ca. bar. ber. bry. ca-a. ca-ca. ca-o. cac. chd. chi. chio. cis. cu-asi. elaps. frm. glo. hg. hg-i. hg-s. hll. hur. hyo. jcr. k-bicr. k-i. kd-o. li-ca. mg-ca. mg-sa. mrl. msc. myris. na-cl. na-sa. ner. nic. ol-a. os. p-x. par. pet. phl. phy. pt. rs-r. rut. sep. smc. sn. sup-n. str-i. vr-v. zn.
BORING. ca-a. ca-ca. ca-o. myris.
CONTRACTIVE. myris.
CUTTING. hg-s.
FALSE SENSATIONS, **Foreign Body.** mg-sa.
GNAWING. hyo. pt.
NUMBNESS. mrl.
PRESSING. alo. hur. hyo. mg-sa. mrl. myris. ner. par. phy. pt. rut. zn.

Like a Plug. smc.
SHOOTING. acon. alo. ba-ca. ber. ca-a. hur. mrl. nic. ol-a.
SMARTING. hg-s. pt.
SWELLING, **Feeling of.** hg-s.
TEARING. al-o. kd-o. mg-ca. mrl. os. phl.
TENSIVE. mrl. pt,
UNDEFINED. chi. hg. ner. sep. snp-n. zn.

ORBIT INFERIORLY.

aps. art-v. au. euph-a. hg-i. hg-s. k-i. mg-cl. na-sa. p. phy. smi. thu.
BRUISED. mg-cl. smi.
GNAWING. k-i.
PRESSING. art-v.
TEARING. p.

ORBIT EXTERNALLY.

au. f-hx. led. li-ca. narth. pt. ptv. sn.
BRUISED. ptv.
PRESSING. led. narth.

ORBIT INTERNALLY.

cit-c. hg. k-bicr. lch. mn-ca. p-x. sep. si-x. thu,
COLDNESS. p-x.
CRAMPY. mn-ca.
PRESSING. cit-c.
SHOOTING. p-x.
SWELLING. hg.
TEARING. mn-ca.

ORBIT POSTERIORLY.

au. dig. rs. smr.
CRAMPY. au,

PRESSING. au
SHOOTING. dig.
UNDEFINED. rs. smr.

ORBITAL INTEGUMENTS.

acon. æsc. æth. aga. al-o. alli. alo. amb. amm-cl. anm.
aps. arn. art-v. as-h. as-o. asc. atp. ba-ca. ber. bi-na. br. bry.
buf. c-bis. ca-a. ca-ca. ca-s. can. can-i. cb-a. cb-v. cch. chi.
cic. cit-c. cle. clv. cmc. cn-sa. con. cph. cr-o. crd. crn.
cro. crt. crt-c. cth. cu. cyc. delph. dig. dl-s. dph. dro. dt.
elaps. ery. euphr. evo. f-hx. fe. glo. glp. grp. grt. gui.
hæm. hg. hg-bicl. hg-s. hll. hpm. hur. hyo. i. irs. jat.
jnp-s. k-bicr. k-ca. k-na. k-o. klm. lac-ac. lac-f. lct. lo-cœ.
ly-b. lyc. mg-ca. mgs-ar. mgs-au. mn-ca. morph-a. mrl.
mtr. myris. n-x. na-ba. na-ca. na-cl. narth. ner. nic. ol-a.
p. p-x. par. pau. pb. ped. phl. phy. pln. pod. pru-l. pt.
rn-b. rn-s. rs. rs-r. rut. s. s-x. sa-l. se. sep. si-x. smc. smi.
sn. so-d. spi. spi-m. spo. spo-f. sr-ca. str. str-i. thu. trg.
trn. trx. vi-t. vr-a. vr-s. vtx. woo. zn. zng.
COLOR **Dark**. acon. aga. anm. art-v. as-h. as-o. ber.
bi-na. buf. c-bis. ca-ca. ca-s. cch. chi. clv. cn-sa. cph. crn.
cu. cyc. dl-s. dph. dt. ery. fe. grp. hæm. hg. hg-bicl. hg-s.
hpm. hur. irs. jat. jnp-s. k-ca. lyc. mrl. mtr. myris. n-x.
na-ca. ner. p. p-x. pb. pod. ptv. rs. rs-r. s. sa-l. sep. smc.
sn. spi. spo-f. sr-ca. str. str-i. trg. trn. trx. vr-a. vr-s. woo.
Green. (myris). vr-a.
Red. ca-s. ery. hg. na-ba. rs. si-x. sr-ca.
Yellow. crt-c. n-x. spi. str.
CREEPING. as-o. sep.
DRAWING. f-hx.
ERUPTIONS, **Boils**. s.
Pimples. ca-s. dl-s. euphr.
Scabs. grp. hg.
Tubercles. p.
Undefined. as-o. ca-ca. ca-s. con. dl-s. hg. ner. pct.
s. si-x. str-i. vtx.
HEAT. as-o. cic. glo. p. rs-v.
HEAVINESS. lac-f.
ITCHING. amb. aps. as-o. ber. can-i. cb-v. con. cr-o.
lyc. p. smi. trg.
MOVEMENTS, **Convulsions**. cic. dph. rut.

PRESSING. arn. elaps. lac-f. mg-ca. phl.
SHOOTING. æth. ber. br. spo.
SMARTING. æth. ber. br. cr-o. mgs-au. n-x. ped.
STIFFNESS. klm.
SWELLING. alli. aps. as-o. elaps, fe. hg-s. n-x. p.
pul. rhe. rs. rs-v. spi-m. spo.
Œdematous. aps. rs. rs-v.
Red. rs.
TEARING. amb. i. lyc.
TENSIVE. al-o. myris.
UNDEFINED. aps. n-x. p.

ORBITAL INTEGUMENTS SUPERIORLY,

(Eyebrows).

ucon. æth. aga. al-o. alli. alo. amb. amm-cl. aps. arn. art-v.
as-h. as-o. asc. atp. ba-ca. ber. br. bry. ca-a. ca-pa. ca-s. can.
cb-a. chi. cic. cit-c. cle. con. cph. crd. cro. crt. crt-c. cth. cu.
delph. dig. dl-s. dro. dt. elaps. eryn. euph. evo. f-hx. fe. glo.
glp. grp. grt. gui. hg. hll. hur. hydr. hyo. i. jcr. jnp-s. k-ca.
k-i. k-na. k-o. lac-ac. lau-c. lch. li-ca. ly-b. mg-ca. mgs-ar.
mn-ca. morph-a. mrl. msc. n-x. na-cl. narth. ner. ol-a. p-x.
par. pau. pb. pet. phl. phy. pln. ppv. pru-l. pt. rho. rn-b. rn-s.
rs. rs-r. rs-v. rut. s. sb-s. sb-t. se. sep. si-x. smc. sn. so-d. spi.
spo. sr-ca. str. str-i. thu. trg. trn. trx. vi-t. vr-v. vtx. zn. zng.
BORING. ca-á.
COLOR **Red.** elaps.
CONTRACTIVE. hll. n-x. so-d.
CRAMPY. hll. narth.
CREEPING. rn-b.
CUTTING. crd. dro.
DRAWING. (alo). atp. cic. dro. grt. hll. k-o. mgs-ar.
narth. pru-l. rs.
ERUPTIONS, **Boils.** na-cl.
Hard. gui. rn-b.
Hot. sn.
Itching. na-cl. se.
Pimples. gui. hur. rn-s. sn. trx.
Hot. sn.
Pressing. sn.
Pressing. se. sn.
Pustules. thu.
Scabs. f-hx. sep.

Tubercles. k-o. sb-s.
  Undefined pain. sb-s.
  White. sb-s.
Undefined. as-o. ba-ca. cle. dl-s. hll. i. k-na. k-o. na-cl. par. s. se. sep. si-x. thu.
  Undefined Pain. sb-s.
Urticaria. f-hx.
Vesicles. se.
White. sb-s.
GNAWING. hyo. vtx.
HAIRS, **Color White.** as-h.
Fall out. aga. hll. k-ca. pb. se.
HEAT : acon. aga. alli. aps. as-o. atp. ber. bry. cit-c. dig. dro. elaps. hg. k-ca. s. sb-t. spi. thu.
HEAVINESS. con.
ITCHING. æth. aga. al-o. alli. aps. ber. chi. k-na. k-o. mgs-ar. na-cl. ol-a. par. s. sb-t. se. si-x. vtx.
MOVEMENTS, **Convulsions.** al-o. art-v. crt-c. glp. grt. hll. ol-a. rut. sep. sr-ca.
Downwards. cb-a.
  Feeling of. can. ol-a.
Upwards, drawn. lch.
NUMBNESS. as-h.
PECKING. pet.
PRESSING. aga. amb. arn. br. ca-s. cb-a. chi. crt. cth. evo. fe. hyo. k-o. morph-a. mrl. ner. p-x. par. phy. rn-b. s. str-i. zng.
SHOOTING. aga. alli. aps. as-o. ba-ca. ber. ca-a. cb-a. cic. cph. crt. elaps. f-hx. glp. hll. ly-b. mn-ca. pet. thu. vi-t. zn.
SMARTING. ber. glo. gui. k-o. par. pet. pt. vtx.
SWELLING. aps. k-ca.
Feeling of. par.
TEARING. al-o. amm-cl. arn. atp. mg-ca. mrl. rs. smc.
TENSIVE. con. dro. ly-b. par. pt.
THROBBING. k-ca. k-o. pet. sr-ca. zn.
TINGLING. cro.
UNDEFINED. delph. hydr. ner. pau. spi.
WRINKLED. dt. str.

ORBITAL INTEGUMENTS INFERIORLY.

æsc. aps. as-h. as-o. atp. atrop. bi-na. bry. cmc. crn. cro. cu. dt. f-hx. glo. hg-s. lct. lo-cœ. mn-ca. mtr. myris. n-x. na-cl.

ner. p. pau. pb. pb-a. pln. ptv. pul. rs. rs-r. rut. s-x. sep. si-x.
spi. spo. str. teu. trn. vtx.

COLOR Dark. as-h. as-o. bi-na. crn. cu. dt. glo. myris.
p. rs. rs-v. trn.

Yellow. n-x. spi.
CONTRACTIVE. cro.
HEAT. cro. f-hx. mn-ca.
ITCHING. vtx.
MOVEMENTS, Convulsions. sep.
SHOOTING. rs.
SMARTING. vtx.
SWELLING. aps. as-o. bry. cmc. dt. lct. mtr. ner. p.
pln. pul. rs-v. str.

Œdematous. lct.
Red. ner. sep.

ORBITAL INTEGUMENTS EXTERNALLY.

f-hx. spi. spo.
SWELLING. spi.

EYELIDS.

ach. acon. æsc. æth. ag. ag-na. aga. al-o. alli. alm. amb.
amm-ca. amm-cl. amph. anan. anm. aph. aps. arn. art-v.
arum-t. as-o. asr. ast. atp. atrop. au. ba-ca. ba-cl. bap. ber.
bi-na. br. bru. bry. buf. bz-x. c-bis. ca-a. ca-ca. ca-o. ca-pa.
ca-s. can. can-i. cap. cast. cb-a. cb-v. cch. ccs. chd. chi. chio.
chlor. cic. cit-c. cl-hx. cle. clv. cmc. cmf. co. con. cop. cph.
cr-o. crn. cro. crot. crt-c. cth. cu. cub. cy-hx. cyc. dig. dl-s.
dph. dph-i. dro. dt. elaps. erig. ery. eryn. eupat. euph. euphr.
f-hx. fe. fe-mgs. fe-pa. frm. glo. glp. gn-l. grc. grp. grt. gui.
gym. hæm. hg. hg-s. hll. hpm. hur. hydr. hyo. i. ind. irs. itu.
jat. jnp-s. k-bicr. k-ca. k-cla. k-i. k-na. k-o. klm. kre. krm.
lac-ac. lac-c. lac-d. lac-f. lam. lau-c. lct. led. lpd. lpt. ly-b.
lyc. men. mg-ca. mg-cl. mgs. mgs-ar. mgs-au. mn-ca. morph-a.
mph. mrl. msc. mtr. myris. n-x. na-ba. na-ca. na-cl. na-sa.
naj. narth. ner. ni-ca. nic. ol-a. os. ox-x. p. p-x. pæo. par. pb.
pet. phl. phy. physo. pim. pln. pnx. pol. ppv. pru-l. pso. ptv.
pul. pul-n. qu-sa. rhe. rho. rn-b. rn-s. rs. rs-r. rut. s. s-x. sa-a.
sa-l. sang. sb-s. sb-t. se. sep. si-x. smb. smc. smi. smr. sn.
so-d. so-o. so-t. spi. spi-m. spo. spo-f. sr-ca. srr. stc. str. str-i.

stry. te. teu. thu. til. trg. trn. trx. tx-b. u-na. urg. urt.
val. vi-o. vi-t. vin. vp-r. vr-a. vr-s. vrb. vsp. vtx. woo. ziz.
zn. zng.

ADHESION of.   ach. acon. æth. ag-na. aga. al-o.
amm-ca. amm-cl. aps. art-v. arum-t. as-o. atp. au. ba-ca. bry.
ca-a. ca-ca. ca-s. cast. cb-a. cb-v. cch. ccs. chd. cic. cl-hx. co.
con. cop. cro. dig. dl-s. dro. dt. erig. (eryn). euph. euphr. fe.
glp. grc. grp. grt. (gym). hg. (hydr). i. k-bicr. k-ca. (k-na).
k-o. kre. led. lpt. ly-b. lyc. mg-ca. mg-cl. mgs-ar. mgs-au.
mn-ca. mrl. mtr. myris. n-x. na-ba. na-ca. na-cl. na-sa. ni-ca.
ol-a. p. p-x. pb. phy. pol. pru-l. pt. pul. pul-n. rhe. rho. rs.
rs-r. rut. s. s-x. sb-s. sep. si-x. smi. sn. spi. spo. str. str-i. thu.
trn. trx. (u-na). vr-a. ziz. zn.

BRUISED.   as-o. chlor. s.
BURSTING.   aps. woo.
COLDNESS.   al-o. asr. br. chlor. grp. hur. k-ca. p-x. rs-r.
COLOR Dark.   as-o. clv. dig. dro. hur. k-ca. n-x. spo-f.
tx-b.
Red.   acon. ag. alli. (alm). anan. aps. as-o. atp. atrop. au.
ba-ca. ba-cl. ber. bi-na. bry. buf. ca-ca. ca-s. can. cb-v. chlor.
cl-hx. cmc. cmf. con. cu. dig. dl-s. dt. euph. euphr. fe. gel.
grp. hg. hll. hur. hyo. i. irs. k-bicr. k-i. k-o. kre. lau-c. lpd.
lyc. mg-cl. mgs. mgs-au. mtr. na-ca. na-cl. ni-ca. p-x. par. pb.
pso. pul. rho. rs. rs-r. s. sa-a. sb-s. sep. (si-x). smi. so-t. spi.
spo. srr. str. str-i. thu. trg. vin. vr-a. vr-s. woo. zn.
White.   acon.
Yellow.   acon.
CONTRACTIVE.   ber. chi. crot. dl-s. euphr. lpt. ner. pb.
physo. rs. sn. str. vi-t.
CRAMPY.   crot. vi-o.
CREEPING.   art-v. chi. k-bicr. pol.
CUTTING.   ca-ca.
DISCHARGE Hard.   k-o. p-x. (sb-s).
Mucus.   acon. æth. ag-na. aga. amm-cl. (aps). ba-ca. bry.
ca-a. ca-ca. dro. erig. euph. euphr. fe. grt. hg. hydr. i. k-bicr.
(k-ca). k-i. k-o. kre. lct. led. lpt. lyc. mg-ca. mgs-ar. mgs-au.
mrl. mtr. n-x. na-ca. (p-x). phy. pol. pul. pul-n. rhe. rs. (sb-s).
spi. str. str-i. vr-a. ziz.
Pus.   dl-s. dt. rs. rut. str-i. trx.
Yellow.   aga. ziz.
DRAWING.   ber. cch. grp. mgs-ar. p. p-x. pt. pul. rhe.
str.
DRYNESS.   acon. al-o. amm. arn. art-v. as-o. asr. ber.
bry. cb-v. chi. cph. cyc. dl-s. dph-i. euph. glp. grp. hpm.

k-bicr. mg-cl. mgs. mgs-ar. mgs-au. mn-ca. mrl. mtr. myris.
pul. rs. s. smi. srr. str. vr-a.

ERUPTIONS Dry. kre.
Encysted Tumors. ca-ca. thu.
Erythema circumscripta. ery.
Granulations. k-bicr.
Herpes. ery. kre. woo.
  Dry. kre.
Hot. smi. woo.
Itching. smi.
Pimples. pet. s. smi.
Pustules. ca-ca. con. lyc. pt. rs. s. se.
  Feeling of. trn.
Scabs. buf. hg. lyc.
Scales. kre. pul.
  Dry. kre.
Shooting. smi.
Smarting. hg-s.
Spongy. (alm).
Styes. amb. aps. au. ca-s. con. cub. dig. dl-s. fe. k-o. lyc.
men. mgs-au. pul. rs. sep. si-x. sn. val.
  Tubercles. (alm). bry. dl-s. k-i. k-o. rn-s.
  Spongy. (alm).
Ulcers. buf. cch. cro. dl-s. k-i. led. lyc. na-cl. p. pul. rs.
si-x. spi. str. str-i.
Undefined. ca-s. hg. k-bicr. sep.
Urticaria. chlor. smi.
  Hot. smi.
  Itching. smi.
  Shooting. smi.
Vesicles. mgs-ar. rs. se.
EVERSION. (alm). aps. atp. hg. spi. str-i.
GNAWING. str-i. vtx.
HÆMORRHAGE. arn. atp. (ery.)
HAIRS Falling out. al-o. aps. buf. chlor.
Inverted.(al-o). na-ba. rs. spi. zn.
  Feeling. (te).
Irregular. chlor. na-ba.
HARDNESS. acon. bry. dl-s. n-x. rn-s. spi. thu.
  Feeling of. dl-s. spi.
HEAT. acon. aga. al-o. alli. amb. aph. aps. art-v. as-o.
asr. atp. ber. bry. buf. bz-x. ca-ca. ca-pa. cap. cb-v. ccs. chd.
chlor. cit-c. cle. con. cro. glo. grp. hg. hydr. itu. k-bicr. k-ca.

k-i. k-o. kre. lau-c. lct. lyc. mgs-au. mrl. n-x. narth.ncr.
ni-ca. p. p-x. pæo. par. phl. phy. pnx. pol. pru-l. pul.
pul-n. rn-s. rs. rs-r. s. sb-t. sep. spi. si-x. smi. sn. so-t. spi.
stc. str. thu. trg. vi-o.

HEAVINESS see UPPER LIDS.

INVERSION. (alm).

ITCHING. acon. al-o. amb. anm. aps. art-v. as-o. atp.
ber. bry. c-bis. ca-a. cb-v. chi. cit-c. cro. crot. (cu). cyc.
dl-s. dph. dro. euph. euphr. grt. hg. hg-s. hur. i. k-bicr.
k-i. k-o. kre. lau-c. lyc. mgs. mgs-ar. mgs-au. mrl. na-ca.
na-cl. narth. ner. ol-a. p. pæo. par. pb. pet. pul. rs. rs-r.
s. sb-t. sep. si-x. smr. spi. spo. str. til. trg. trn. tx-b. vin.
vr-a. vtx. zn.

LOOSENESS, Feeling of. spi.

MOVEMENTS. Closing. acon. æth. ag. ag-na. aga.
al-o. alm. alo. amm-ca. amm-cl. aps. arn. art-v. arum.
as-o. atp. atrop. ba-ca. bap. bru. bry. c-bis. ca-ca. ca-pa.
ca-s. can. cb-a. cb-v. chd. chi. chlor. cit-c. cl-hx. cld. cof.
(cop). cph. cro. crt. cth. cu. cy-hx. dig. dl-s. dph. dt. elaps.
ery. euph. fe. gel. glo. glp. grt. hg. (hg-bicl.) hg-s. hll.
hur. hyo. (hyp). ind. jnp-s. k-na. k-o. kre. lac-ac. lac-c.
lac-f. lau-c. lch. li-ca. lpd. ly-b. lyc. (mg-cl). mg-sa.
mgs-au. mrl. mtr. myris. na-ca. na-cl. (na-sa). narth. ner.
ox-x. p-x. pb. phl. physo. pnx. ppv. pru-l. pt. ptv. qu-sa.
rs. rs-r. rut. s. s-x. sa-l. sb-t. sep. smb. snp-n. spi. (spo).
srr. (stach). str. str-i. thu. trx. tx-b. urg. vi-o. vi-t. vr-a.
vr-s. vrb. zn.

Spasmodically. acon. al-o. amb. anm. as-o. atp.
br. bry. ca-ca. (ca-i). ca-s. chd. chi. cic. con. cop. cro.
(crot). cyc. dl-s. dt. euph. euphr. fe. (grp). hæm. hg. hg-bicl.
hyo. (hyp). ind. k-ca. kre. (lyc). mrl. mtr. n-x. na-ba. na-ca.
na-cl. nic. p. pb. pru-l. pt. (rho). rs. s. sb-t. sep. si-x. spi.
spo. str-i. sym. urg. vi-o. vi-t.

Convulsions. æsc. aga. al-o. amb. anan. anm. art-v.
as-o. ast. atp. ber. bry. c-bis. ca-ca. chd. cph. cro. crot. cth.
cu. (dt). glp. grt. hg. hll. hyo. i. ind. jat. k-bicr. k-o. kre.
lac-f. men. mgs-ar. mtr. na-ca. na-cl. ol-a. pb. pet. pol. ppv.
pt. pul. rhe. rho. rs. rut. s. se. sep. si-x. smc. so-d. str. str-i.
thu. vi-o. vr-a. vrb. woo.

Opening Wide (spasmodically). acon. alm. anm.
atp. bru. bry. chi. cit-c. cof. con. cph. (cu). cy-hx. (dl-s).
dol. dt. dt-t. eupat-p. f-hx. fe. glp. hll. hyo. lau-c. lch.
lyc. mtr. na-cl. narth. p-x. pb. pod. ppv. pru-l. s. sb-s. sb-t.
smb. (spo). str-i. urg. vr-a.

Outwards Drawn. cph. cro. mtr. rhe. rut.

Winking. ag-na. aga. amm-ca. anan. ast. atp. buf. ca-ca. ca-s. cb-a. chd. chi. con. cro. (cu). dl-s. dph. euphr. f-hx. glo. k-o. lau-c. mrl. (myris). n-x. p-x. pet. ppv. (pt). sb-s. smc. sn. spi.

NUMBNESS. mrl. pb.

PARALYSIS. acon. ag-na. aga. al-o. amb. amm-ca. anan. anm. art-v. as-o. atp. ba-ca. bar. br. bry. ca-ca. ca-s. cap. cb-a. cb-v. chd. chlor. con. cro. cu. cy-hx. dro. (dt). elaps. eug. euph. fe. gel. grp. hg. hll. hyo. k-ca. k-o. li-ca. lpd. ly-b. lyc. men. mg-ca. mg-cl. mrl. mtr. myris. n-x. na-ba. na-ca. na-cl. nic. p. pæo. pb. pet. physo. pnx. pol. ppv. pul. rs. s. s-x. sa-l. sep. si-x. so-d. spi. srr. str. thu. trg. trn. vi-t. vr-a. zn.

Closing Difficult. acon. cy-hx. eug. myris. na-ba. ppv. (sa-l).

Opening Difficult. acon. ag-na. aga. (al-o). amb. amm-ca. anan. anm. art-v. as-o. atp. ba-ca. bap. br. bry. ca-ca. ca-s. cap. cb-a. cb-v. chd. chlor. con. cro. cu. cy-hx. dro. (dt). elaps. euph. fe. gel. hg. hll. hyo. k-ca. k-o. li-ca. ly-b. lyc. men. mg-ca. mg-cl. mrl. mtr. myris. n-x. na-ba. na-ca. na-cl. nic. p. pæo. pb. ped. pet. physo. pnx. ppv. ptv. pul. rs. s. s-x. sa-l. sep. si-x. so-d. spi. srr. str. thu. trg. trn. vi-t. vr-a. zn.

PRESSING. al-o. amb. amm-ca. aps. art-v. atrop. bry. ca-s. can. cro. cu. cyc. dt. euph. grp. k-ca. lyc. mph. msc. myris. n-x. na-cl. pol. rhe. s. si-x. smi. sn. spi. spo. str. vr-a.

SHOOTING. acon. aps. arn. as-o. ber. cyc. hg. hll. hur. k-bicr. lau-c. mgs-ar. mgs-au. narth. p-x. s. so-t. spi. str-i. trx. tx-b. vr-a. zng.

SMALL. can-i. kre. pb. rho.

Feeling. gui. kre.

SMARTING. acon. æth. aps. atrop. ber. bry. ca-ca. ca-s. cb-v. (chd). cit-c. cle. cmf. co. cr-o. cro. cth. dig. dro. frm. glp. k-ca. k-o. kre. lau-c. led. mgs-au. ol-a. p-x. pet. phy. pln. pnx. pul. pul-n. rs. rs-r. s. si-x. so-t. spi. str. str-i. thu. trn. val. vr-a. vr-v. vtx. ziz. zn.

STIFFNESS. al-o. chlor. klm. men. rs. s. spi. vr-a.

SWEAT. ca-pa.

SWELLING. acon. ag. ag-na. aga. al-o. alli. anan. aps. arn. as. as-o. atp. au. ba-ca. ba-cl. bry. buf. ca-ca. ca-s. cch. chd. chlor. cl-hx. cln. clv. con. cph. crot. cu. cyc. dt. euph. euphr. fe. grp. hg. hg-bicl. hll. hyo. i. k-bicr. k-ca. k-o. kre. lyc. mg-ca. mg-cl. mn-ca. mtr. n-x. na-ca. ni-ca. p.

pb. phy. pol. pso. pul. rho. rs. rs-r. rut. s. sa-a. sb-t. sep.
spi-m. spo. srr. str. str-i. thu. til. urt. urt-u. val. vp-r. woo.

Bag-like. k-ca.

Dark. phy.

Hard. acon. thu.

Œdematous. aps. as-o. crot. i. k-bicr. k-i. pb. phy.
rs-r. sa-a. urt. urt-u.

Red. acon. phy. thu.

Watery. pul.

Feeling of. acon. ber. (ccs). chd. cro. cyc. gel. hg-s.
k-o. men. myris. rs. rs-r. sa-l. thu. val. vr-v.

TEARING. ber. bry. can. cch. i. k-na. mg-ca. pb. smc.
str. zn.

TENSIVE. acon. as-o. cth. dl-s. hg-s. lyc. mrl. myris.
n-x. s. s-x.

THROBBING. buf. cch. cph. cro. euphr. hur. k-ca. men.
mg-ca. mgs-ar. mtr. rhe. rs. rs-r. s. woo.

TINGLING. art-v. pol.

UNDEFINED. as-o. atrop. ca-ca. (ca-s). (cb-a). chi. grp.
(hg). (k-bicr). lyc. mgs-ar. mn-ca. p. pb. pnx. rs. s. si-x. spi.
(spo-f). str-i. val. zn.

WRINKLED. (chio).

UPPER EYELID.

acon. æth. ag. ag-na. aga. al-o. alli. alo. amb. amm-ca.
amm-cl. amph. anan. anm. aps. arn. art-v. arum-t. as-o. asr.
atp. au. ba-ca. ba-cl. bap. ber. br. bru. bry. buf. e-bis. ca-ca.
ca-o. ca-s. can. can-i. cap. cb-a. cb-v. cch. chd. chi. chio. cic.
cit-c. cl-hx. cld. cle. cmf. co. cof. con. cop. cph. crd. crn.
cro. crot. crt-c. cth. cu. cy-hx. cyc. dig. dl-s. dph. dph-i. dro.
dt. elaps. ery. eug. euph. euphr. f-hx. fe. fe-mgs. frm. gel.
glo. glp. gn-l. grp. grt. hæm. hg. hg-s. hll. hur. hyo. ind.
jup-s. k-bicr. k-ca. k-cla. k-i. k-na. k-o. kre. krm. lac-ac.
lac-c. lac-d. lac-f. lau-c. lch. li-ca. lpd. lpt. ly-b. lyc. men.
mg-ca. mg-cl. mgs-ar. mgs-au. mn-ca. morph-a. mrl. msc. mtr.
myris. n-x. na-ba. na-ca. na-cl. na-sa. naj. narth. ner. nic.
ol-m. os. ox-x. p. p-x. pæo. par. pb. pet. phl. physo. pim. pnx.
pol. ppv. pru-l. pt. ptv. pul. qu-sa. rhe. rho. rs. rs-r. rut. s.
sang. sb-s. sb-t. sep. si-x. smb. smc. smi. sn. so-d. so-o. so-t. spi.
spo. srr. str. str-i. stry. te. teu. thu. trg. trn. trx. tx-b. urg.
vi-o. vi-t. vr-a. vr-s. vr-v. vrb. vsp. vtx. ziz. zn.

COLDNESS. grp.

COLOR, Dark. str-i.
Red. acon. ca-s. hg. k-bicr. k-o. s. teu. zn.
CONTRACTIVE. bry. dl-s. euphr.
CREEPING. asr. par.
CUTTING. thu.
DRYNESS. acon. arn. cb-v. glp. n-x. str-i. vr-a.
ERUPTIONS, Hard. dl-s.
Herpes. bry. rs. sep.
Hot. c-bis.
Itching. c-bis.
Pimples. ca-s. cth. lyc. msc. n-x. s.
Pustules. c-bis. ca-s. chd.
   Hot. c-bis.
   Itching. c-bis.
Rhagades. anan.
Scabs. co.
Styes. al-o. fe. hg. k-o. p-x. pul. s. trg. ziz.
Tubercles. dl-s. k-i. k-o. n-x.
EVERSION. anan. atp. str-i.
HARDNESS. acon.
HEAT. alli. bry. ca-ca. can-i. co. k-bicr. lyc. p. p-x. trg.
HEAVINESS. acon. al-o. anan. aps. arum-t. as-o. atp. ba-ca. ber. br. c-bis. ca-ca. ca-o. ca-s. can. chd. cit-c. cl-hx. cph. cr-o. crn. cro. crot. crt-c. dig. dl-s. dph. dph-i. ery. euph. euphr. fe. frm. gel. glo. grp. grt. hg. hg-s. hll. hur. ind. jnp-s. k-bicr. k-na. k-o. lac-c. lac-d. lac-f. lpd. ly-b. lyc. mrl. mtr. na-ca. na-sa. narth. ner. ol-m. ox-x. p-x. phl. physo. pnx. ppv. pru-l. pt. ptv. pul-n. qu-sa. rs. rs-r. s. sep. si-x. spi. spo. str. str-i. thu. trn. trx. tx-b. vi-o. vi-t. vr-a. vr-s. vr-v. zn.
ITCHING. alli. art-v. ba-ca. bry. cb-a. dl-s. f-hx. glp. k-bicr. lyc. n-x. na-ba. si-x. vtx.
MOVEMENTS, **Convulsions.** aga. al-o. amph. arum-t. as-o. asr. atp. bry. ca-ca. cb-a. cl-hx. con. crd. cro. cy-hx. jnp-s. lau-c. lch. mg-cl. mn-ca. mrl. par. rho. s. so-t. vr-a.
   Feeling of. lch.
Upward drawn. acon. lch.
NUMBNESS. narth.
PRESSING. ca-s. can. cb-a. cb-v. chd. dl-s. fe-mgs. k-o. lac-f. lyc. msc. mtr. na-ba. narth. p. rhe. s. si-x. sn. spi. str. trx. vr-a.
SHOOTING. ba-ca. br. ca-o. ca-s. cb-a. cyc. glp. mgs-ar. mn-ca. sang. si-x. spi. trg. vr-a.

SMALL. na-ba.
SMARTING. ca-s. co. crn. gn-l. k-o. pim. trg. vtx.
STIFFNESS. hg-s. krm. rs. spi. vr-a.
SWELLING. acon. al-o. aps. (as-o). bry. ca-s. cyc. hg.
hg-bicl. k-bicr. k-ca. k-o. mg-cl. morph-a. msc. myris. n-x.
na-ca. s. sep. si-x. str-i. teu. thu. zn.
Feeling of. al-o. can-i. k-o. vi-o.
TEARING. al-o. can. k-ca. k-o.
TENSIVE. acon. amm-ca. cth.
THROBBING. ba-ca. br. cl-hx. lau-c. mn-ca.
UNDEFINED. as-o. ca-o. cmf. cth. k-cla. lpt. pnx. spi.

LOWER EYELID.

ag. aga. al-o. alm. amm-cl. aps. arn. as-o. asc. asr. atp.
au. bry. c-bis. ca-ca. ca-s. cb-v. cch. chd. chi. cic. cit-c.
clv. cro. cth. dig. dph. dro. euph. euphr. fe. fe-mgs. fe-pa.
glo. grp. hur. i. ind. jnp-s. k-bicr. k-i. k-o. lam. lau-c.
led. lyc. mg-ca. mgs. mgs-au. mn-ca. mtr. myris. na-ca.
na-cl. ner. ol-a. p. p-x. pet. phy. pol. ppv. pru-l. pul. rn-b.
rph. rs. rut. s. s-x. sep. si-x. sn. spi. spo. trg. zn.
COLOR, **Dark**. glo.
Red. as-o. atp. bry. dig. glo. grp. k-i. lau-c. mg-ca.
na-cl. p-x. s. sep. si-x. trg.
CUTTING. spi.
DRAWING. grp. rut.
DRYNESS. pet.
ERUPTIONS, **Pimples.** al-o.
Pustules. na-cl. pol.
Styes. grp. p. pol. rs.
Tubercles. au. bry. ca-ca. thu.
  Undefined pain. bry.
Ulcers. cch. na-cl.
Undefined pain. bry.
HEAT. chd. ind. k-bicr. k-o. ner.
HEAVINESS. k-o.
ITCHING. k-o. lam. ner. ol-a. pet. rut. s-x.
MOVEMENTS, **Convulsions.** amm-cl. cic. cth. grp.
hg. i. ind. k-i. lyc. mg-ca. mgs. p-x. pol. rut. s. sep.
Downwards drawn. phy.
PRESSING. bry. cit-c. cro. sep.
SHOOTING. al-o. aps. cro. cth. dph. jnp-s. s-x.
SMARTING. al-o. asc. ca-ca. led. rs. s-x.

SWELLING. as-o.· atp. au. bry. ca-ca. dig. euphr. fe-mgs. glo. mg-ca. mgs-au. p-x. ppv. rs. sep. trg. u-na.
Œdematous. bry. hur. rph. u-na.
Feeling of. cit-c.
TEARING. mg-cl.
TENSIVE. myris.
THROBBING. atp. mg-ca. pol.

TARSAL EDGES.

acon. æth. ag. ag-na. alm. amm-ca. anan. aps. arn. art-v. arum-t. as-o. ast. atp. ba-ca. ber. bry. c-bis. ca-ca. ca-s. can-i. cb-v. cch. ccs. chd. chlor. cle. cln. cmc. con. cth. dig. dl-s. dph. dt. eupat. euphr. grp. grt. hg. hg-bicl. hg-s. hur. ind. jat. jnc. k-bicr. k-na. k-o. kre. krm. lac-d. lau-c. lch. li-ca. lo-cœ. lyc. mgs-ar. mgs-au. mph. mrl. mtr. myris. na-ba. na-cl. narth. ni-ca. ox-x. p. p-x. pd. pnx. pol. pru. pru-l. ptv. pul. rhe. rn-s. rs. rs-r. s. sb-t. se. sep. si-x. smc. spi. spo-f. srr. str. str-i. trn. val. vr-s. woo. zn.
COLDNESS. p-x.
COLOR, **Dark.** spo-f.
Red. acon. æth. ag. as-o. ast. atp. c-bis. ca-ca. cb-v. cch. chd. cle. cmc. dig. dl-s. dt. eupat. euphr. grp. hur. k-bicr. mgs-au. mrl. na-ba. pul. spi. val. vr-s. woo.
DISCHARGE, **Foam.** ber.
Hard. ag-na. ca-ca. dl-s. grp. k-na. ox-x. pol. s.
Mucus. æth. aps. hg. pol. str-i.
Pus. as-o. euphr. mrl. pul.
White. ber.
DRYNESS. arn. as-o. cln. mtr. pd. rs.
ERUPTIONS, **Granulations.** aps.
 Feeling of. k-bicr.
Itching. ca-ca. se.
Moist. ca-ca.
Pimples. na-cl.
Scabs. con. hg. sb-t. srr. woo.
Tubercles. hg-s. srr.
Ulcers. anan. cle. con. euphr. hg. mrl. na-ba. s. spi. woo.
 Undefined. ca-ca.
Vesicles. se. ,
GNAWING. str-i.
HARDNESS. na-ba. rs. spi. spo-f.

HEAT. aps. art-v. as-o. bry. c-bis. cch. ccs. dph. hg. hg-bicl. k-bicr. k-o. lau-c. mph. ni-ca. pol. ptv. pul. rn-s. rs-r. str.

ITCHING. acon. amm-ca. art-v. bry. ca-ca. can-i. cb-v. chd. chlor. con. dl-s. grt. hg. hur. jat. jnc. k-bicr. kre. mgs-ar. narth. pnx. pru. rs-r. se. str. trn.

PRESSING. se. smc.

SHOOTING. dph. hur. narth. ni-ca.

SMALL. woo.

Feeling. lac-d.

SMARTING. acon. aps. arn. bry. ccs. cle. cln. cth. dig. hur. jat. kre. lau-c. li-ca. na-ba. pnx. rs-r. s. spi. str. str-i. val.

SWELLING. ag. arum-t. con. kre. lch. na-cl. ni-ca. pul. s.

Feeling of. ccs. val.

TEARING. bry. cle.

UNDEFINED. as-o. p.

UPPER TARSAL EDGE.

art-v. ba-ca. dl-s. hg-s. krm. lo-cœ. mgs-ar. myris. pol. pru-l. rhe. (spi).

COLOR **Red.** myris.

DRAWING. pru-l.

ERUPTIONS, **Vesicles.** mgs-ar.

FALSE SENSATIONS, **Sand.** (spi).

HEAT. art-v. pol. rhe.

ITCHING. art-v. ba-ca. dl-s.

PRESSING. rhe.

SHOOTING. hg-s.

SMARTING. krm.

LOWER TARSAL EDGE.

alm. ber. chd. dph. hur. ind. jnp-s. mtr. na-cl. pul. rut. sep. thu.

COLOR **Red.** chd. ind. mtr. pul.

CREEPING. ber.

DRAWING. ber.

ERUPTIONS, **Pimples.** na-cl. thu.

HEAT. dph. sep.

ITCHING. dph. rut.
SHOOTING. dph. jnp-s.
SMARTING. ber.
SWELLING. chd. mtr. pul.
THROBBING. ber.

EYELIDS, INNER SURFACE.

æth. ag-na. arn. as-o. atp. ba-ca. ber. ca-o. chd. chlor.
cit-c. co. con. dig. eupat. glp. hg-bicl. hur. hydr. ind. k-bicr.
k-o. lo-i. mrl. mtr. n-x. na-ba. (na-sa). ol-a. p-x. pol. ppv.
pul. pul-n. rhe. rs. rs-r. s. smr. so-t. spo-f. str-i. thu. vr-a.
zn. zng.

APPEARANCE **Velvety**. con.
COLDNESS. p-x.
COLOR, **Red**. ag-na. as-o. atp. ba-ca. ber. ca-o. chlor.
con. cph. dig. glp. hg-bicl. hydr. k-bicr. mrl. na-ba. ol-a.
ppv. pul. rs. rs-r. s. smr. so-t.
Yellow. dig.
CREEPING. chi.
DISCHARGE, **Mucus**. æth. pol. str-i.
Tenacious. eupat.
DRYNESS. arn. mtr. n-x. ol-a. s.
ERUPTIONS, **Blisters**. (na-sa). thu.
Granulations. k-bicr.
Pimples. hur.
Ulcers. na-ba.
HARDNESS. spo-f.
HEAT. ber. con. pul-n. rhe. s.
ITCHING. k-o. vr-a.
PRESSING. n-x. rhe.
SHOOTING. zng.
SMARTING. arn. lo-i. s. vr-a.
SOFTNESS. rs. thu.
SWELLING. æth. con. rs.
Red. rs.
TENSIVE. s.
WRINKLED. ag-na. zn.

UPPER EYELIDS, INNER SURFACE.

co.
SMARTING. co.

LOWER EYELIDS, INNER SURFACE.

chd. ind. rs.
COLOR, **Red**. chd. ind.
SMARTING. rs.

PUNCTA LACHRYMALIA.

acon. aps. as-o. atp. grp. hg-s. hur. na-cl.
ITCHING.· hur.
OCCLUSION. acon. as-o. atp. grp. na-cl.
SMARTING. hur.

PUNCTA LACHRYMALIA.—UPPER EYELID.

hg-s.
SHOOTING. hg-s.

CANTHI.

acon. æsc. æth. ag. ag-na. aga. al-o. amm-ca. amm-cl.
anan. aps. arn. art-v. arum-t. as-o. as-ters. asr. atp. au. ba-a.
ba-ca. ber. bi-na. bru. bry. buf. bz-x. ca-a. ca-ca. ca-s. cast.
cb-a. cb-v. cch. chd. chi. cic. cit-c. cl-hx. cle. cof. con. cop.
cot. cph. cr-o. crd. crot. crt. crt-c. dig. dl-s. dph. elaps. ery.
eug. euph. euphr. f-hx. fe-mgs. frm. glo. glp. grc. grp. grt.
gui. hæm. hg. hg-a. hg-s. hll. hyo. i. ind. irs. k-bicr. k-ca. k-cla.
k-i. k-na. k-o. kre. lac-d. lam. lau-c. lch. led. lo-cœ. ly-b.
lyc. men. mg-ca. mg-cl. mgs. mgs-ar. mgs-au. mrl. msc.
mtr. n-x. na-ba. na-ca. na-cl. ner. ni-ca. ol-a. p. p-x. par.
pb. pb-a. pet. phl. phy. pnc. pol. ppv. pru. pru-l. pt. pul.
rho. rn-b. rn-s. rs. rs-r. rut. s. s-x. sa-l. sang. sb-s. sb-t.
sep. si-x. smc. smi. sn. so-o. spi. spo. sr-ca. str. str-i. teu.
thu. til. trg. trn. trx. urg. val. vi-t. vr-a. vr-s. zn.
  BORING. thu.
  COLOR, **Dark.** pb.
  Red. acon. ag-na. aga. al-o. as-o. [bi-na. ,bru. crt.
euphr. grc. hg-a. hg-s. ly-b. mg-ca. mtr. na-cl. p., pul. s.
str. str-i.
  CRAMPY. msc.
  CREEPING. cop. pt.

DISCHARGE, **Hard**. aga. bi-na. ca-ca. cof. cph. dig. dl-s. euph. grp. gui. k-o. pol. sb-s. str. thu.

Mucus. as-ters. bi-na. ca-a. cof. dig. dl-s. euphr. grp. hll. k-bicr. k-i. k-o. kre. lch. lyc. mtr. n-x. na-ca. par. pol. sb-s. vi-t.

Pus. art-v. buf. dl-s. grp. grt. mtr. pul. str.

Thin. pet.

White. lch.

Yellow. k-bicr. str.

DRYNESS. euph.

ERUPTIONS, **Ulcers**. buf. euph. hg. k-ca. na-cl. p. s. sb-s.

HEAT. aga. al-o. amm-cl. asr. au. ba-ca. buf. ca-ca. cb-v. cle. dl-s. hg-a. hll. k-na. mg-ca. mrl. na-ca. na-cl. ol-a. p. p-x. par. pnc. pul. s. sep. si-x. sn. sr-ca. str. thu.

ITCHING. æth. ag. ag-na. aga. al-o. aps. arn. art-v. ber. bru. bry. bz-x. ca-a. ca-ca. cb-v. cl-hx. cle. con. crt. crt-c. euph. f-hx. hg-a. hll. hyo. i. k-bicr. k-ca. k-o. lam. lyc. mg-ca. mgs. na-ba. na-cl. pb-a. pnc. pru. pt. pul. s. vr-a.

LACHRYMATION. pet. thu.

MOVEMENTS, **Closing Spasmodically**. crot.

Convulsions. crt. hyo.

PRESSING. aga. ca-a. cb-v. cch. dl-s. grt. hll. mg-cl. msc.

SCRAPING. pru-l.

SHOOTING. aga. al-o. ber. ca-a. ca-ca. con. crot. dl-s. mgs-ar. na-cl. p-x. pet. sb-t. sn. vr-a.

SMARTING. al-o. aps. asr. ber. cast. cb-v. cch. cl-hx. dl-s. dph. fe-mgs. hg. hll. hyo. k-ca. mgs-ar. pb. pnc. rn-b. rn-s. s. sb-s. sep. si-x. str. thu.

SWELLING. aga. ca-a. si-x.

Feeling of. rs.

TEARING. cast. hyo. men.

TENSIVE. ner.

THROBBING. ca-ca. k-cla.

UNDEFINED. aga. si-x.

EXTERNAL CANTHUS.

acon. æth. aga. alo. amm-cl. anan. art-v. arum-t. as-o. asr. ba-ca. ber. bry. ca-a. ca-ca. ca-s. cb-a. cb-v. cch. chd. chi. cl-hx. co. con. cot. cph. crt-c. dig. dl-s. euph. euphr. fe-mgs. frm. glo. grc. grp. hg. hg-s. hyo. k-bicr. k-ca. k-na.

lau-c. lch. lct. lo-cœ. lyc. mgs. mgs-ar. mn-ca. msc. mtr. n-x. na-ba. na-ca. na-cl. ni-ca. p. p-x. pnc. pol. pru-l. pul. rn-b. rn-s. rs. rs-v. rut. s. s-x. sa-l. sb-s. sep. si-x. smc. smi. sn. spi. spo. sr-ca. stach. str. str-i. thu. til. trn. trx. urg. vr-s.

COLDNESS. asr. ni-ca.

COLOR, **Red**. ber. ca-ca. grp. hg. k-bicr. rn-b. s. str.

CONTRACTIVE. euph.

CUTTING. ca-s.

DISCHARGE, **Hard**. chi. cph. dl-s. vr-s.

Mucus. al-o. as-o. ba-ca. ca-s. cch. chi. cph. dl-s. lyc. mgs-ar. na-cl. pul. rut. sep. str-i. vr-s.

ERUPTIONS, **Rhagades**. grp.

Ulcers. anan. ca-a. ca-ca. lyc. sb-s. zn.

FALSE SENSATIONS, **Sand**. aga. al-o. ba-ca. con. crt-c. n-x. str-i.

Water. ni-ca.

HÆMORRHAGE. grp.

HEAT. art-v. cb-a. dig. dl-s. k-bicr. k-ca. k-na. pnc. s. sep. spi. sr-ca. urg.

ITCHING. æth. art-v. bry. euph. hg-s. hyo. lo-cœ. mgs. na-ba. pnc. pul. s. sb-s. sep. til. trn. urg.

LACHYMATION. arum-t.

MOVEMENTS, **Closing.** grp. stach.

Convulsions. ba-ca. lau-c. na-cl.

NUMBNESS. acon.

PRESSING. ba-ca. ca-ca. chi. con. dl-s. lch. n-x. p-x. pul. s-x. str-i.

SHOOTING. ba-ca. ca-a. dl-s. hg-s. k-ca. s. str-i.

SMARTING. ag-na. ca-ca. ca-s. cb-a. cb-v. cch. co. dig. grc. grp. k-bicr. k-ca. k-na. lau-c. lct. lyc. mgs-ar. mn-ca. mtr. rn-b. rs. sep. str. str-i. zn.

SWELLING. anan. grp. rn-b.

TEARING. amm-cl. dl-s. str-i.

TENSIVE. dl-s. grt.

THROBBING. ba-ca. lau-c.

UNDEFINED. (fe-mgs). rs-r.

INTERNAL CANTHUS.

æsc. æth. ag-na. aga. al-o. anan. arn. art-v. as-o. asr. atp. au. ba-a. ba-ca. ber. br. bru. bry. buf. ca-a. ca-ca. ca-s. cb-a. cb-v. chd. cic. cit-c. cl-hx. cle. cof. con. cr-o. crd. dig. dl-s. dph. elaps. ery. eug. euphr. glo. glp. grc. grp. grt.

hæm. hg. hg-cy. hg-s. hll. hyo. ind. irs. k-bicr. k-cla. k-i. k-na. k-o. lac-ac. lac-d. lct. led. lo-cœ. lyc. men. mg-ca. mg-cl. mgs. mgs-ar. mgs-au. msc. mtr. n-x. na-ba. na-ca. na-cl. ner. ni-ca. nic. ol-a. p. p-x. par. pb. pet. phl. phy. ppv. pru-l. pul. rho. rs. rs-r. rut. s. s-x. sa-l. sang. sb-s. sb-t. sep. si-x. smc. smi. sn. so-o. spi. spo. sr-ca. str. str-i. teu. thu. trg. trx. val. vr-a. zn.

COLOR, **Dark**. au. pb. smi.

Red. ag-na. aga. au. ber. cle. eug. glo. grp. grt. hæm. hg. mg-ca. na-ca. rs. str. teu. val.

CONTRACTIVE. anan. eug.

CRAMPY. eug.

DISCHARGE, **Hard**. dl-s. euphr. hll. par. rs.

Mucus. aga. al-o. art-v. cof. con. dl-s. euphr. hyo. lyc. mg-ca. ni-ca. p. pul. rho. rs. rut. sb-s. si-x. thu. zn.

Pus. buf. ca-ca. grp. na-cl. p.

Tenacious. lac-ac.

Thin. k-i.

DRYNESS. al-o. asr. ber. mtr. na-cl. rs. str.

ERUPTIONS, **Blisters**. k-bicr.

Boils. bry.

Pustules. bry.

 Soft. bry.

Rhagades. zn.

Soft. bry.

Styes. na-cl. s. sn.

Ulcers. buf.

FALSE SENSATIONS, **Pellicle**. k-o.

Sand. al-o. dig. (spi.) trx.

HEAT. æsc. aga. art-v. asr. au. ba-ca. ber. buf. ca-ca. dig. glo. glp. grp. hll. irs. k-bicr. k-o. mg-ca. na-cl. nic. p. p-x. par. pet. phl. pru-l. rho. sb-t.

ITCHING. æth. art-v. atp. br. bru. ca-a. con. cr-o. dl-s. dph. glo. grc. grt. ind. k-o. led. lyc. mg-ca. mgs. mgs-ar. n-x. na-ba. na-cl. ol-a. p-x. pb. phl. phy. pul. rs-r. rut. sep. sn. spi. sr-ca. str. str-i. zn.

MOVEMENTS, **Closing Spasmodically**. eug.

Convulsions. k-cla.

PRESSING. ber. cb-a. lyc. na-cl. p-x. pet. pul. rho. rs-r. trg. zn.

SCRAPING. pru-l.

SHOOTING. aga. anan. arn. atp. ca-a. ca-ca, cle. con. crd. dl-s. elaps. eug. grp. grt. ind. men. na-ca. p-x. phl. pru-l. pul. sb-t. sn. vr-a.

SMARTING. al-o. atp. bry. cl-hx. con. cr-o. dig. dl-s. dph. grp. grt. hg-s. hll. ind. k-ca. k-o. lct. mg-ca. mgs-au. ni-ca. ol-a. p. phy. pul. rut. s. sb-t. sep. spi. str. teu. zn.
SWELLING. ag-na. aga. ca-ca. hg. k-i. na-cl. pet. ppv.
TEARING. atp. k-na. men.
TENSIVE. ba-a. grt. hg-cy. ner.
THROBBING. ca-ca.
UNDEFINED. al-o. atp. dig. k-i. na-cl. so-o. trg.

CARUNCULA LACHRYMALIS.

ag-na. aga. (alm). bry. ca-ca. dl-s. hæm. hur. k-bicr. ppv. pul. str. zn.
COLOR, **Red**. ag-na. hæm. hur.
ERUPTIONS, **Spongy**. (alm).
      Tubercles. (alm).
      Spongy. (alm).
SWELLING. ag-na. aga. ppv.

LACHRYMAL GLAND.

aga. anan. arn. br. (cu). dl-s. grp.
ERUPTIONS, **Ulcers**. anan.
PRESSING. arn. dl-s.
SWELLING. aga. grp.
TEARING. dl-s.
UNDEFINED. (fe-mgs).

LACHRYMAL BONES.

hg. k-bicr. lch. si-x.
SWELLING. hg.

LACHRYMAL SAC.

(alm). ca-ca. chd. dl-s. f-hx. grp. na-ca. na-cl. pet. pul. rut. s. si-x. sn. trg.
ERUPTIONS, **Abscess**. na-ca. pul.
Fistula. (alm). ca-ca. chd. dl-s. f-hx. grp. pet. pul. rut. s. si-x. sn. trg.
SWELLING. na-cl. pet.
UNDEFINED. na-cl.

I. C. GENERAL CHARACTER, SEQUENCE,

and DIRECTION.

PERIODICAL.

acon. amb. amm-ca. aph. arn. as-o. atp. ba-ca. ber. c-bis.
ca-ca. ca-s. cac. chd. chi. clv. con. cro. dig. dl-s. dt. euphr.
fe-mgs. grp. hg. hyo. k-bicr. k-na. k-o. lyc. n-x. na-ca. na-cl.
na-sa. narth. ni-ca. p. pæo. pb. pet. phl. physo. pnx. pul. rho.
rn-s. rs. rut. s. sb-s. sb-t. sep. si-x. smb. smc. smi. spi. spo-f.
srr. str. thr. vr-a. vr-s. woo.

OBJECTS IMAGINARY. **Vibrations.** thr.
Visions Terrible. smb.
PHOTOPHOBIA. as-o. na-cl. si-x.
SIGHT IMPAIRED. acon. amm-ca. atp. ba-ca. ca-ca.
cac. chd. chi. clv. con. cro. dig. dl-s. dt. euphr. fe-mgs. grp.
hg. hyo. k-na. k-o. lyc. na-ca. na-cl. p. pb. pet. physo. pul. rs.
rut. s. sb-s. sb-t. sep. si-x. smc. spi. srr. vr-a. woo.

EYEBALL. **Color, Red.** as-o. k-o. na-cl.
Discharge. s.
Dryness. rho.
Heat. amb. amm-ca. as-o. narth. rho. spi. vr-s.
Lachrymation. as-o. na-cl.
Pressing. arn. ca-s. s. si-x.
Small. sep.
Tearing. as-o. ber. ca-ca.
Tensive. spi.
Throbbing. ca-ca. p.
IRIS. **Pupils Contracted.** na-cl.
ORBIT CIRCUMFERENCE. **Pressing.** arn.
ORBIT SUPERIORLY. **Shooting.** ber.
ORBITAL INTEGUMENTS. **Pressing.** phl.
EYELIDS. **Adhesion of.** s.
Heat. aph.
Movements, Closing Spasmodically. na-cl.
UPPER EYELIDS. **Itching.** pæo.
EYELIDS, INNER SURFACE. **Color, Red.** as-o.
Pressing. n-x.
CANTHI. **Smarting.** rn-s.

PERIODICAL—ALTERNATE DAYS.

amb. as-o. smi.
EYEBALL. **Heat.** amb.
Lachrymation. smi.

PERIODICAL—EVERY DAY.

as-o. fe-mgs. spi.
OBJECTS IMAGINARY. **Blue.** fe-mgs.
Bright. fe-mgs.
Circles. fc-mgs.
     Blue. fe-mgs.
     Bright. fe-mgs.
     Zigzags. fe-mgs.
Zigzags. fe-mgs.
SIGHT IMPAIRED. fe-mgs.

PERIODICAL—FROM 4 A.M. TO 3 P.M.

spi.

PERIODICAL.—FROM 10 A.M. TO 3 P.M.

as-o.

PERIODICAL—EVERY NIGHT.

(dt).

PERIODICAL.—EVERY FORENOON.

dt. na-cl. p. s.
OBJECTS IMAGINARY. **Veil.** dt.
SIGHT IMPAIRED. dt.
EYEBALL. **Color Red.** na-cl.
Lachrymation. na-cl.
Throbbing. p.
EYELIDS. **Adhesion of.** s.
Movements, Closing Spasmodically. na-cl.

PERIODICAL—AT 7 A.M.

na-cl.
PHOTOPHOBIA. na-cl.
IRIS. **Pupils Contracted.** na-cl.

PERIODICAL—EVERY NOON.

vr-a.

PERIODICAL—EVERY AFTERNOON.

as-o. asr. ca-ca. (dt). rho. s. si-x.
EYEBALL. **Pressing.** s. si-x.
EYELIDS. **Heat.** aph.

PERIODICAL—FROM 3 TO 4 P.M., TO 9 TO 10 P.M.

ca-ca.
EYEBALL. **Tearing.** ca-ca.

PERIODICAL—AT 4 P.M.

as-o.
PHOTOPHOBIA. as-o.
EYEBALL. **Color, Red.** as-o.
Heat. as-o.
Lachrymation. as-o.
EYELIDS, INNER SURFACE. **Color Red.** as-o.

PERIODICAL—AT 5 P.M.

asr.
EYEBALL. **Color, Red.** asr.
Lachrymation. asr.
CANTHI. **Heat.** asr.

PERIODICAL—AT 6 P.M.

rho.
EYEBALL. **Heat.** rho.

PERIODICAL—EVERY HALF-HOUR.

hg.
SIGHT IMPAIRED. hg.

PERIODICAL—SYNCHRONOUS with PULSE.

pnx. si-x.
OBJECTS **Appear Moving Up and Down.** si-x.
Vibrating. pnx.

GRADUALLY INCREASE and DECREASE.

as-o. dig. k-bicr. lyc. myris. na-cl. ner.
OBJECTS IMAGINARY. **Vibrations Bright.** dig.
PHOTOPHOBIA. na-cl.
SIGHT IMPAIRED. lyc.
EYEBALL. **Color, Red.** na-cl.
Lachrymation. na-cl.
IRIS. **Pupil Contracted.** na-cl.
ORBIT SUPERIORLY. **Contractive.** myris.
Pressing. ner.
EYELIDS. **Movements, Closing Spasmodically.—**
na-cl.

GRADUALLY COME, SUDDENLY GO.

pul.

SUDDENLY COME, GRADUALLY GO.

hg-s.

SUDDENLY COME and GO.

dig. hg-s. na-ba.
EYEBALL. **Cutting.** na-ba.

CHANGING CHARACTER or PLACE in EYES.

aga. amb. atp. ba-ca. ber. bru. ca-a. ca-ca. ca-s. can. cb-a.
ccs. chd. chio. cic. cl-hx. con. cot. cro. crot. cu. cy-hx. dl-s.
dt. (ery). eryn. f-hx. gn-l. grp. jnp-s. k-bicr. k-ca. k-o. kre.
lam. lau-c. men. mg-ca. mgs. mgs-ar. msc. n-x. na-ba. na-cl.
na-sa. ner. p. p-x. pb. pnx. pol. pru-l. pul. qu-sa. s. sb-t. sep.
si-x. smb. smc. smi. sn. spi. spo. sr-ca. str-i. thu. trg. trn. trx.
u-na.
OBJECTS APPEAR **Blue then Grey.** atp.
Blue then White. atp.
Bright then Red. atp.
Red then Blue. atp.
OBJECTS IMAGINARY. **Plain White to which
Spots Bright descend, then Plain Bright to which
Spots White descend.** p-x.
Vibrations Bright Red, then Flames Red. f-hx.

SIGHT IMPAIRED. **Presbyopia then Myopia.** dt.
EYEBALL.   **Coldness then   False   Sensations,**
Sand. ·f-hx.
      then **Shooting.** mgs-ar.
Color Red then Lachrymation. grp.
Drawing then Lachrymation. grp.
Eruptions, Blisters then Granulations. sb-t.
False Sensations, Wind (cold) then Sand. f-hx.
Heat then Coldness. chd.
      then **Color Red.** sr-ca.
      then **Shooting.** sr-ca.
Itching then Color Red. kre.
      then **False Sensations, Sand.** kre.
      then **Heat.** cb-a. k-bicr. kre.
      then **Lachrymation.** cb-a. k-o.
      then **Pressing.** ca-ca. cb-a. kre. trg.
      then **Smarting.** kre.
      then **Undefined.** k-bicr.
Lachrymation then Dryness. s.
Movements Convulsions then Itching. na-cl.
Pressing then Color Red. kre.
      then **Lachrymation.** ca-s. grp. kre.
            Hot. grp. kre.
      then **Shooting.** k-ca.
Shooting then Color Red. n-x.
      then **Pressing.** spo.
Smarting then Lachrymation. s.
Tearing then Lachrymation. mg-ca.
Undefined then Color Red. crot.
IRIS.   **Pupils Contracted then Dilated.** aga-p. atp.
can. cic. cl-hx. cu. dl-s. jnp-s. k-o. lam. lau-c. men. pb.
pnx. pol. pul. smb. smc. sn. trx.
Dilated   then   Contracted. aga. atp. ca-a. cy-hx.
ner. p-x. qu-sa.
   ORBIT.   **Shooting then Pressing.** ba-ca.
TARSAL EDGES.   **Sensitive then Drawing.**· ber.
      then **Throbbing.** ber.
Tingling then Drawing. ber.
      then **Throbbing.** ber.
EYELIDS, INNER SURFACE.   **Smarting then**
Dryness. s.
   CANTHI.   **Color Red then Itching.** bru.
OBJECTS IMAGINARY, then SIGHT IMPAIRED. p.
Mist Red then EYEBALL **Lachrymation.** (ery).

' **Flames Red** then EYEBALL **Lachrymation.** spi.
   ,,   then IRIS **Pupils Dilated.** spi.
SIGHT IMPAIRED then SIGHT DAZZLED. na-cl.
 then EYEBALL **Appearance Dim.** dt.
 then ,, **Color Red.** kre.
 then ,, **Lachrymation.** ca-ca. dt. kre.
       p-x. spi.
 then ,,   ,, **Hot.** kre.
 then ,, **Pressing.** dt.
 then ,, **Smarting.** dt.
 then IRIS **Pupils Dilated.** spi.
EYEBALL **Heat** then OBJECTS ' IMAGINARY,
Flames Red. spi.
Shooting then   ,,   **Mist.** k-ca.
Appears Staring, then SIGHT IMPAIRED. cic. msc.
Heat then.   ,, spi.
Lachrymation then ,, cro.
Pressing then ,, ,, cro. (sep).
Shooting then ,, ,, k-ca.
Undefined then ,, ,, con. cro.
Color Red then LENS **Cataract.** atp. n-x.
Appearance Staring then IRIS **Pupils Contracted.**
msc.
 Itching, then EYELIDS **Adhesion of.** k-bicr.
 Sensitive, then UPPER EYELIDS **Shooting.** gn-l.
 Undefined then ,,   ,, gn-l
 Gnawing, then CANTHI **Discharge.** kre.
 Heat then . ,, ,, kre.
 Itching then ,, ,, kre.
ORBIT **Shooting,** then EYEBALL **Lachrymation,
Feeling of.** ba-ca.
 Pressing, then ORBIT SUPERIORLY **Pressing
Down.** chio.
EYELIDS **Movements Closing,** then OBJECTS
IMAGINARY, **Flames Red.** spi.
     then SIGHT IMPAIRED. spi.
 Adhesion then EYEBALL **Lachrymation.** smi.
str-i.
 Movements Closing then ,, **Appearance
Staring.** lau-c.
lau-c.   ,,   then ,, **Upward-looking.**
  Opening Spasmodically then ,,
False Sensations, Sand. f-hx.

EXTERNAL CANTHUS **Pressing then EYELIDS Adhesion**. pul.
INTERNAL CANTHUS **Heat then LOWER EYE-LID Heat**. k-bicr.

ALTERNATING in CHARACTER or PLACE in EYES.

ba-a. ba-ca. buf. c-bis. ca-ca. can. chi. cic. cl-hx. clf. crb-x.
cro. lyc. physo. pnx. si-x. smi. so-n. str-i. thu.
OBJECTS APPEAR **Near and Distant**.' cic.
PHOTOPHOBIA **with EYEBALL Color Red**. si-x.
      ,, **with** ,, **Lachrymation**. si-x.
SIGHT IMPAIRED. **Myopia with Presbyopia**. lyc.
  ,,   ,, **with EYEBALL Pressing**. cro.
EYEBALL **Color Red with PHOTOPHOBIA**. si-x.
Lachrymation with ,, si-x.
Pressing with SIGHT IMPAIRED. cro.
IRIS. **Pupils Contracted and Dilated**. ba-a. ba-ca.
buf. can. chi. cic. cl-hx. clf. crb-x. physo. pnx. so-n. str-i.
EYELIDS. **Heat with Pressing**. smi.

ALTERNATELY in EITHER EYE.

acon. amb. atp. chio. cu. glp. lyc. na-sa. rn-b.
EYEBALL. **Dryness**. atp.
Heat. acon. atp. cu.
Pressing. na-sa. rn-b.
Shooting. lyc.
Smarting. cu.
Tearing. amb.
Tensive. glp.
ORBIT SUPERIORLY. **Undefined**. chio.

RIGHT then LEFT.

aga. alm. *as-o. ber. chd. *chi. chio. cot. cph. cro. cund.
fe-mgs. hg-bini. hg-s. *k-ca. lac-ac. lch. menth. mg-cl. n-x.
*na-cl. *s. sep. str-i.
OBJECTS IMAGINARY. **Blue**. fe-mgs.
Bright. fe-mgs.
Circles. fe-mgs.
  Blue. fe-mgs.
  Bright. fe-mgs.
  Red. fe-mgs.
Zigzags. fe-mgs.

E

Red. fe-.mgs
Zigzags. fe-mgs.
SIGHT IMPAIRED. *chi.
EYEBALL. **Boring.** ber.
Color Red. *as-o. cph. hg-bini. n-x.
False Sensations, Sand. lch.
Movements, Convulsions. aga. lac-ac.
Pressing. *as-o. chd. menth.
Shooting. . ber. chd.
Smarting. cot.
Tearing. chd.
Undefined. str-i.
LENS. **Cataract.** *p.
ORBIT SUPERIORLY. **Drawing.** chio.
Smarting. hg-s.
Swelling, Feeling of. hg-s.
ORBITAL INTEGUMENTS. **Swelling.** *k-ca.
EYELIDS. **Movements, Convulsions.** cro.
LOWER EYELIDS. **Itching.** alm.
EYELIDS, INNER SURFACE. **Color Red.** cph.
INTERNAL CANTHUS. **Itching.** mg-cl.
FORWARDS. **Orbit Superiorly Pressing.** na-cl.
DOWNWARDS. **Orbit Superiorly Pressing.** chio.
TO HEAD—ANTERIORLY. **Eyeball Boring.** ber.
                    Shooting. ber.
RIGHT OBJECTS IMAGINARY, **Pyriform body**,
then LEFT OBJECTS APPEAR **Confused.** cund.
     then LEFT OBJECTS IMAGINARY, **Mist.** cund.
RIGHT EYEBALL **Shooting then** LEFT EYEBALL
Color Red. n-x.

LEFT then RIGHT.

     aga. ba-ca. *cph. *cro. *crot. dig. f-hx. glo. *li-ca. *mg-ca.
na-cl. *na-cl. na-sa. rs. *rs. smi. *spi. thu. *zn.
     OBJECTS, FALSE APPEARANCE of. **Part Visible.**
*li-ca.
     OBJECTS IMAGINARY. **Vibrations Bright.** dig.
SIGHT IMPAIRED. *li-ca.
EYEBALL **Color Red.** *spi.
Eruptions, Pterygium. *zn.
Heat. na-cl.
Itching. na-sa.

Lachrymation. aga. ba-ca. *spi.
  Appearance of. *cro.
  Feeling of. ba-ca. *cro.
Pressing. ba-ca. smi. *spi.
Shooting. *cph. *spi. thu.
LENS. **Cataract.** *mg-ca.
ORBIT. **Pressing.** thu.
Tensive. thu.
EYELIDS. **Movements Closing.** ba-ca.
Swelling. *rs.
UPPER EYELIDS. **Swelling.** *crot. rs.
Œdematous. *crot. rs.
Red. *crot. rs.
TARSAL EDGES. **Discharge Pus.** *crot. rs.
                 White. *crot. rs.
                 Yellow. *crot. rs.
FORWARDS. **Eyeball Pressing.** *spi.
                 Shooting. *spi.
EYEBALL to JAW. **Undefined.** f-hx.
LEFT SIGHT DAZZLED then RIGHT OBJECTS
IMAGINARY, **Veil Crooked.** *na-cl.
LEFT INTERNAL CANTHUS **Bruised, then** LEFT
ORBIT SUPERIORLY **Bruised.** glo.

ANTERO—POSTERIORLY—FORWARDS.
(Within—Outwards).

    acon. al-o. alli. alo. anan. asr. ast. atp. au. ber. br. bry.
ca-ca. ca-o. ca-s. can. can-i. cb-v. cl-hx. cmc. con. crd. (cro).
crt-c. cth. dl-s. dro. (dt). gel. glo. glp. gui. gym. hll. k-i.
k-na. k-o. lau-c. lch. led. ly-b. lyc. mg-ca. mg-cl. mg-sa.
mgs-ar. mrl. mtr. n-x. na-ba. na-ca. na-cl. narth. p. p-x.
pan. par. pol. ppv. pru-l. pso. ptv. pul. rho. rn-b. rs. s.
sang. scu. sep. si-x. snc. spi. str. str-i. thu. trg. val. vi-t. zng.
    EYEBALL. **Pressing.** (as if eyes would come out,
&c.) acon. al-o. alo. anm. asr. atp. au. ber. bry. ca-ca. ca-o. ca-s.
can. can-i. cb-v. cmc. con. crd. crt-c. cth. dl-s. glo. gui.
gym. hll. k-i. k-na. k-o. lau-c. lch. led. lyc. mg-ca. mg-cl.
mg-sa. mgs-ar. mrl. mtr. na-cl. narth. p. p-x. par. pol. pru-l.
pso. ptv. pul. rn-b. rs. sang. scu. sep. si-x. spi. str. str-i.
thu. trg. val. zn.
    Shooting. anm. au. ca-ca. cl-hx. dro. gel. na-ca. s. sep.
si-x. val. vi-t.
    Tearing. alli. anm. atp. ca-ca. p-x. si-x

Tensive. glp.
Undefined. ast.
EYEBALL SUPERIORLY. **Pressing.** au.
EYEBALL INTERNALLY. **Pressing.** au.
ORBIT. **Tearing.** atp.

ANTERO—POSTERIORLY—BACKWARDS.

(Without—Inwards.)

acon. aga. amb. aps. arn. ast. atp. au. bap. bi-na. bry.
ca-ca. ca-s. can. chd. chi. chio. cit-c. (con). cor. dph. dt.
grp. hæm. hg-s. hyp. k-ca. k-o. kre. lac-f. ly-b. mn-ca. na-ba.
na-sa. p. p-x. pb. pet. pnx. s. sa-l. si-x. smc. spi. teu.
zn.
EYEBALL. **Drawing.** ast. ca-s. ly-b. pb. s. si-x.
Pressing. acon. aga. amb. ast. atp. au. bap. bi-na.
bry. ca-ca. can. chd. cit-c. cor. hæm. hg-s. k-ca. k-o. kre.
na-ba. p-x. pnx. smc. spi. teu. zn.
  Like a Plug. chi.
Shooting. aps. arn. atp. p. pet.
ORBIT. **Pressing.** atp. chd.
UPPER EYELIDS. **Pressing.** acon.

VERTICALLY—DOWNWARDS.

ath. atp. au. bap. bry. cb-a. cb-v. chd. chi. chio. cit-c.
gel. hll. k-o. lac-f. ner. par. rn-b. s. smc. snp-n. spi. trg.
zn. zng.
EYEBALL. **Pressing.** ath. bap. cb-v. chd. chio. rn-b.
s. smc. snp-n.
Scraping. pul.
Shooting. cb-a.
EYEBALL INTERIORLY. **Pressing.** chio.
ORBITAL INTEGUMENTS. **Pressing.** lac-f.
EYELIDS. **Swelling.** as-o.
TARSAL EDGES. **Cutting.** zng.
 ORBITAL INTEGUMENTS SUPERIORLY **to** TAR-
SAL EDGES. **Cutting.** trg.

VERTICALLY.—UPWARDS.

acon. amm-cl. arn. atp. bi-na. chio. cmc. euph-a. krm. nic. vr-s.
EYEBALL. **Boring**. ber.
False Sensations, Sand. amm-cl.
Pressing. arn. bi-na. chio.
Shooting. ber.
Undefined. acon.
EYEBALL INTERIORLY. **Pressing**. chio.
EYEBALL to ORBITAL INTEGUMENTS SUPE-
RIORLY. **Undefined**. acon.
EYEBALL to EYELIDS. **Drawing**. chd.
UPPER TARSAL EDGE to ORBIT. **Shooting**. nic.

LATERALLY—LENGTHWAYS.

cr-o. dro. gel. na-ba. p-x.
EYEBALL. **Shooting**. gel.
EYELIDS. **Shooting**. p-x.

LATERALLY—OUTWARDS (To External Canthi).

alo. arn. bap. (con). euph-a. hg-s. i. lch. na-ca. p-x. rs.
EYEBALL. **Drawing**. arn.
Pressing. bap. p-x.
ORBIT SUPERIORLY. **Cutting**. hg-s.
ORBITAL INTEGUMENTS SUPERIORLY. **Draw-ing**. alo.

LATERALLY—INWARDS (To Internal Canthi).

cub. nic. pet. rho. s-x. spo.
EYEBALL. **Shooting**. cub.

OBLIQUELY.

dro.

ALTERNATING with HEAD.

atp. dt. phl. trg.
OBJECTS IMAGINARY. **Vibrations**. trg.
Zigzags. trg.
SIGHT IMPAIRED. phl.

EYEBALL. **Appearance Wild**. dt.
ORBIT. **Pressing—Backwards**. atp.
Tearing—Forwards. atp.

ALTERNATING with EARS.

atp. cic.
OBJECTS FALSE APPEARANCE of. **Black**. cic.
Multiplied. cic.
ORBIT. **Pressing—Backwards**. atp.
Tearing—Forwards. atp.

ALTERNATING with FACE.

kre.

ALTERNATING with ABDOMEN.

cic. euphr. hg-bini. kre.
EYEBALL. **Color Red**. hg-bini.
Heat. hg-bini.
Movements, Convulsions. cic.
Undefined. euphr.

ALTERNATING with URINARY ORGANS.
kre.

ALTERNATING with GENITAL ORGANS.
kre.

ALTERNATING with CHEST.

kre. rn-b.
EYEBALL. **Pressing**. rn-b.

ALTERNATING with BACK.

hg-bini.
EYEBALL. **Color Red**. hg-bini.
Heat. hg-bini.

ALTERNATING with ARMS.

atp. hg-bini.
SIGHT IMPAIRED. atp.
EYEBALL. **Color Red**. hg-bini.
Heat. hg-bini.

ALTERNATING with LEGS.

atp.
SIGHT IMPAIRED. atp.

To HEAD.

acon. aga. anan. as-o. atp. ba-ca. ber. br. buf. ca-o. cb-v.
cch. ccs. cic. cit-c. cmc. cmf. crt-c. cth. euph-a. glo. grp. hg-s.·
hur. k-o. kre. lac-ac. lac-f. lch. li-ca. ly-b. lyc. nic. par. pau.
phy. s. sang. spi. spo-f. thu. trg. trn. u-na. vr-v. woo.
EYEBALL. **Boring.** ber.
Cutting. cit-c.
Drawing. aga. crt-c. grp.
Heaviness. glo.
Pressing. aga. cit-c. kre. nic.
Shooting. ber. ca-o. s. spi. thu. trg.
Tensive, like a thread. par.
Throbbing. br. ccs.
Undefined. acon. ccs. spo-f. woo.
ORBIT, CIRCUMFERENCE. **Shooting.** k-o.
ORBIT, SUPERIORLY. **Shooting.** pau.
Throbbing. buf.
EYELIDS. **Swelling.** as-o.
INTERNAL CANTHUS. **Contractive.** anan.
Shooting. anan.

To HEAD—ANTERIORLY.

acon. aga. atp. ber. br. ca-o. ccs. cit-c. cth. hur. lac-ac. lac-f.
ly-b. lyc. sang. spo-f. trg. vr-v.
EYEBALL. **Boring.** ber.
Drawing. aga.
Pressing. aga. cit-c.
Shooting. ber. ca-o.
Throbbing. br.
Undefined. ccs. spo-f.
ORBIT. **Undefined.** hur.
ORBIT SUPERIORLY. **Shooting.** acon. cth.

To HEAD—SUPERIORLY.

cmf. kre. phy. trg.
EYEBALL. **Pressing.** kre.
Shooting. trg.
Undefined. cmf.

To HEAD—TEMPLES.

acon. ba-ca. br. ccs. crt-c. glo. hg-s. lac-f. lch. li-ca. spo-f.
EYEBALL. **Drawing**. crt-c.
Heaviness. glo.
Throbbing. ccs.
Undefined. spo-f.
ORBIT SUPERIORLY. **Shooting**. acon.

To HEAD—LATERALLY.

cit-c. trn.
EYEBALL. **Pressing**. cit-c.

To HEAD—POSTERIORLY.

cch. ccs. cic. cmc. cmf. lch. nic. spi. thu. u-na.
EYEBALL. **Pressing**. nic.
Shooting. spi. thu.

To EARS.

ba-ca. dl-s. elaps. hg-s. li-ca.

To NOSE.

alli. ba-ca. ca-o. chd. cit-c. k-o. ni-ca. sa-l.
EYEBALL. **Drawing**. chd.
ORBIT SUPERIORLY. **Tearing**. ca-o.

To NOSE—ROOT.

chd.
EYEBALL. **Drawing**. chd.

To NOSE—POINT.

sa-l.

To FACE.

acon. aga. ca-o. cl-hx. cor. f-hx. jcr. k-bicr. lyc. i. mgs. spi.
ORBIT. **Shooting**. acon.
UPPER EYELIDS. **Drawing**. cl-hx.
Shooting. cl-hx.
INTERNAL CANTHUS. **Tearing**. ca-o.

To FACE—JAWS.

mgs.

To FACE—UPPER JAW.

aga. f-hx. k-bicr.

To FACE—LOWER JAW.

jcr.

To FACE—UPPER LIP.

ca-o.

To TEETH.

acon. hg-bicl. lac-ac. lyc.
ORBIT. **Shooting**. acon.

To TEETH—UPPER.

hg-bicl.

To ABDOMEN.

mgs.

To CHEST.

mgs.

To BACK.

as-o. mgs. rs. trg.

To BACK—NECK.

trg.
EYEBALL. **Tensive like a Thread**. trg.

To LEGS.

mgs.

To LEGS—HIPS.

mgs.

To WHOLE BODY.

acon. cit-c.
EYEBALL. **Undefined.** cit-c.
EXTERNAL CANTHUS. **Numbness.** acon.

I D. RIGHT SIDE, (Right Eye).

acon. æsc. aga. al-o. alli. alm. alo. amb. amm-ca. amm-cl.
amph. anan. aps. arn. arum-t. asc. asr. ast. atp. atrop. au.
bap. bar. ber. br. bry. buf. c-bis. ca-a. ca-ca. ca-pa. cac. cb-a.
cb-v. cch. ccs. chd. chio. cic. cis. cit-c. cl-hx. cld. cle. cmc.
cmf. cof. con. cop. cot. cph. cr-o. crb-x. cro. crt. cth. cu.
cund. cyc. delph. dig. dl-s. dro. dt. elaps. ele. erig. ery. eug.
f-hx. fe-mgs. fe-pa. frm. gel. glo. glp. grp. gui. gym. hg.
hg-bini. hg-i. hg-s. hur. hyp. i. irs-f. jcr. k-bicr. k-ca. k-i. k-na.
k-o. klm. kre. krm. lac-ac. lac-f. lau-c. lch. li-ca. lo-cœ. lo-i.
lpd. ly-b. lyc. mg-ca. mg-cl. mg-sa. mgs. mll. mn-ca. mrl.
mtr. myris. n-x. na-ba. na-ca. na-cl. na-sa. naj. narth. ner.
ni-ca. nic. ol-a. p. p-x. pæo. par. pau. pb. pet. phl. phy.
pim. pnc. pnx. pol. ppv. pru-l. pso. pt. ptv. pul. qu-sa. rho.
rn-b. rs. rs-r. rś-v. rut. s. s-x. sa-l. sang. sb-s. sb-t. sep. si-x.
smc. smi. sn. so-o. so-t. spi. spi-m. spo. spo-f. sr-ca. str. str-i.
te. teu. thr. thu. trg. trn. trx. tx-b. u-na. urg. urt. val. vi-t.
vr-a. vr-s. vsp. xan. ziz. zn. zng.
　OBJECTS, FALSE APPEARANCE of. **Blue.** ni-ca.
Confused. eug. rs-r.
Multiplied. (mtr).
Small. thu.
OBJECTS IMAGINARY. **Black.**　cund. p. (qu-sa).
(si-x).
　Blue. cund. elaps.
　Bright. ca-ca. cit-c. na-sa. ol-a.
　Circles. cit-c.
　Crystals with Black tips. cund.
　Curls. cund.
　Feathers. al-o.
　Figures. myris.
　　At side of Visual Ray. myris.
　Green. na-sa.
　Halo. cmc.
　　Red. cmc.
　Horns Black. cund.
　Leaf White. na-sa.

Low down. cit-c.
Mist. au. cit-c. cund. mg-ca. na-sa. ol-a.
Moving. cund.
Moving with Eye. ca-ca. (qu-sa).
Near Eye. na-sa.
Pyriform body. cund.
  Blue. cund.
  Red. cund.
Red. cmc. cund.
Serpentine bodies. cund.
  Black. cund.
  Moving. cund.
Moving. cund.
Side of Visual Ray at. cit-c. myris.
Spots, Black. (qu-sa). (si-x).
      Moving with Eye. (qu-sa).
  Bright. cit-c. ol-a.
    Low down. cit-c.
    Moving with Eye. ca-ca.
    Side of Visual Ray, at. cit-c.
  Low down. cit-c.
  Moving with Eye. ca-ca.
  Side of Visual Ray, at. cit-c.
Star Bright. ca-ca. na-sa.
    Moving with Eye. ca-ca.
    Near Eye. na-sa.
  Green. na-sa.
    Near Eye. na-sa.
  Moving with Eye. ca-ca.
  Near Eye. na-sa.
    Yellow. na-sa.
    Near Eye. na-sa.
Threads. con. cund. pol.
Veil Black. p.
  Blue. elaps.
  Crooked. na-cl.
  White. elaps.
Vibrations. chd. dig. trg.
  White. elaps. na-sa.
  Yellow. na-sa.
SIGHT IMPAIRED. aps. (atp). cit-c. con. cph. cro.
cund. elaps. eug. k-o. krm. mg-ca. n-x. na-ca. na-sa. ol-a. p.
qu-sa. rut. str-i. trn.

EYEBALL. **Boring.** ber. cof.
Bruised. ly-b. ptv. smi.
Bursting. lau-c.
Coldness. asr. cro. dt. li-ca. par. pt. s.
Color Dark. k-bicr.
    Red. al-o. aps. atp. ca-ca. cb-a. ccs. con. cot. cph. dt. eug. hg-bini. hg-s. hur. lac-f. lau-c. n-x. p. sep. vr-a. zn.
    Contractive. krm. n-x. spi. urg.
    Like a Cord. amph.
Cutting. (atp). cl-hx. s. vi-t. zn.
Discharge Hard. sb-s.
    Mucus. al-o. aps. euph. k-na. p.
    Undefined. s.
Drawing. arn. ccs. crt. cth. hg-s. vr-s.
Dryness. atp. cr-o. ppv. sa-l.
Eruptions, Styes. ca-ca. cth. .na-cl.
False Sensations, Hair. nic.
    Mucus. euph.
    Pellicle. k-o.
    Sand. amph. dt. lo-cœ. lyc. pt. rs. sep. sr-ca. teu. zn.
    Water. dt.
    Wind. asr. cro.
Gnawing. kre.
Hard. cit-c.
Heat. alo. amb. aps. cu. dig. dro. k-bicr. lo-cœ. ly-b. na-sa. pb. rs-v. sang. sep. spi. te. teu.
    Heaviness. aps. lpd. trn.
Itching. aga. asc. chd. dt. f-hx. lch. ly-b. na-sa. spi. zn.
    Lachrymation. aps. atp. br. cb-v. con. crb-x. dt. ery. hg-bini. hg-s. k-o. lac-f. lo-cœ. na-sa. (s). sa-l. sang. sep. so-t. te. teu. (trg).
    Hot. atp. k-na. na-sa. spi.
Motion in, Jumping, like something. dt.
    Passing round, like something. rs.
    Undulation. pt.
Movements, Convulsions .æsc. krm. lac-ac. sa-l. thu. trg. zn.
    Squinting. (alm). dt. hyo. pb. spi-m.
    Inwards. (alm). hyo. pb.
Paralysis. k-o.
Pressing. aga. alo. arum-t. au. bry. cch. ccs. chd. cit-c. cmf. con. crt. f-hx. glo. glp. k-o. klm. myris. na-sa. pul. rho. rn-b. rs. smi. spi. spo. thu. trg. val. zn.

Projecting. arn.
Feeling. cmc.
Shooting. acon. aga. as-o. atp. ber. c-bis. ca-a. ca-ca.
chd. cic. cld. cyc. grp. gym. hur. k-ca. k-o. lac-f. li-ca. lpd.
mg-cl. mn-ca. n-x. na-cl. pso. rho. s. spi. spo. str-i. trg.
trn. trx. vi-t. zn.
Hot. rho.
Smarting. al-o. anan. aps. cmc. cot. cu. gym. k-i. kre.
krm. lo-cœ. lo-i. lyc. na-ca. p. pb. pim. pt. rho. rn-b. rs.
sep. (trg). urt.
Swelling. anan. ele. k-ca. p.
Chemosis. vsp.
Œdematous. chio.
Veins of. mg-ca.
Feeling of. cmc.
Tearing. aga. amb. as-o. ca-a. cch. cro. hyp. k-ca. lyc.
mg-cl. mrl. pnc. thu. val.
Tensive. au. glp. k-o. zn.
Throbbing. atp. bry. c-bis. pet. thr. thu. trg.
Undefined. anan. bap. erig. f-hx. gel. (hg-bini). mll.
na-sa. sa-l. sang. str-i. trn. urt. vsp. vr-v. zn.
EYEBALL SUPERIORLY. **False Sensations, Sand.**
lo-cœ. spi.
Pressing. ast. dl-s.
Shooting. cot.
Swelling. br. si-x.
Undefined. alli.
EYEBALL INFERIORLY. **Crampy.** aga.
Pressing. sep.
EYEBALL EXTERNALLY. **Bruised.** vr-a.
Color Dark. k-bicr.
False Sensations, Sand. dt.
Heat. p-x. sn.
Shooting. p-x.
Smarting. sn.
EYEBALL INTERNALLY. **Color Red.** ca-ca. ery. mtr.
Heat. trx.
Swelling. ca-ca.
Undefined. li-ca.
EYEBALL POSTERIORLY. **Pressing.** glo. sep.
Undefined. spo-f.
EYEBALL INTERIORLY. **Drawing.** vr-s.
Pressing. glo.
Shooting. as-o. lac-f.

Smarting. ,m-b.
Undefined. as-o. li-ca.
EYEBALL CIRCUMFERENCE. **Undefined.** gel.
EYEBALL CENTRE. **Shooting.** lac-f.
CORNEA. **Eruptions Pustule.** dig.
                       With Red Areola. dig.
  Ulcers. aps.
Opacity. (rs).
IRIS. **Color Discolored.** atp. (rs).
       Green. (rs).
Pupil Contracted. atp. nic.
  Dilated. atp. mn-ca. p-x. pru-l. rho.
  Insensible. (rs).
  Irregular. (rs).
LENS. **Cataract.** amm-ca. con. (rs). s.
ORBIT. **Boring.** frm. lo-cœ.
Drawing. atp. li-ca. sn.
Heaviness. hur.
Pressing. acon. atp. f-hx. glo. glp. ppv. su. thu.
Shooting. f-hx. glo. nic.
Smarting. hg-i.
Tearing. k-ca. zn.
Tensive. thu.
Throbbing. hur. li-ca. trg.
Undefined. hg-i. hur. ziz.
ORBIT CIRCUMFERENCE. **Drawing.** li-ca.
Tearing. cl-hx.
Throbbing. li-ca.
ORBIT SUPERIORLY. **Boring.** elaps. ol-a.
Bruised. glo.
Bursting. dl-s. na-cl.
Contractive. acon.
Drawing. chio. k-i. li-ca.
Heaviness. cac.
Motion in, Undulation. pt.
Pressing. amm-cl. bry. vr-v.
Shooting. bry. cis.
Smarting. hg-s.
Swelling, Feeling of. hg-s.
Tearing. acon. amm-cl. bar. k-i. phl.
Throbbing. amm-cl. li-ca. na-cl. sn.
Undefined. chio. dl-s. jcr. (na-cl). pet. rs-r.
ORBIT INFERIORLY. **Pressing.** na-sa. phy. thu.
Shooting. na-sa.

Softness, Feeling of. na-sa.
Undefined. (au). hg-i. (thu).
ORBIT EXTERNALLY. **Crampy.** pt.
Drawing. li-ca.
Tearing. au.
Throbbing. li-ca.
ORBIT INTERNALLY. **Boring.** thu.
Swelling. k-bicr. si-x.
Throbbing. k-bicr.
ORBITAL INTEGUMENTS. **Color Red.** dt.
Heat. k-bicr.
Swelling. dt.
Tearing. cch.
Tensive. myris.
ORBITAL INTEGUMENTS SUPERIORLY. **Bruised.**
pt.
Contractive. bry. rho.
Crampy. aga.
Creeping. phl. rn-b.
Drawing. k-i.
Eruptions, Boils. ca-pa. i.
  Hard. gui.
  Pimples. asc. gui.
      Hard. gui.
      Smarting. asc.
      Undefined pain. gui.
  Smarting. asc.
  Undefined pain. gui.
Heat. f-hx. hg.
Itching. aps. f-hx. rho. spi.
Movements, Convulsions. k-ca.
Numbness. ppv.
Pressing. dig. grp. k-ca. lau-c. ol-a. thu. zn.
Shooting. mn-ca. nic. ol-a. thu. trn.
Smarting. aps.
Swelling, Feeling of. aps.
Tearing. bar. k-ca. phl.
Tensive. i.
Undefined. chd. delph. jcr. li-ca. str.
ORBITAL INTEGUMENTS INFERIORLY. **Color
Dark.** s-x.
Contractive. si-x.
Cutting. atrop.
Drawing. lo-cœ.
Movements, Convulsions. n-x.

Shooting. pau.
Swelling. myris.
Tearing. teu.
EYELIDS. **Adhesion of.** ca-ca. euph. k-na. na-ba. na-ca. p. s.
   Color Red. k-ca. k-o. p. pol. s. vsp.
   Discharge Mucus. sb-s.
     Pus. s.
   Drawing. cb-v.
   Heat. hg. k-na. narth. ner. s. sn.
   Itching. aps. asc. cro. k-na. na-ca. p.
   Movements, Closing. (chi). dig. (grp). k-o. mg-cl. (pb). pnx. (vr-a). zn.
       Spasmodically. hyp. lyc.
    Convulsions. s. trg.
    Open wide. buf. dl-s. na-cl.
    Winking. pt.
Paralysis, Opening difficult. myris.
Shooting. aps. s. sn.
Smarting. k-na. s.
Swelling. k-o. lyc. p. pol. (sep). vsp.
   Red. vsp.
   Feeling of. trx.
Tensive. myris. ner.
UPPER EYELID. **Boring.** ptv.
Color Red. acon. crot. na-ca. rs. sep.
Drawing. cb-v.
Eruptions. Boils. ca-pa.
   Herpes. trn.
   Pimples. trn.
   Pustules. cth. lyc.
   Vesicles. br.
Hardness. acon. rs.
Heat. alli. cit-c. cle. cmf. ner. p-x. rs. s. sn. spi.
Heaviness. p-x. pnx.
Itching. al-o. aps. p. pæo. pru-l. rs. rs-r. vsp. zn.
Movements, Convulsions. al-o. aps. atp. ba-ca. bar. ca-ca. cch. chd. chi. cit-c. cop. frm. krm. lac-ac. n-x. na-cl. par. pb. pnc. pol. rho. smi. thu. trn.
       Feeling of. dt.
Numbness. naj.
Paralysis. al-o. pnx. rs.
Pressing. chd. hyo. lyc. na-ca. na-cl. p. p-x. pol. rs. thu. trg. trx.

Shooting. bar. chd. cyc. irs-f. pæo. rs. sn. spi.
  Hot. os.
Smarting. bar. rs. zn.
Swelling. acon. cmf. crot. k-ca. k-o. na-ca. p. rs. sep. vsp.
  Air-like. p.
  Hard. acon.
  Œdematous. atp. crot. rs.
  Red. acon.
  Feeling of. rs.
Tearing. al-o. ba-ca. zn.
Tensive. acon.
Throbbing. cth. mn-ca. p. s.
Undefined. xan.
LOWER EYELID, **Contractive.** rs.
Cutting. cit-c.
Eruptions Pustules. chio.
  Styes. fe-pa. pol. so-o.
  Ulcers. na-cl.
Heat. alm. cit-c. pru-l. rn-b. si-x. sn.
Itching. alm. hg-s. hur. krm.
Movements, Convulsions. aga. ars. cth. krm. narth.
Pressing. hg-s. p-x.
Scraping. si-x.
Shooting. cth. hg-s. sn. zn.
Smarting. aps. c-bis. dro. na-cl. rn-b. si-x.
Swelling. chio.
  Œdematous. chio.
Throbbing. asr. pol. pru-l. rho. rs.
TARSAL EDGES. **Discharge.** crot. rs.
  Pus. crot. rs.
  White. crot. rs.
  Yellow. crot. rs.
Heat. narth.
Itching. k-ca.
Scraping. p.
UPPER TARSAL EDGE. **Discharge.** s
  Hard. s.
Dryness. li-ca.
Eruptions, Tubercles. thu.
  Vesicles. pol.
  Warts. sb-t.
Itching. spi.
Shooting. spi.
Smarting. li-ca. lo-cœ.

Swelling. s.

Tingling. par.

LOWER TARSAL EDGE. **Eruptions, Pimples.** au.

   Smooth. au.

   Tubercles. au.

        Smooth. au.

Heat. alm.

Itching. alm.

Smarting. hur.

EYELIDS, INNER SURFACE. **Color Red.** cph.

Shooting. cit-c.

CANTHI. **Discharge, Mucus.** gui.

Itching. asc.

Movements, Convulsions. lch.

Scraping. pru-l.

Undefined. sa-l.

EXTERNAL CANTHUS. **Bruised.** vr-a.

Coldness. asr.

Color Red. na-ba.

Cutting. k-i.

Discharge, Mucus. euph. na-ba. sb-s.

Dryness. thu.

Eruptions, Pustules. alo.

False Sensations, Sand. s-x. (spi). thu.

Heat. dl-s. glo. na-ca. ol-a. sn. spi.

Itching. al-o. bry. ca-ca. euph. frm. na-cl. tx-b. urg.

Movements, Convulsions. pol. ppv.

Pressing. cb-v.

Shooting. cl-hx. dl-s. k-ca. rn-s. sn.

Smarting. ag-na. cb-v. cch. cot. frm. p. rn-b. rn-s. rs.

Swelling. br.

Tearing. au.

Undefined. sa-l.

INTERNAL CANTHUS. **Boring.** thu.

Coldness. li-ca.

Color Red. amm-ca. ery. mg-ca. pet. pt. sb-t. zn.

Creeping. pt.

Discharge, Mucus. na-ca. zn.

   Pus. zn.

Dryness. al-o.

Eruptions, Styes. na-cl.

False Sensations, Sand. bar. rho. s-x. thu. trx.

Hæmorrhage. mtr.

Heat. au. cit-c. cle. f-hx. gel. hg-s. hur. mg-ca. narth. pru-l. sb-t. trx.

Itching. al-o. au. ca·ca. cl-hx. f-hx. hg-s. k-o. lpd. mg-cl. nic. p.

Movements, Convulsions. krm. s-x. sn.

Pressing. amph. cb-v. chd. cic. dl-s. hg-s. hll. ppv. rho. smc. sn. trx. zn.

Shooting. chd. cit-c. f-hx. hg-s. mg-cl. pru-l. spi. thu.

Smarting. cb-v. cl-hx. k-bicr. mg-ca. mg-sa. s. sb-t. sep. sn.

Swelling. pet. si-x. smi.

Tearing atp. krm. lyc.

Throbbing. chd. rs-r. s-x.

Undefined. k-o. sa-l. sang.

CARUNCULA. **Smarting.** bry.dl-s. k-bicr. pul. str. zn.

Swelling. ca-ca.

LACHRYMAL GLAND. **Swelling.** br. si-x.

LACHRYMAL BONE. **Swelling.** k-bicr. si-x.

Throbbing. k-bicr.

LACHRYMAL SAC. **Swelling.** si-x.

PERIODICAL. **Eyeball Shooting.** c-bis.

  Smarting. rho.

  Throbbing. c-bis.

Eyeball Externally. Bruised. vr-a.

Eyeball Posteriorly. Undefined. spo-f.

External Canthus. Heat. dl-s.

SUDDENLY COME and GO. **Eyeball Pressing.** dig.

ALTERNATING in EYE. **Eyeball Shooting with Throbbing.** c-bis.

  Throbbing with Sensitiveness. thu.

CHANGING CHARACTER or PLACE. **Objects Imaginary, Mist, then Star Bright Green Yellow Near Eye.** na-sa.

Eyeball Contractive, then Lachrymation. aga.

                     then Smarting. aga.

False Sensations, Pellicle, then Shooting. k-o.

Shooting, then Heat. p-x.

Tensive, then Shooting. k-o.

Throbbing then Sensitive. thu.

Orbit Inferiorly, Sensitive then Pressing. na-sa.

  Shooting-Backwards   **then**   ,,   na-sa.

  Softness, Feeling of   **then**   ,,   na-sa.

Lower Eyelid. Swelling, then Eruptions, Pustules. chio.

Objects Imaginary, Star Bright Green Yellow Near Eye, then Eyeball Pressing. na-sa.

Sight Impaired, then Objects Imaginary, Star Bright Green Yellow Near Eye. na-sa.

Eyeball Pressing, then Sight Impaired. sep.

Moving Body in, then Orbit Superiorly Sensitive. cb-a.

Smarting, then External Canthus Smarting. cot.

Eyelids, Movements, Winking, then Orbit Superiorly Sensitive. cb-a.

Pressing-Forward, then Orbit Circumference, Pressing. na-ba.

Upper Eyelid, Movements, Drawn-Down, -then Orbit Superiorly Sensitive. cb-a.

Eyeball to Jaw Shooting, then Eyeball to Abdomen, Chest, Neck, Legs, Drawing. mgs.

FORWARDS. **Eyeball, Pressing.** cmc. pul. str-i. zng.

Shooting. rho.

Tearing. ly-b.

Orbit, Pressing. ppv.

Orbit Superiorly, Pressing. dl-s.

Lower Eyelid, Tearing. na-ca.

BACKWARDS. **Eyeball, Pressing.** cit-c.

Shooting. atp. grp. hyp. lac-f.

Undefined. sa-l.

Orbit Inferiorly, Shooting. na-sa.

Orbital Integuments Superiorly, Shooting. mn-ca.

DOWNWARDS. **Eyeball, Pressing.** au. bry. cit-c.

Shooting. gel.

Orbit, Drawing. atp.

Orbit Superiorly, Pressing. chio.

Eyelids, Swelling. vsp.

UPWARDS. **Eyeball, Boring.** ber.

Drawing. vr-s.

Shooting. ber.

Upper Eyelid, Pressing. krm.

INWARDS. **Eyeball, False Sensations, Sand.** s-x.

Shooting. rho.

Orbital Integuments Superiorly, Shooting. nic.

ALTERNATING with HEAD. **Orbit, Pressing.** atp.
To HEAD. Eyeball, Drawing. trg.
  Shooting. s. trg.
Orbital Integuments Superiorly, Drawing. cb-v.
To FOREHEAD. Eyeball, Shooting. lac-f. trg.
  Tearing. lac-f.
  Throbbing. ly-b.
Orbit Superiorly, Undefined. vr-v.
To VERTEX, Eyeball, Shooting. trg.
To TEMPLE. Eyeball, Shooting. lac-f.
  Throbbing. lac-f.
  Orbital Integuments Superiorly, Undefined.
li-ca.
  Punctum Lachrymale, Undefined. hg-s.
To OCCIPUT. Eyeball, Pressing. nic.
  Shooting. cic. spi.
  Throbbing. ccs.
  Undefined. cmc. cmf.
  Orbit, Shooting. u-na.
To EAR. Orbital Integuments Superiorly, Un-
defined. li-ca.
  Eyelids, Boring. elaps.
  External Canthus, Heat. dl-s.
  Internal Canthus, Drawing. hg-s.
To NOSE. Eyeball, Undefined. alli.
  External Canthus, Drawing. k-o.
To TIP of NOSE. Internal Canthus, Undefined.
sa-l.
To FACE. Internal Canthus, Tearing. i.
To UPPER JAW. Eyeball, Undefined. f-hx.
To LOWER JAW. Eyeball, Drawing. jcr.
To ABDOMEN. Eyeball, Drawing. mgs.
To CHEST. Eyeball, Drawing. mgs.
To NECK. Eyeball, Drawing. mgs.
To HIP. Eyeball, Drawing. mgs.
DIAGONALS with OTHER ORGANS. cld. cro. dro.
frm. li-ca. n-x. na-sa. thu. trg. trn.
  With LEFT HEAD. Eyeball, Shooting. trn.
  With LEFT EAR. Eyeball, Dryness. thu.
  Heat. dro.
  Itching. na-sa.
  Shooting. n-x.
Lower Tarsal Edge, Heat. thu.

With LEFT TEETH. **Eyeball, Tearing.** cro.
With LEFT GENITALS. **Eyeball, Dryness.** thu.
Lower Tarsal Edge, Heat. thu.
With LEFT ARM. **Eyelids, Movements, Convulsions.** trg.
With LEFT LEG. **Eyeball, Shooting.** cld.
Eyelids, Movements, Convulsions. trg.
Before LEFT HEAD. **Eyeball, Pressing.** trg.
Before LEFT EAR. **Orbit, Boring.** frm.
Before LEFT LEG. **Eyeball, Pressing.** trg.
After LEFT HEAD **Orbital Integuments Superiorly, Undefined.** li-ca.

I. E. LEFT SIDE (Left Eye).

ach. æsc. ag. ag-na. aga. al-o. alli. alm. amm-cl. amph. aps. arn. art-v. as-o. asc. asr. ast. atp. au. ba-a. ba-ca. ba-cl. bar. blt. br. bry. c-bis. ca-a. ca-ca. cb-a. cb-v. cch. ccs. chd. chi. chio. cis. cit-c. cl-hx. cle. cnv-d. con. cop. cor. cot. cph. cr-o. crb-x. cro. crt. crt-c. cth. cu. cu-asi. cund. cyc. dl-s. dph. dro. dt. ecb. elaps. ele. eryn. (eupat). euph. euph-a. euphr. f-hx. frm. frm-s. glo. glp. grc. gym. hg. hg-bini. hg-bicl. hg-s. hll. hur. hydr. i. itu. jat. jnp-s. k-bicr. k-ca. k-cla. k-na. k-o. klm. krm. lac-cg. lac-d. lac-f. lau-c. lch. lct. led. li-ca. lo-cœ. lo-i. lpd. lyc. men. mg-ca. mg-sa. mgs. mgs-au. mim. msc. myris. n-x. na-ba. na-cl. na-sa. narth. ner. ni-ca. nic. ol-a. ox-x. p. p-x. pan. pau. pb. pb-a. pd. ped. pet. phl. phy. plb. pln. pod. pol. pru-l. pt. ptv. pul. rhe. rho. rmx. rn-b. rs. rs-r. rut. s. s-x. sa-l. sa-mgs. sang. sb-s. se. (sep). si-x. smc. smi. sn. snc. snp. snp-n. so-o. so-t. spi. spo. sr-ca. str. str-i. stry. te. teu. thu. trg. trn. trx. tx-b. u-na. urg. urt. vi-t. vr-a. vr-s. vr-v. zn. zng.
    OBJECTS FALSE. APPEARANCE **of. Black.** na-cl.
Confused. cund.
Multiplied. atp. (mtr).
Small. pet.
White. cop. rn-b.
    OBJECTS IMAGINARY. **Black.** aga. atp. ca-ca. k-o s. zn.
Blue. dt.
Bright. cph. dig. dt. str. vr-a.
Brown. aga.

Circles Black. s.
  Bright. cph.
  Variegated. cph.
Far off. dt.
Green. zn.
Grey. lch.
Halo Green. zn.
  Variegated. atp.
Mist. ag-na. cund. ly-b. pt. s.
Moving. k-o. lch.
Moving with Eye. s.
Rays. atp.
Side of Visual Ray at. dt. str.
Spots Black. aga. atp. ca-ca. k-o. s.
          Moving. k-o.
          Moving with Eye. s.
  Blue. dt.
  Bright. dt. vr-a.
          Far off. dt.
          Side of Visual Ray at. dt.
  Brown. aga.
  Far off. dt.
  Grey. lch.
          Moving. lch.
  Moving. k-o. lch.
  Moving with Eye. s.
  Side of Visual Ray, at. dt.
Stripe Black. zn.
Variegated. atp. cph.
Veil. smi.
Vibrations Bright. dig. dt. str.
          Side of Visual Ray at. str.
SIGHT DAZZLED. na-cl.
SIGHT IMPAIRED. ag-na. amm-cl. as-o. atp. ca-ca.
cb-a. hg. ly-b. na-ba. na-cl. narth. pt. rmx. rn-b. si-x. smi.
EYEBALL. **Appearance Dim.** as-o. chd. s.
Boring. ber. euph-a. s.
Bruised. s. str.
Bursting. mg-ca.
Coldness. æsc. nic. trn.
Color Red. al-o. alli. as-o. atp. cnv-d. cop. eryn. glo.
hg-bini. hur. led. mim. pau. pb. phy. plb. pod. rn-b. rs. str.
str-i. te. teu. thu. trg.

Contractive. ag. amph. jnp-s. lch. lpd. n-x. ppv.
 Vertically. lch.
Crampy. chd. cit-c. k-cla.
Creeping. na-sa.
Cutting. cr-o. cund. i. s.
Discharge Corrosive. u-na.
 Mucus. cb-a. cb-v. eryn.
 Pus. eryn. na-sa. pb. (spi). u-na.
Drawing. alli. alo. f-hx. nic. pt. s.
Dryness. sa-mgs.
Eruptions, Granulations. eryn.
 Pterygium. ca-ca.
 Pustules. k-bicr.
 Styes. dl-s. lyc. pul.
False Sensations, Hairs. k-na. trn.
 Mucus. aps.
 Pellicle. s.
 Sand. al-o. as-o. cb-a. dl-s. dt. f-hx. hur. k-bicr.
mg-sa. na-sa. ox-x. p-x. rhe. rs. sa-mgs. smi. zng.
 Water, Cold. trn.
Gnawing. s.
Heat. æsc. al-o. bry. c-bis. chd. cit-c. crb-x. cu. dro.
glo. gym. k-ca. klm. led.'myris. na-ba. s. spo. trx. vr-s.
 Heaviness. acon. pd. trn.
Itching. ag-na. aps. ca-ca. chd. elaps. f-hx. hg-bicl.
hur. na-sa. sn. spi. sr-ca.
 Lachrymation. alli. amph. chd. dt. euph. hg-s. k-ca.
lac-f. lpd. (ly-b). pau. phy. plb. pul. rs-r. rut. s. s-x. (sep).
si-x. snp. stry. thu. trg. u-na.
 Cold. trg.
 Hot. al-o. ca-ca. spi.
 Feeling of. hg-s.
Movements, Convulsions. aga. al-o. aps. as-o. lac-cg.
se. trg. zn.
 Squinting. art-v. ca-ca. cyc.
 Inwards. art-v. ca-ca. cyc.
 As if Turned Round. chi.
Numbness. s.
Pressing. acon. al-o. as-o. asr. c-bis. cb-v. ccs. chd.
chio. cit-c. cle. eryn. hg-bini. hydr. lch. na-sa. ner. pan. pol.
rn-b. s. smi. sn. spi. str-i. teu. urt. vr-v. zng.
 Shooting. æsc. al-o. alli. atp. ber. br. chd. chi. cis.
dro. dt. elaps. frm-s. glo. hg-bini. hur. i. k-bicr. lac-f. mgs

myris. pau. phy. pul. s. sb-s. si-x. sn. snc. snp. snp-n. spi.
spo. trn. vr-v. zn.

Smarting. ag-na. al-o. cb-v. cot. cu. (eupat). lac-f.
mg-ca. n-x. ner. p. pod. rn-b. s. si-x. snp-n. u-na. vi-t. zn.

Stiffness. ca-ca.

Swelling. cb-v. ele. eryn.

Chemosis. atp.

Veins of. atp. pru-l.

Feeling of. aga. chd. cit-c. rs. rs-r.

Tearing. au-cl. cb-v. cch. chd. dro. k-ca. ni-ca. ol-a.
pb. s. smc. spo.

Tensive. dro. glp. lyc. nic. sn. spi.

Laterally like a Thread. s.

Throbbing. as-o. ca-ca. cl-hx. hur. lau-c. na-cl. pb.

Undefined. alli. au. br. cb-v. (eupat). gym. hg-bini.
lac-cg. lyc. pd. ppv. s. sa-l. sang. snp-n. str-i.

EYEBALL SUPERIORLY. **False Sensations,
Sand.** dl-s. hg. 'phy.

Heat. thu.

Pressing. as-o. chd. sr-ca. thu.

Shooting. as-o. i. snc.

EYEBALL INFERIORLY. **False Sensations, Sand.**
men.

Pressing. aps.

Shooting. zn.

Smarting. zn.

EYEBALL EXTERNALLY. **Boring.** i.

False Sensations, Sand. rs.

Heat. spi.

Pressing. i. spo.

EYEBALL INTERNALLY. **Color Red.** k-bicr

Eruptions, Pustule. k-bicr.

White with Red Areola. k-bicr

Heat. thu.

Pressing. rut.

EYEBALL POSTERIORLY. **Crampy.** au.

Pressing. au.

Undefined. asc. pd.

EYEBALL INTERIORLY. **Drawing.** alli.

Pressing. cis. chd. pol.

Smarting. lac-f.

Swelling, Feeling of. chd.

Undefined. lac-cg.

EYEBALL CIRCUMFERENCE. **Heat.** æsc. spo.
Shooting. æsc.
EYEBALL ROUND CORNEA. **Color Red.** thu.
EYEBALL CENTRE. **False Sensations, Sand.** rs.
Shooting. k-bicr. lac-f.
CORNEA. **Color Dark.** k-bicr.
  White. k-bicr.
Eruptions, Pustules. k-bicr. p.
             With Red Areola. k-bicr.
Opacity. atp. k-bicr.
Shooting. k-bicr.
CHAMBERS of EYE. **Discharge, Pus.** atp.
IRIS. **Pupil Contracted.** ag-na. as-o. rho.
  Dilated. cb-a. dt. nic. rho.
  Insensible. ag-na.
  Irregular. nic. s.
LENS. **Cataract.** mg-ca.
ORBIT. **Contractive.** spi.
Gnawing. s.
Heat. cit-c.
Heaviness. hur.
Pressing. aga. aps. bry. cit-c. spi. thu.
Shooting. ba-ca. itu.
Smarting. cu-asi.
Tearing. aga.
Tensive. thu.
Throbbing. as-o. ba-a. bry. glo. hur. sn.
Undefined. asc. li-ca. s.
ORBIT CIRCUMFERENCE. **Bruised.** na-cl.
Pressing. na-cl. narth. rho.
Shooting. aps. rho.
Tearing. phl.
Undefined. narth. os.
ORBIT SUPERIORLY. **Boring.** cu-asi.
Crampy. p-x.
Drawing. al-o. chio. sn.
Pressing. msc. myris. p-x. sn. str-i.
  Like a Plug, &c. hll. na-sa.
Shooting. hur. k-bicr.
Smarting. cu-asi.
Tearing. chd.
Throbbing. myris.
Undefined. chio. frm. hg-i. k-bicr. msc.

ORBIT INFERIORLY. **Boring.** euph-a.
Bruised. alm.
Pressing. aps.
Smarting. hg-s.
Swelling, Feeling of. hg-s.
Tearing. na-sa.
Throbbing. na-sa.
ORBIT EXTERNALLY. **Heat.** f-hx.
Throbbing. sn.
ORBIT INTERNALLY. **Broken, as if.** lch.
Bruised. lch.
Creeping. sep.
ORBITAL INTEGUMENTS. **Drawing.** pt. spo.
Heat. aps. dl-s.
Itching. aps.
Pressing. dl-s. dph.
Shooting. spo.
Swelling, Feeling of. aps.
ORBITAL INTEGUMENTS SUPERIORLY. **Boring.**
(ca-a).
  Bruised. pln.
  Contractive. p-x.
  Crampy. arn.
  Creeping. cro.
  Drawing. ca-a. n-x. rho.
  Eruptions, Granulations. eryn.
    Hard. rn-s.
    Pimples. k-ca. rho. rn-s.
      Hard. rn-s.
    Scabs. spo.
      Undefined Pain. spo.
      Yellow. spo.
    Tubercles. thu.
    Undefined Pain. spo. thu.
    Yellow. spo.

Heat. aga. alli. aps. men. narth. str.
Itching. br. pru-l. vi-t. vr-v.
Movements, Convulsions. k-o. zn.
  Downwards—Drawn. elaps.
        Feeling of. ol-a.
Pressing. acon. ca-a. jnp-s. msc. sb-s. thu. trx.
Shooting. aps. (ca-a). ol-a. rs-r. sb-s. thu. vi-t. zn.
Smarting. aps. dro. k-ca. ner.

Tearing. jnp-s. thu. trg. zn.
Tensive. hll.
Throbbing. aga.
Undefined. amm-cl. chd. crt-c. elaps. lac-cg. msc. rs-v. (thu).
ORBITAL INTEGUMENTS INFERIORLY. **Drawing.** atp.
Heat. hg-s. pb-a. rut.
Itching. na-cl. spo.
Movements, Convulsions. æsc.
Shooting. pb. ptv. spo.
Smarting. na-cl. ptv.
ORBITAL INTEGUMENTS EXTERNALLY. **Itching.** f-hx.
Movements, Convulsions. f-hx.
Tensive. spo.
EYELIDS. **Adhesion of.** cb-a. cb-v. chd. eryn. gym. k-ca. na-ba. na-sa. pb. rs. (spi). u-na.
Bruised. s.
Color, Red. atp. s. u-na.
Cutting. s.
Discharge, Mucus. k-ca.
Dryness. zn.
Eruptions, Styes. elaps. s.
Smarting. s.
Smarting. s.
Heat. al-o. asr. dro. rs-r. trx. zn.
Itching. aps. chi. hur. na-ca. ped.
Movements, Closing. atp. buf. chd. (chi). euph. grp. na-sa. (pb). sep. thu. tx-b. urg. (vr-a).
Spasmodically. rho. spo.
Convulsions. cb-v. k-o. lyc. mg-ca. p. phl. s. sb-s. trg.
Paralysis. ag-na. al-o. ba-cl. pb.
Opening Difficult. al-o.
Shooting. tx-b.
Smarting. aps. k-o.
Swelling. aga. arn. atp. cb-v. p. s..
Tensive. dro. ner.
Throbbing. cro.
UPPER EYELID. **Color, Red.** arn. atp. chio. crot. crt. lch. rs. so-o.
Contractive. so-t.

Cutting. dl-s. hg.
Dryness. crt. zn.
Eruptions, **Blisters**. arn.
  Pimples. hg. trg.
  Pustules. chd.
  Scabs. te.
  Styes. u-na.
  Tubercles. lch.
  Undefined Pain. hg-s.
  Vesicles. arn. lch.
Hairs feel Inverted. te.
Heat. bar. bry. ca-a. chd. crt. hg-bicl. k-o. lau-c. men.
phl. zn.
Heaviness. cit-c. k-o.
Itching. alli. bry. chd. chi. chio. lch. mg-cl. ner. pb.
te.
Movements, Convulsions. ach. cb-v. cl-hx. dph. jat.
lac-f. mg-ca. narth. ni-ca. nic. ol-a. rho. rs. sr-ca.
  Pressing. as-o. (chd). jnp-s. narth. te. zn.
  Shooting. ag. aga. au. ba-ca. bar. chd. cro. krm. ner.
spi. zn.
  Smarting. au. c-bis. dro. k-o. phl. te.
  Swelling. asr. chio. cit-c. crot. p. rs. te. trg. urg.
    OEdematous. as-o. chio. crot. rs. te.
    Red. te.
  Tearing. ba-ca. hg-bicl.
  Tensive. ach. men.
  Throbbing. asr. rs. so-t. stry.
  Undefined. (atp).
  Wrinkled. chio.
− LOWER EYELID. **Color, Dark**. arn.
    Red. ca-ca.
  Contractive. cro.
  Creeping. aga.
  Drawing. bar. cch.
  Eruptions, Pimples. bry.
    Pustules. al-o.
    Styes. cch. p. rs.
  Heat. cro. hg. k-o. phl. sep. sn. spo.
  Itching. aga. al-o. alm. euph. grc. hur. phl. trg.
  Movements, Convulsions. amm-cl. ccs. chi. hg. hur.
lyc. mg-ca. sep. thu. zn.
    Downwards-Hanging. grp.

Pressing. mgs-au. p-x. rs. zn.
Shooting. ca-ca. cro. hg-s. k-i. p. rs-r.
Smarting. hur. phl.
Swelling. ca-ca. cch. hg.
  Œdematous. arn.
  Feeling of. rs-r.
Tearing. ba-ca. na-ca. phl.
Tensive. bar. phl.
Throbbing. ca-ca. chi. cth.
Undefined. cro.
TARSAL EDGES. **Color Red.** atp. hur.
Discharge Pus. atp. crot. rs.
  White. crot. rs.
  Yellow. crot. rs.
Heat. atp. chd.
Itching. bry. hur.
Pressing. atp.
Swelling. atp.
Undefined. aps.
UPPER TARSAL EDGE. **Heat.** cit-c.
  Itching. zn.
  Pressing. pol.
  Shooting. cit-c.
LOWER TARSAL EDGE. **Cutting.** spi.
  Eruptions, Ulcers. cch.
  Pressing. zn.
EYELIDS, INNER SURFACE. **Color Red.** cit-c.
  Eruptions, Ulcers. cit-c.
  Shooting. cit-c.
LOWER EYELIDS, INNER SURFACE. **Shooting.** chd.
PUNCTUM LACHRYMALE. **Color Red.** atp. hur.
Discharge, Pus. atp.
Heat. atp.
Itching. hur.
Pressing. atp.
Smarting. hur.
Swelling. atp.
Undefined. aps.
CANTHI. **False Sensations, Sand.** aga.
Itching. chd. lo-i.
Pressing. si-x.
Shooting. ag. blt.

Smarting. hll. lct.
Swelling. aga.
EXTERNAL CANTHUS. **Color Red.** rn-b. str.
Contractive. euph.
Discharge, Hard. rs.
  Mucus. rs. str.
Drawing. spo.
Dryness. thu.
Eruptions, Dry. tx-b.
  Herpetic. tx-b.
  Red Areola with. tx-b.
  Ulcers. k-ca.
False Sensations, Sand. aps. rs. str-i.
Heat. aga. chd. pru-l. thu. trx.
Itching. ca-a. ca-ca. cb-v. cl-hx. rs.
Movements, Convulsions. na-cl. ni-ca. p.
Pressing. aga. smc. thu.
Shooting. amph. chd. elaps. n-x. ni-ca. ol-a. pru-l. spo
trx. urg.
Smarting. bry. cl-hx. k-ca. rn-b. sep. ,
Swelling. rn-b.
Tearing. chi.
Tensive. spo.
Throbbing. na-cl.
Undefined. sa-l.
INTERNAL CANTHUS. **Bruised.** glo.
Bursting. au.
Color Red. atp. ca-ca. chd. hg-s. na-ba. pru-l. rs. sep.
Contractive. aga.
Creeping. ach.
Discharge, Mucus. na-ba. rs.
Drawing. spo.
False Sensations, Sand. aga. chd.
Heat. asr. chd. cle. con. rs-r. sep. sn.
Itching. aps. bar. cb-v. chd. f-hx. k-o. lch. lo-cœ. na-cl.
os. pru-l. sep. spi.
Movements, Closing. aga.
  Convulsions. lac-d.
Pressing. aga. euphr. si-x. sn.
Scraping. pb.
Shooting. aga. al-o. au. blt. ca-ca. cb-a. chd. cle. ccb.
hg-s. n-x. na-ca. pru-l. rs-r. sn. spo. thu.
Smarting. aps. cb-a. cb-v. dl-s. lo-cœ. ox-x. rs-r. sa-l.

Swelling. aga. hg-s. sep. sn.
  Feeling of. rs.
Tearing. ni-ca.
Undefined. atp. hg-s. hur. lac-d. sa-l.
CARUNCULA. **Swelling.** aga.
LACHRYMAL BONE. **Broken as if.** lch.
Bruised. lch.
PERIODICAL. **Objects Imaginary, Mist.** s.
Eyeball, Creeping. na-sa.
  Shooting. spi.
  Tearing. ni-ca.
Orbit Superiorly, Undefined. k-bicr.
ALTERNATE DAYS. **Sight Impaired.** as-o.
Eyeball, Appearance Dim. as-o.
  Color Red. as-o.
  Pressing. as-o.
  Throbbing. as-o.
FROM 4 A.M. TO 3 P.M. **Eyeball, Color Red.** spi.
  Lachrymation Hot. spi.
  Undefined. spi.
FROM 10 A.M. TO 3 P.M. **Orbit Superiorly, Throbbing.** as-o.
EVERY NIGHT. **Eyeball, Pressing-Forward.** (dt).
EVERY NOON. **Objects Imaginary, Spots Bright.** vr-a.
EVERY AFTERNOON. **Eyeball, Pressing-Forward.** (dt).
GRADUALLY INCREASE and DECREASE. **Sight Impaired.** as-o.
  Eyeball, Appearance Dim. as-o.
    Color Red. as-o.
    Pressing. as-o.
    Throbbing. as-o.
  Orbit Superiorly, Shooting. k-bicr.
    Throbbing. as-o.
    Undefined. k-bicr.
SUDDENLY COME and GO. **Orbit Inferiorly, Smarting.** hg-s.
  Swelling, Feeling of. hg-s.
SUDDENLY COME, GRADUALLY GO. **Orbit Inferiorly Smarting.** hg-s.
    Swelling, Feeling of. hg-s.

CHANGING CHARACTER or PLACE. **Eyeball,**
Color Red, then Discharge Pus. eryn.
   Drawing then Pressing. rho.
   False Sensations, Hair, then Pressing. ccs.
   Pressing, then Discharge Pus. eryn.
   Shooting, then Lachrymation. snp.
    then Numbness. s.
   Swelling, then Discharge Pus. eryn.
   Tearing then Shooting. thu.
Eyeball Superiorly, Throbbing, then Pressing.
amb.
    Tingling, then   ,,   amb.
  Orbit, Shooting, then Pressing. ba-ca.
Upper Eyelids, Swelling, then Color Red. chio.
    then Itching. chio.
    then Wrinkled. chio.
Punctum Lachrymale, Heat then Pressing. atp.
Internal Canthus, Itching then Pressing. pru-l.
Eyeball, Color Red, then Eyelids, Adhesion of.
eryn.
    Lachrymation, then   ,,   u-na.
    Pressing, then   ,,   eryn.
    Swelling, then   ,,   eryn.
  Orbit, Shooting, then Eyeball, Lachrymation,
Feeling of. ba-ca.
    then Eyelids, Movements, Closing. ba-ca.
  FORWARDS. **Eyeball, Drawing.** alo.
   Pressing. al-o. (dt). gym. lau-c.
   Shooting. pan. sep. snc.
   Tearing. chd.
  Orbit Superiorly, Drawing. alo.
  BACKWARDS. **Eyeball, Shooting.** chio. dt.
  DOWNWARDS. **Eyeball, Pressing.** bry. chd. ner.
spi.
  Orbit Superiorly, Pressing. chio.
  UPWARDS. **Eyeball, Boring.** ber.
   Shooting. ber. br.
   Throbbing. br.
  Orbit Inferiorly, Boring. euph-a.
  Orbital Integuments Inferiorly, Drawing. atp.
  External Canthus, Shooting. cmc.
       G

LENGTHWAYS. Eyeball, Cutting. cr-o. na-ba.
  Heat. dro. na-ba.
  Tearing. dro.
  Tensive. dro. na-ba.
Eyelids, Heat. dro.
  Tensive. dro.
OUTWARDS. Eyeball, Cutting. i.
  False Sensations, Sand. rs.
  Shooting. i.
Orbit Superiorly, Shooting. k-bicr.
Orbit Inferiorly, Boring. euph-a.
Orbit Internally to Eyeball, Bruised. lch.
INWARDS. Orbital Integuments, Drawing. spo.
  Shooting. spo.
OBLIQUELY. Orbit Superiorly, Cutting. dro.
To HEAD. Eyeball, Shooting. atp.
Orbit, Boring. euph-a.
To FOREHEAD. Eyeball, Tearing. ccs.
Undefined. lac-cg.
Orbit Superiorly, Shooting. ber.
  Tearing. ber.
Upper Eyelid, Shooting. br.
  Throbbing. br.
To VERTEX. Eyeball, Shooting. phy.
To TEMPLE. Eyeball, Undefined. ba-ca.
Orbit Internally, Bruised. lch.
Upper Eyelid, Shooting. br.
        Throbbing. br.
To SIDE of HEAD. Eyeball, Shooting. trn.
To OCCIPUT. Eyeball, Tearing. cch.
Orbit Internally, Bruised. lch.
To EAR. Eyeball, Undefined. ba-ca.
To NOSE. Internal Canthus, Tearing. ni-ca.
To FACE. Eyeball, Shooting. mgs.
        Undefined. f-hx.
Orbit, Drawing. cor.
    Pressing. spi.
Orbit Superiorly, Undefined. k-bicr.
To JAWS. Eyeball, Shooting. mgs.
To UPPER JAW. Eyeball, Shooting. aga.
Orbit Superiorly, Undefined. k-bicr.
To TEETH. Eyeball, Undefined. lac-cg.

To NECK. **Orbit, Undefined.** rs.
DIAGONALS **with** OTHER ORGANS. ber. f-hx.
pet. trg.

With RIGHT FACE. **Eyeball, Drawing.** f-hx.
With RIGHT ARM. **Eyeball, Undefined.** trg.
Before RIGHT EAR. **Eyeball, Undefined.** pet.
To RIGHT HEAD. **Orbit Superiorly, Shooting.** ber.

SECTION II. CONDITIONS.

A. AGGRAVATIONS.

DAY. (Sunrise to Sunset).

ag-na. al-o. amb. amm-ca. as-o. au. c-bis. cop. cro. dt. ery. euphr. grc. hur. k-bicr. lct. led. ly-b. lyc. na-cl. na-sa. p. p-x. pul. sb-t. sep. smi. sn. so-d. str-i. vr-s. zn.

OBJECTS, FALSE APPEARANCE of. amm-ca. ly-b.
Black. amm-ca.
Inverted. ly-b.
Moving. amm-ca.
OBJECTS IMAGINARY. ag-na. sb-t.
Bright. sb-t.
Figures. ag-na.
Flashes, Bright. sb-t.
PHOTOPHOBIA. grc. na-cl. (p-x). sep.
SIGHT IMPAIRED. amm-ca. as-o. lct. sn. so-d.
EYEBALL. al-o. as-o. au. c-bis. dt. ery. euphr. k-bicr. lyc. p. pul. smi. str-i. zn.
Appearance, Dim. (as-o).
Color, Dark. (c-bis).
 Red. (as-o). (dt). na-cl.
Discharge. ery. p. (vr-s).
 Mucus. ery. p. (vrs).
False Sensations. (al-o). (dt). k-bicr.
 Sand. (al-o). (dt). k-bicr.
Heat. k-bicr. (lct).
Itching. (euphr).
Lachrymation. al-o. (dt). lyc. na-cl. smi. (str-i). zn.
 Hot. str-i.
Movements. (cop). (na-cl).
 Convulsions. (cop).
Pressing. (as-o). k-bicr. (na-sa). (pul).
Shooting. (hur).
Sunken. c-bis.
Tearing. amb.
Throbbing. (as-o). (cro). p.
Undefined. (au).

EYEBALL EXTERNALLY. dt.
IRIS. lct. na-cl.
Pupils Contracted. na-cl.
  Dilated, lct.
ORBIT. na-sa. pul.
ORBIT SUPERIORLY. na-sa.
ORBITAL INTEGUMENTS. amb. c-bis.
Color, Dark. c-bis.
Tearing. amb.
EYELIDS. cro. hur. lct. na-cl. vr-s.
Adhesion of. vr-s.
Heat. lct.
Movements, Closing. na-cl.
                    Spasmodically. na-cl.
Throbbing. cro.
TARSAL EDGES. hur.
Shooting. hur.
CANTHI. vr-s.
EXTERNAL CANTHUS. vr-s.
Discharge, Mucus. vr-s.
RIGHT. cop. dt. pul.
Eyeball, Color Red. dt.
  Lachrymation. dt.
  Pressing. pul.
Eyeball Externally, False Sensations, Sand. dt.
Orbit, Pressing. pul.
Upper Eyelid, Movements, Convulsions. cop.
LEFT. al-o. as-o. au. na-sa.
Sight Impaired. as-o.
Eyeball, Appears Dim. as-o.
  Color Red. as-o.
  False Sensations, Sand. al-o.
  Pressing. as-o.
  Throbbing. as-o.
  Undefined. au.
Orbit Superiorly, Pressing. na-sa.

FORENOON. (**Morning, Sunrise to Noon**).

. ach. acon. ag-na. aga. al-o. alli. alm. amb. amm-ca.
amm-cl. aps. art-v. arum-t. as-o. atp. ba-ca. ber. bry. ca-a.
ca-pa. ca-s. cap. cb-a. cb-v. ccs. chd. chi. cit-c. cl-hx. cmf.
cof. con. cop. cr-o. cro. cth. dig. dl-s. drm. dro. dt. elaps.

erig. ery. eug. euph. fe-mgs. frm. frm-s. gel. glo. glp. grc.
grp. gua. gym. hg. hg-i. hll. hydr. k-bicr. k-ca. k-na. k-o.
kre. krm. lch. lct. led. li-ca. lpd. ly-b. lyc. mg-ca. mg-cl.
mg-sa. mgs. mgs-ar. mgs-au. mn-ca. mph. mrl. mtr. myris.
n-x. na-ba. na-ca. na-cl. na-sa. ni-ca. ol-a. ox-x. p. p-x.
par. pb. pet. phl. phy. pnx. pod. pol. pru-l. pt. pul. pul-n.
rhe. rho. rn-b. rs. rs-r. rut. s. s-x. sb-s. sb-t. se. sep. si-x.
smc. smi. spi. spo. sr-ca. str. str-i. te. thu. trg. trn. trx. urg.
val. vr-a. vr-s. ziz. zn.

OBJECTS, FALSE APPEARANCE of. dig. ery. gel.
gua. lpd. ly-b. lyc. mg-ca. mtr. p.

  Inverted. gua.

  Moving. ery. gua. lpd. ly-b. lyc. mg-ca. p.

    Circularly. ery. lpd. ly-b. lyc. mg-ca.

    From Below Upwards. gua.

    Downwards. lpd.

    Vibrating. p.

  Multiplied. gel.

  White. dig.

OBJECTS IMAGINARY. ag-na. amm-cl. ba-ca. ca-ca.
ca-s. cb-v. cit-c. dt. ery. fe-mgs. frm-s. hg. k-o. lch. lct.
ly-b. na-ba. ni-ca. pul. trg. zn.

  Blue. dt. fe-mgs.

  Bright. ag-na. ca-ca. ca-s. cb-v. cit-c. dt. ery. fe-mgs.
na-ba. pul. trg.

  Circles. cit-c. fe-mgs. pul.

    Blue. fe-mgs.

    Bright. cit-c. fe-mgs. pul.

    Red. fe-mgs.

    Zigzags. fe-mgs.

  Flames. ag-na. ca-s. ery.

  Flashes, Bright. ag-na. ery.

  Halo. trg.

  Mist. amm-cl. ba-ca. (cit-c). frm-s. k-o. lct. ly-b. ni-ca.
trg. zn.

  Red. fe-mgs.

  Spirits. ca-s.

  Spots. ca-ca. dt. ery. lch.

    Blue. dt.

    Bright. ca-ca. dt. ery.

    Yellow. lch.

  Threads. (ery).

  Veil. dt.

Vibrations, ca-ca. cb-v. cit-c. (dt). na-ba.

   Bright. ca-ca. cb-v. cit-c. (dt). na-ba.

Water. hg.

Yellow. lch.

Zigzags. fe-mgs.

PHOTOPHOBIA. (dt). k-na. na-sa. phy. pnx. sb-s. si-x. str. str-i.

SIGHT DAZZLED. s.

SIGHT IMPAIRED. amm-cl. ba-ca. bry. cap. cb-v. chd. cit-c. drm. dt. ery. glp. k-o. lct. ly-b. lyc. mtr. na-ba. na-cl. na-sa. ni-ca. p. pet. pul. s. s-x. sep. str. trg. trn. val. zn.

EYEBALL. ach. ag-na. aga. al-o. alli. amb. amm-ca. amm-cl. aps. art-v. as-o. atp. ba-ca. ber. bry. ca-a. ca-ca. cap. cb-a. cb-v. chd. cl-hx. cmf. con. cr-o. cro. dig. dl-s. ery. eug. euph. frm. frm-s. glp. grc. grp. gym. hg. hll. k-bicr. k-ca. k-na. k-o. kre. krm. lch. led. li-ca. ly-b. lyc. mg-ca. mg-cl. mn-ca. mph. mrl. mtr. myris. na-ca. na-cl. na-sa. ni-ca. ox-x. p. p-x. par. pb. phl. pod. pol. pru-l. pt. pul. rs. s. s-x. sb-s. sb-t. se. sep. si-x. smc. smi. spi. str. str-i. te. thu. trg. trn. trx. val. zn.

 Appearance Dim. mtr.

 Boring. aps.

 Bruised. (smi).

 Bursting. (na-sa).

Color Red. (acon). atp. bry. (ery). eug. (hg). rs. sep. (str).

Discharge. ach. ag-na. aga. al-o. amm-cl. art-v. as-o. atp. ba-ca. ber. bry. ca-a. (cb-a). cb-v. chd. cl-hx. (cof). dig. dl-s. (euph). glp. grp. hg. (hll). k-bicr. k-ca. k-na. k-o. kre. krm. led. ly-b. lyc. mg-ca. mg-cl. mn-ca. mrl. na-ca. na-cl. ni-ca. ox-x. p. (p-x). par. pb. pol. pru-l. pul. rs. s. s-x. sb-s. sep. si-x. str. str-i. trx. zn.

 Hard. atp. (hll). p-x. (sb-s).

 Pus. atp.

Drawing. myris. pol.

Dryness. ag-na. ber. dl-s. (grp). lch. (li-ca). lyc. mg-ca. (mg-cl). (mgs). (mgs-ar). p. si-x.

False Sensations. k-na. na-cl. pul. (s-x). si-x.

 Sand. k-na. na-cl. pul. (s-x). si-x.

Gnawing. (str-i).

Hardness. (acon).

Heat. ag-na. al-o. (alm). amm-cl. cap. cl-hx. frm-s. (glp). grc. grp. (hg). (k-bicr). k-na. krm. lch. mg-ca. mph.

(n-x). na-sa. (ol-a). (phl). (pol). pul. s. sep. (si-x). (smi). (sr-ca). val.

Heaviness. (glo). k-bicr. (sep).

Itching. (alm). amm-ca. (dl-s). frm-s. grp. (hg). (k-o). (na-cl). (sep). (te).

Lachrymation. al-o. amm-cl. ca-ca. cap. cb-v. (con). cr-o. (dig). (dl-s). (ery). hg. k-bicr. k-na. k-o. (kre). krm. lch. mg-ca. (na-cl). na-sa. ni-ca. p. phl. pru-l. s. sep. te. zn.

   Hot. con. dig. dl-s. kre. na-cl.

   Appearance of. ca-ca.

Movements. (ca-pa). cit-c. (cop). (li-ca). mgs-au. (na-cl). (pod). (s). (sep). (spo).

   Convulsions. mgs-au. (s).

   Squinting, Feeling of. pod.

Paralysis. (ag-na). (amb). art-v. (ba-ca). (ca-s). (con). (k-ca). (mg-ca). (n-x). (na-ba). (ni-ca). (pet). s-x. (si-x).

Pressing. ach. ag-na. aga. amb. atp. bry. ca-ca. cmf. dl-s. (glp). grp. (k-ca). k-na. k-o. (lct). lyc. mph. (na-ba). pt. sb-t. (spi). (str).

Scraping. (si-x).

Shooting. (alli). aps. (bry). (cb-a). (con). cro. hll. na-sa. (p). sb-s. se. (sep). smc. (str-i). thu. (trn).

Smarting. al-o. amm-ca. (cb-a). gym. (hll). k-bicr. (k-o). (krm). li-ca. rs. (si-x). str. (str-i). (te). val.

Stiffness. ca-ca.

Swelling. (acon). ba-ca. (ca-ca). chd. (elaps). k-bicr. (k-ca). mtr. (phy). (rs-r). (s). sep. (te).

   Dark. (phy).

   Hard. (acon).

   Œdematous. (te).

   Red. (acon). (te).

   Feeling of. cmf. (k-o). mg-ca. ni-ca. (val).

Tearing. lyc. mg-ca. (na-sa). (pb). smc. (str-i).

Tensive. (acon). (s-x).

Throbbing. (na-sa). pb.

Undefined. (alli). (chi). cmf. ery. frm. (hg-i). (k-bicr). na-ca. p-x. s. (sep). smi. (trg). zn.

EYEBALL SUPERIORLY. cmf.

Undefined. cmf.

EYEBALL INTERNALLY. ery.

EYEBALL ANTERIORLY. sb-s.

Shooting. sb-s.

EYEBALL INTERIORLY. cmf.

Undefined. cmf.

IRIS. pnx. pul. val.
Pupil Contracted. pnx.
      Dilated. pul. val.
ORBIT. bry. chi. hg-i. k-bicr. k-ca. lct. na-sa. smi.
Pressing. k-ca. lct.
ORBIT CIRCUMFERENCE. **na-sa.**
Bursting. na-sa.
ORBIT SUPERIORLY. bry. chi. hg-i. k-bicr.
Undefined. chi.
ORBIT INFERIORILY. na-sa. smi.
Bruised. na-sa.
ORBITAL INTEGUMENTS. elaps. na-cl.
Swelling. elaps.
ORBITAL INTEGUMENTS SUPERIORLY. na-cl.
Itching. na-cl.
EYELIDS. ach. acon. ag-na. aga. alm. amb. aps. art-v.
as-o. atp. ba-ca. ca-ca. ca-pa. ca-s. ccs. chd. cit-c. con. cop.
dig. dl-s. erig. glo. grp. hg. hg-s. hydr. k-bicr. k-ca. k-o. kre.
led. li-ca. mg-ca. mg-cl. mgs. mgs-ar. mn-ca. mtr. n-x. na-ba.
na-cl. na-sa. ni-ca. p. p-x. pb. pet. phl. phy. pol. pul. pul-n.
rs. rs-r. s. s-x. sb-s. sep. si-x. smi. spo. str. str-i. te. thu. trn.
val. ziz. zn.
  Adhesion. ach. aga. as-o. atp. ca-ca. ccs. chd. cop. dig.
dl-s. erig. grp. hydr. k-bicr. k-ca. k-o. kre. led. mg-ca. mn-ca.
mtr. na-sa. ni-ca. p. phy. pul. pul-n. rs. (s). (sb-s). si-x. smi.
str. str-i. thu. trn. ziz. zn.
  Discharge. k-bicr. mg-ca. si-x.
    Hard. p-x.
  Dryness. grp. mg-cl. mgs. mgs-ar.
  Heat. grp. k-bicr. n-x. phl. smi.
  Movements, Closing. ca-pa. (cop). li-ca. (na-cl). (s).
sep. (spo).
      Spasmodically. cop. na-cl. s. sep. (spo).
  Paralysis. ag-na. amb. art-v. ba-ca. ca-s. con. k-na.
mg-ca. n-x. na-ba. ni-ca. pet. s-x. si-x.
  Swelling. ba-ca. chd. k-ca. s.
    Feeling of. k-o.
  Tearing. pb.
  Tensive. s-x.
  Undefined. sep.
UPPER EYELIDS. acon. ag-na. amb. art-v. ba-ca.
ca-s. cit-c. con. glo. k-ca. k-na. mg-ca. n-x. na-ba. ni-ca. pet.
s-x. sep. si-x. str. te.
  Color Red. acon.
  Heaviness. glo. sep.

Pressing. str.
Swelling. acon.
Tensive. acon.
LOWER EYELID. alm. aps. ca-ca. rs-r. si-x.
Itching. alm.
Swelling. ca-ca. rs-r.
TARSAL EDGES. alm. hg. hg-s. li-ca. pol. str. str-i.
val.
Color Red. hg.
Gnawing. str-i.
Heat. hg-s. pol.
Itching. hg.
Smarting. str. str-i. val.
Swelling, Feeling of. val.
UPPER TARSAL EDGE. pol.
Heat. pol.
LOWER TARSAL EDGE. alm.
CANTHI. aga. as-o. cb-a. cof. con. dl-s. ery. hll. k-bicr.
k-o. lyc. ni-ca. ol-a. p. pul. s. s-x. sb-s. sep. si-x. sr-ca. str.
str-i. zn.
Smarting. si-x.
EXTERNAL CANTHUS. as-o. ol-a. pul. s-x. sb-s.
sr-ca. str. str-i.
Discharge. as-o. pul. str. str-i.
Heat. sr-ca.
Shooting. str-i.
Tearing. str-i.
INTERNAL CANTHUS. aga. cb-a. cof. con. dl-s. ery.
hll. k-bicr. k-o. lyc. ni-ca. p. pul. sb-s. sep. str. zn.
Discharge. aga. cof. dl-s. lyc. ni-ca. p. pul. sb-s. zn.
Hard. hll.
Dryness, str.
Heat. k-bicr.
Itching. dl-s. sep.
RIGHT then LEFT. alm.
Lower Eyelid, Itching. alm.
TO FACE. k-bicr.
RIGHT. acon. alli. alm. aps. bry. cit-c. ery. eug. euph.
glp. hg-i. k-o. krm. li-ca. na-ba. na-sa. ol-a. s. s-x. sb-s. sep.
si-x. spi. trn.
Sight Impaired. chd. cit-c.
Eyeball, Color Red. eug.
Discharge. euph. sb-s.
Hard. sb-s.

Heat. na-sa.
Itching. k-o.
Lachrymation. ery. na-sa.
Pressing. glp. na-ba. spi.
Shooting. alli. trn.
Smarting. krm.
Undefined. alli.
Eyeball Internally, Color Red. ery.
Orbit Superiorly, Pressing. bry.
Shooting. bry.
Undefined. hg-i.
Eyelids, Adhesion of. s. sb-s.
Discharge, Hard. sb-s.
Movements, Convulsions. s.
Upper Eyelid, Color Red. acon. sep.
Movements, Convulsions. cit-c.
Swelling. acon. sep.
Hard. acon.
Red. acon.
Tensive. acon.
Lower Eyelid, Heat. si-x.
Scraping. si-x.
Smarting. aps.
Upper Tarsal Edge, Dryness. li-ca.
Smarting. li-ca.
Lower Tarsal Edge, Heat. alm.
Itching. alm.
External Canthus, Discharge. sb-s.
False Sensations, Sand. s-x.
Heat. ol-a.
Internal Canthus, Color Red. ery.
Itching. k-o.
Smarting. k-o.
LEFT. alm. cb-a. dt. hll. k-bicr. na-sa. pb. phy. rs.
sep. spo. str. te. trg.
Objects Imaginary, Blue. dt.
Bright. dt.
Spots, Blue. dt.
Bright. dt.
Vibrations Bright. dt.
Eyeball, Discharge. cb-a.
Tearing. pb.

Throbbing. pb.
Undefined. trg.
Orbit Superiorly, Undefined. k-bicr.
Orbit Inferiorly, Tearing. na-sa.
   Throbbing. na-sa.
Eyelids, Adhesion of. rs.
  Movements, Closing. sep.
              Spasmodically. spo.
Swelling. phy.
  Dark. phy.
Upper Eyelid, Itching. te.
  Smarting. te.
  Swelling. te.
     Œdematous. te.
     Red. te.
Lower Eyelid, Itching. alm.
Canthi, Smarting. hll.
Internal Canthus, Color Red. str.
  Heat. sep.
  Shooting. cb-a.
  Smarting. cb-a.
  Swelling. sep.
To Face. Orbit, Undefined. k-bicr.

AFTERNOON. (Evening, Noon to Sunset).

ach. ag. aga. al-o. alli. alm. alo. amm-ca. amm-cl. amph.
aph. aps. art-v. arum-t. asr. (atp). bar. ber. bry. ca-ca.
ca-s. can-i. cb-a. cb-v. ccs. chd. chi. cit-c. cl-hx. cmc. cmf.
co. con. cop. cor. cph. cr-o. cro. crt. cth. cu. cub. dig. dl-s.
dph. dro. dt. ery. eug. euph. euphr. f-hx. fe. frm. frm-s.
gel. glo. glp. grc. grp. hg. hg-bini. hg-s. hur. i. ind. k-bicr.
k-ca. k-cla. k-i. k-na. k-o. klm. krm. lch. led. ly-b. lyc.
mg-ca. mg-cl. mgs. mgs-ar. mgs-au. mn-ca. mph. mrl. myris.
n-x. na-ba. na-ca. na-cl. na-sa. narth. ner. ni-ca. nic. ol-a.
os. ox-x. p. p-x. pb. pd. pet. pol. pru-l. pt. ptv. pul. pul-n.
rhe. rho. rmx. rn-b. rs. rs-r. rut. s. sang. sb-t. scr-m. se.
sep. si-x. smc. smi. so-t. spi. spo. spo-f. srr. str. str-i. te.
thu. til. trg. trm. trn. trx. u-na. val. vi-t. vr-a. vtx. woo.
zn. zng.
  OBJECTS, FALSE APPEARANCE **of.**   al-o. amm-ca.
cb-v. dt. hg. lyc. rs-r. sep.

Confused. dt.

Moving. al-o. amm-ca. hg. lyc. sep.

  Circularly. al-o. amm-ca. sep.

  Vibrating. hg. lyc.

Small. cb-v.

Strange. rs-r.

OBJECTS IMAGINARY. al-o. art-v. ber. can-i. con. cro. dt. ery. eug. f-hx. fe. grp. krm. lch. mn-ca. na-sa. nic. ol-a. p. p-x. sb-t. scr-m. smi. til. trn. val.

Black, ery.

Bright. dt. ery. eug. f-hx. mn-ca. ol-a. sb-t. til. trn. val.

  Circles. f-hx. mn-ca.

    Bright. mn-ca.

  Cyphers. p-x.

  Far off. (dt).

  Figures. can-i.

  Flames. ery. eug.

  Flashes, Bright. ery. f-hx.

  Leaf. (na-sa).

    White. (na-sa).

  Light. val.

  Mist. ol-a. p.

  Semicircle. dt.

    Bright. dt.

  Spots. dt. ery. krm. ol-a. sb-t.

    Black. ery.

    Bright. dt. ery. ol-a. sb-t.

      Far off. (dt).

    Far off. (dt).

    White. krm.

  Stars. trn.

  Stripes. dt.

    Bright. dt.

      Vertical. dt.

    Vertical. dt.

  Variegated. ery.

  Veil. al-o. art-v. ber. cro. fe. lch. nic. ol-a. p. scr-m. (smi).

  Vertical. dt.

  Vibrations. f-hx. til.

    Bright. f-hx. til.

  White. krm. (na-sa).

Zigzags. con. grp.

PHOTOPHOBIA. (atp). ca-s. cb-a. hg. k-bicr. p. p-x. trg. zng.

SIGHT DAZZLED. hg.

SIGHT IMPAIRED. al-o. alm. art-v. ber. cb-a. cro. dph. dt. fe. frm. k-bicr. lch. (na-ba). na-ca. narth. ni-ca. nic. ol-a. (os). p. pul. sang. scr-m. sep. (smi). str-i. thu. trg. trn. woo. zn.

Presbyopia. dt.

Sensation as if Axis of Vision was Moved Backwards and Forwards. os.

EYEBALL. ach. aga. al-o. alli. alo. amm-ca. amm-cl. aps. art-v. arum-t. asr. (atp). bar. bry. ca-ca. ca-s. cb-a. cb-v. ccs. chd. chi. cit-c. cl-hx. cmc. cmf. con. cor. cph. cro. crt. cu. cub. dig. dl-s. dph. (dt). ery. eug. euph. f-hx. fe. frm-s. gel. glo. grc. grp. hg. hg-bini. hg-i. hg-s. i. k-bicr. k-ca. k-cla. k-i. k-o. klm. krm. lch. led. lyc. mg-cl. mn-ca. mph. mrl. myris. na-ba. na-ca. na-cl. na-sa. ni-ca. nic. ol-a. ox-x. p-x. pb. pd. pet. pol. pru-l. pt. ptv. pul. rho. rmx. rn-b. rs. s. sang. sb-t. se. sep. so-t. spi. spo. srr. str-i. te. thu. trg. trn. val. vtx. woo. zn. zng.

  Boring. pul.

  Bruised. lyc. s.

  Bursting. pol.

  Coldness. hg-s. lyc. s.

  Color, Red. al-o. asr. (atp). chi. cor. cph. dig. (euph). hg-bini. k-cla. lyc. rs. s. (thu). woo. zn.

  Contractive. aga. krm. rs. woo.

  Creeping. (chi). (cop).

  Cutting. ca-ca. hg. (k-i). pul. (s).

  Discharge. (aga). ca-s. euph. grc. k-i. (lch). mg-cl. na-ca. (p). pb. (rs). sep.

    White. lch.

  Drawing. (crt). klm.

  Dryness. al-o. (art-v). bar. ca-ca. cit-c. cro. dl-s. (grp). lyc. mn-ca. na-cl. na-sa. ni-ca. pd. pru-l. (pul). (rs). spi. (str-i). trg.

  False Sensations. art-v. (bry). ca-ca. ccs. (chd). chi. cor. fe. gel. k-bicr. ni-ca. (nic). (ox-x). sang. (te).

    Hairs. sang. (te).

  Sand. art-v. (bry). ca-ca. ccs. (chd). chi. cor. fe. gel. k-bicr. ni-ca. (nic). (ox-x). (sang).

    Smoke. sang.

  Heat. aga. al-o. (alli). amm-ca. amm-cl. (aph). (art-v).

asr. bar. ber. bry. ca-ca. cl-hx. dl-s. eug. (f-hx). (glp).
(grp). hg-bini. hg-s. k-bicr. k-i. k-o. krm. led. (mg-ca). mg-cl.
mn-ca. mph. na-ba. na-cl. na-sa. ni-ca. nic. ol-a. p-x. pol.
pru-l. pul. (pul-n). rho. rs. rut. (s). sb-t. (sep). spi. thu.
(trx). vtx. zn.

Heaviness. (cr-o). (s).

Itching. (alli). (bar). ca-ca. (cr-o). cu. (f-hx). fe. grc.
grp. (hur). (ind). k-bicr. (mg-ca). (ol-a). (p). pd. pru-l.
(pul). rn-b. (rs-r). s. (si-x). srr. (str). (te). (trm).

Lachrymation. alli. asr. (atp). chi. cub. eug. hg. (lyc).
(na-sa). ni-ca. (p). (pul). rs. s. sep. so-t. str-i. trg. zn.

Hot. (na-sa). pul.　　　　　　　　　＼

Appearance of. trg.

Feeling of. myris.

Movements. (al-o). (cro). (dig). (glo). (myris). (na-ca).
(na-cl). (s). (smc).

Convulsions. (cro). na-cl. (s).

Drawn-Down Feeling. (ol-a).

Paralysis. cro. i. lyc.

Pressing. (al-o). (alo). (art-v). bry. ca-ca. cb-v. (cit-c).
cmc. cmf. con. cor. crt. dl-s. (dt). ery. (f-hx). (glo). (glp).
grp. hg-s. klm. led. lyc. mph. (n-x). na-ba. (na-cl). ni-ca.
pet. pol. ptv. rn-b. (rs). s. si-x. spo. (str-i). (te). val. zn.

Shooting. ach. (acon). (ag). aps. (bar). (cld). (f-hx).
(frm-s). (krm). (lau-c). lyc. (ol-a). p. pru-l. pul. (s). se. spo.
thu. (trn). (u-na). zng.

Cold. s.

Smarting. (acon). al-o. cl-hx. cmc. (cr-o). (cro). (dig).
dl-s. gel. hg-s. (hur). (k-ca). lyc. (ol-a). (p). p-x. (pul).
(rn-b). s. (str). zn.

Swelling. woo.

Feeling of. arum-t. (hg-s). myris.

Tearing. ca-ca. (k-ca). (krm). na-ba. p.

Tensive. (ner).

Throbbing. (na-cl).

Undefined. (ccs). chi. (cmf). dig. dph. (k-cla). lyc. mrl.
(pd). pt. rmx. (trn).

EYEBALL INFERIORLY. glp.

Heat. glp.

EYEBALL EXTERNALLY. rn-b.

Pressing. rn-b.

EYEBALL INTERIORLY. al-o.

Smarting. al-o.

CORNEA. thu.

Color Red. . thu.
IRIS. thu.
Pupil Dilated. thu.
ORBIT. cit-c. con. glp. hg-s. lau-c. u-na.
Pressing. cit-c. con.
Shooting. lau-c.
ORBIT INFERIORLY. hg-s.
ORBITAL INTEGUMENTS. alli. cr-o. hg-s. k-ca. ol-a. rn-b. s.
Itching. cr-o.
ORBITAL INTEGUMENTS SUPERIORLY. alli. k-ca. ol-a. rn-b. s.
Itching. alli.
Pressing. rn-b.
ORBITAL INTEGUMENTS INFERIORLY. hg-s.
EYELIDS. acon. ag. aga. al-o. alli. aph. art-v. arum-t. (atp). bar. chi. cmf. cr-o. cro. dig. euph. glo. glp. grp. hur. k-cla. k-i. krm. myris. n-x. na-ca. na-cl. ol-a. p. p-x. pul. pul-n. rs. s. smc. str-i. te. thu. trx.
Adhesion of. aga. euph. rs.
Color Red. euph.
Discharge. euph.
Dryness. art-v. glp. rs.
False Sensations, Hair. (te).
Heat. aph. art-v. grp. k-i. p-x. pul. thu.
Itching. p. pul.
Movements, Closing. (al-o). dig. glo. (na-ca).
                 Spasmodically. al-o. na-ca.
            Convulsions. cro. na-cl. s.
            Winking. cro. (myris). smc.
Paralysis. cro.
Pressing. art-v. n-x. s.
Shooting. acon. thu.
Smarting. acon. cr-o. cro. pul.
Swelling, Feeling of. myris.
UPPER EYELIDS. ag. al-o. alli. bar. cmf. cr-o. cro. dig. glo. k-cla. krm. na-ca. rs. s. smc. str-i. te.
Dryness. str-i.
Heat. alli.
Heaviness. cr-o. s.
Itching. alli.
Undefined. cmf. k-cla.
LOWER EYELID. arum-t. dig. ol-a.

Itching. ol-a.
Smarting. dig.
Swelling, Feeling of. arum-t.
TARSAL EDGES. (atp). hur. thu.
Color, Red. (atp).
Heat. thu.
Itching. thu.
Shooting. thu.
Smarting. hur.
EYELIDS, INNER SURFACE. chi. pul-n.
Creeping. chi.
Heat. pul-n.
CANTHI. ag. aga. art-v. asr. bar. cl-hx. cop. f-hx. glp.
ind. k-i. krm. lyc. mg-ca. na-cl. ner. ol-a. p. pul. rn-b. rs.
rs-r. s. str. thu. trm.
Creeping. cop.
Discharge. k-i.
Heat. asr. mg-ca. p-x.
Itching. mg-ca.
EXTERNAL CANTHUS. cl-hx. k-i. lyc. na-cl. pul.
rn-b. s.
Heat. s.
Itching. pul.
Shooting. s.
Smarting. lyc.
INTERNAL CANTHUS. aga. art-v. bar. f-hx. glp.
ind. krm. na-cl. ner. ol-a. p-x. pru-l. rs. rs-r. str. thu. trm.
Discharge. aga. rs.
Dryness. na-cl.
Heat. art-v. f-hx. glp: p-x. thu.
Itching. ind. ol-a. pru-l. rs-r. str.
Pressing. na-cl.
Smarting. ol-a. str.
Tensive. ner.
CHANGING CHARACTER or PLACE. spo.
Eyeball, Shooting then Pressing. spo.
FORWARDS. (dt). pol. str-i. val.
Eyeball, Pressing. pol. str-i. val.
BACKWARDS. cit-c. hg-s.
Eyeball, Pressing. hg-s.
DOWNWARDS. cit-c.
To HEAD. ccs. u-na.
To FOREHEAD. ccs.

Eyeball, Undefined. ccs.
To OCCIPUT. u-na.
RIGHT. al-o. alo. bar. cit-c. cld. crt. f-hx. glo. glp.
k-i. krm. lyc. na-sa. nic. ol-a. p. pul. rn-b. rs. sep. si-x.
str-i. trm. trn. u-na. zn.
　Objects Imaginary. na-sa.
　　　　　　　Leaf White. na-sa.
　　　　　　　White. na-sa.
Sight Impaired. pul. trn.
Eyeball Discharge. p.
　Drawing. crt.
　Dryness. pul.
　False Sensations, Sand. nic.
　Heat. na-sa. ol-a. sep.
　Itching. si-x.
　Lachrymation. lyc. s.
　　　　　Hot. na-sa.
　Pressing. al-o. alo. cit-c. crt. f-hx. glo.
　Shooting. cld.　　　　　-
　Smarting. p. zn.
　Undefined. trn.
Orbit, Pressing. glp.
Upper Eyelid, Shooting. bar.
　Undefined. rs.
External Canthus, Cutting. k-i.
　Smarting. rn-b.
Internal Canthus, Heat. pru-l.
　Itching. f-hx. trm.
　Shooting. f-hx. pru-l.
　Tearing. krm.
Forwards. Eyeball, Pressing. str-i.
Backwards. Eyeball, Pressing. cit-c.
Downwards. Eyeball, Pressing. cit-c.
To Occiput. Orbit, Shooting. u-na.
LEFT. aga. al-o. bar. ca-ca. chd. cl-hx. dt. frm-s. hg-s.
k-ca. krm. na-ba. na-cl. ol-a. ox-x. pd. rs. s. smi. te. trn.
trx. zn.
　Objects Imaginary. Bright. dt.
　　　　　　　　Far off. dt.
　　　　　　　　Spot Bright. dt.
　　　　　　　　　　　　Far off. dt.
　　　　Veil. smi.
Sight Impaired. na-ba. smi.

Eyeball, Cutting. s.
  False Sensations, Hairs. te.
             Sand. chd. ox-x.
  Itching. ca-ca. ol-a.
  Movements, Convulsions. al-o.
  Pressing. rs. zn.
  Shooting. frm-s. ol-a. trn.
  Tearing. k-ca.
  Undefined. pd.
Orbit Inferiorly, Smarting. hg-s.
  Swelling, Feeling of. ˙ hg-s.
Orbital Integuments Superiorly, Movements, Drawn-Down Feeling. ol-a.
  Smarting. k-ca.
Orbital Integuments Inferiorly, Heat. hg-s.
Eyelids, Heat. trx.
Upper Eyelid, Itching. te.
  Pressing. te.
  Shooting. ag. krm.
Canthi, Shooting. ag.
External Canthus, Smarting. cl-hx.
           Throbbing. na-cl.
Internal Canthus, Itching. bar.
Forwards. Eyeball, Pressing. (dt).

NIGHT. · (Sunset to Sunrise).

acon. æth. ag. ag-na. al-o. (alm). amm-ca. amm-cl. anm. aps. art-v. as-o. atp. au. ba-ca. ca-ca. ca-s. cast. cb-v. ccs. cd-sa. chd. (cic). cmf. cn-sa. co. cr-o. cro. crt-c. dl-s. dt. ery. eug. euph. euphr. f-hx. fe. fe-mgs. gel. glo. glp. grc. hg. hyo. k-bicr. k-ca. k-o. kre. krm. led. lpd. lyc. mg-cl. mll. mrl. mtr. myris. n-x. na-ca. na-cl. ol-a. p. pb. phy. pol. pul. rho. rn-s. rs. rs-r. rut. s. sb-t. sep. si-x. sn. spo. srr. str. str-i. trn. vr-a. zn.

OBJECTS, FALSE APPEARANCE of. amm-ca. dl-s. myris.
  Closer Together. myris.
  Far, too. myris.
  Moving. amm-ca. dl-s.
      Circularly. amm-ca. dl-s.
  Oblique. myris.
OBJECTS IMAGINARY. acon. amm-ca. dl-s. dt. fe-mgs. na-cl. p. s. spo.
  Blue. dt.

2 H

Bright. amm-ca. dl-s. (dt). fe-mgs. na-ca. spo.

Circles. fe-mgs.

    Blue. fe-mgs.

    Bright. fe-mgs.

    Red. fe-mgs.

    Zigzags. fe-mgs.

Cyphers. s.

Flames. spo.

Flashes, Bright. dt. na-ca.

Green. dt.

Low Down. dt.

Moving. dt.

Moving with Eye. dt.

Red. fe-mgs.

• **Spots**. amm-ca. dt.

    Blue. dt.

    Bright. amm-ca. dt.

    Green. dt.

        Low Down. dt

        Moving. dt.

    Low Down. dt.

    Moving. dt.

Stripes. dl-s. dt. na-ca.

    Blue. dt.

        Moving with Eye. dt.

        Vertical. dt.

    Bright. dl-s. dt. na-ca.

        Vertical. dl-s.

    Green. dt.

        Moving with Eye. dt.

        Vertical. dt.

    Moving with Eye. dt.

    Vertical. dl-s. dt.

Vertical. dl-s. dt.

Visions. acon. p.

Zigzags. fe-mgs.

PHOTOPHOBIA. gel.

SIGHT IMPAIRED. mll.

EYEBALL. acon. ag-na. al-o. amm-cl. anm. aps. as-o. atp. ca-ca. ca-s. cast. cb-v. ccs. chd. cmf. cn-sa. co. cph. cr-o. dl-s. dt. ery. eug. euph. euphr. fe. gel. glo. glp. grc. hg. k-bicr. kre. krm. led. lyc. mg-cl. ol-a. pb. phy. pul. rho. rn-s. rs. rs-r. s. sep. si-x. sn. srr. str-i. trn. zn.

Appearance Dim. ca-s.

Bruised. anm.

Color Red. ag-na. eug.

Cutting. (cr-o).

Discharge. al-o. aps. (ba-ca). ca-s. cast. cb-v.,chd. (cic). cn-sa. (cro). dl-s. (dt). euph. euphr. fe. glp. grc. hg. krm. led. lyc. mg-cl. (n-x). ol-a. phy. (pol). pul. rho. rs. rs-r. (s). sep. si-x. sn. (spo). str-i.

 Pus. rho.

Dryness. lyc. s.

Eruptions. (sb-t).

 Scabs. (sb-t).

False Sensation. ca-ca. (dt). k-bicr.

   Sand. ca-ca. (dt). k-bicr.

Heat. al-o. amm-cl. kre. rs. trn. zn.

Heaviness. (crt-c). (trn).

Itching. (dt). k-bicr. srr. zn.

Lachrymation. amm-cl. (aps). eug. gel. (k-na). rn-s. (s). zn.

 Hot. zn.

Movements. acon. (al-o). (aps). (ca-s). (cro). (na-cl).

 Convulsions. acon. (al-o). (aps). (cro).

  Feeling of. (dt).

Paralysis. (anm). (cb-v). (cro). (lpd). (mrl). (sep).

Pressing. anm. ca-ca. co. (dt). ery. glo. kre. rs.

Shooting. (ag). as-o. (atp). (k-o). (s). (trn).

Smarting. gel. (k-ca). (s). (si-x).

Swelling. pb.

Tearing. (ccs). (k-ca).

Throbbing. as-o.

Undefined. (cmf). co. pb. zn.

EYEBALL, ROUND CORNEA. thu.

Color Red. thu.

IRIS. (alm). pb.

Pupils, Dilated. (alm). pb.

ORBIT. crt-c. k-ca. k-o. zn.

Shooting. k-o.

ORBIT SUPERIORLY. zn.

Undefined. zn.

ORBITAL INTEGUMENTS SUPERIORLY. trn.

EYELIDS. æth. al-o. anm. aps. au. ba-ca. ca-s. cb-v. chd. cro. dl-s. dt. euph. euphr. k-ca. led. lpd. lyc. mg-cl. mrl. na-cl. phy. pul. rs. s. sb-t. sep. si-x. sn. spo. str-i.

 Adhesion of. æth. al-o. aps. au. ba-ca. cb-v. chd. cro.

dl-s. dt. euph. euphr. led. lyc. mg-cl. phy. pol. rs. sep. si-x. sn. spo. str-i.

Movements, Closing. (ca-s). (na-cl).

                Spasmodically. ca-s. na-cl.

Paralysis. anm. cb-v. cro. lpd. mrl. sep.

    Opening Difficult. anm. cb-v. cro. mrl. sep.

Smarting. k-ca. si-x.

UPPER EYELID. al-o. cro. dt.

Movements, Convulsions. al-o. cro.

TARSAL EDGES. dl-s. sb-t.

Discharge. dl-s.

Eruptions, Scabs. sb-t.

EYELIDS, INNER SURFACE. s.

Dryness. s.

Smarting. s.

CANTHI. ag. lyc. pol.

Discharge. lyc. pol.

FORWARDS. (dt).

·BACKWARDS. atp.

LENGTHWAYS. cr-o.

To HEAD. ccs. cmf. trn.

To FOREHEAD. ccs.

To SIDE OF HEAD. trn.

To OCCIPUT. cmf.

RIGHT. aps. atp. crt-c. dt. eug. k-ca. n-x. s. trn.

Eyeball, Color Red. eug.

        Discharge. aps. n-x. s.

        False Sensations, Sand. dt.

        Heaviness. trn.

        Itching. dt.

        Lachrymation. aps.

        Undefined. f-hx.

Orbit, Heaviness. crt-c.

    Tearing. k-ca.

Orbital Integuments Superiorly, Shooting. trn.

Upper Eyelid, Movements, Convulsions, Feeling of. dt.

    Backwards. Eyeball, Shooting. atp.

    To Occiput. Eyeball, Undefined. cmf.

LEFT. ag. aps. as-o. cr-o. dt s. trn.

Objects Imaginary, Blue. dt.
      Bright. dt.
      Spots Blue. dt.
        Bright. dt.
Eyeball, Cutting. cr-o.
  Lacrymation. s.
  Movements, Convulsions. aps.
  Pressing. (dt).
  Shooting. s. trn.
Canthi, Shooting. ag.
Forwards. Eyeball, Pressing. (dt).
Lengthways. Eyeball, Cutting. cr-o.
To Forehead. Eyeball, Tearing. ccs.
To Side of Head. Eyeball, Shooting. trn.

BEFORE MIDNIGHT. (Sunset to Midnight).

al-o. atp. dt. ery. f-hx. frm. k-ca. na-sa. os. os-x. rut. s. sep. smi.
OBJECTS, FALSE APPEARANCE of. os-x. smi.
  Confused. os-x.
  Large, too. os-x.
  Red. smi.
OBJECTS IMAGINARY. al-o. dt. ery. k-ca. na-sa. os. rut. s. sep.
  Black. dt.
  Blue. dt.
  Bright. dt. ery. k-ca. (na-sa).
  Flashes, Bright. ery.
  Green. dt. na-sa. rut.
  Halo. al-o. os. rut. s.
    Green. rut.
    Red. s.
    Variegated. os.
  Mist. (na-sa). sep.
  Moving with Eye. dt.
  Near Eye. (na-sa).
  Rays. k-ca.
  Red. s.
  Spots. dt.
    Black. dt.
      Moving with Eye. dt.

Blue. dt.
Bright. dt.
Moving with Eye. dt.
Stars. (na-sa).
  Bright. (na-sa).
      Near Eye. (na-sa).
  Green. (na-sa).
    Near Eye. (na-sa).
  Near Eye. (na-sa).
  Yellow. (na-sa).
      Near Eye. (na-sa).
Stripes. dt.
  Blue. dt.
    Vertical. dt.
  Green. dt.
    Vertical. dt.
  Vertical. dt.
Variegated. os.
Vertical. dt.
Vibrations. (dt).
      Bright. (dt).
PHOTOPHOBIA. dt.
SIGHT IMPAIRED. (na-sa). sep.
EYEBALL. atp. f-hx. na-sa. smi.
Heaviness. (na-sa).
Pressing. na-sa. smi.
Sensitive. (na-sa).
Shooting. (na-sa).
Smarting. atp.
Softness, Feeling of. (na-sa).
Undefined. (f-hx). (frm).
ORBIT. frm. na-sa.
ORBIT SUPERIORLY. frm.
ORBIT INFERIORLY. na-sa.
EYELIDS. na-sa.
UPPER EYELID. na-sa.
Heaviness. na-sa.
BACKWARDS. na-sa.
CHANGING CHARACTER or PLACE. na-sa.
Objects Imaginary, Mist, then Star Bright Green Yellow Near Eye. na-sa.
OBJECTS IMAGINARY then EYEBALL. na-sa.
SIGHT IMPAIRED then OBJECTS IMAGINARY. na-sa.

RIGHT. na-sa.
Objects Imaginary, Bright. na-sa.
    Green. na-sa.
    Mist. na-sa.
    Near Eye. na-sa.
    Star. na-sa.
       Bright. na-sa.
          Near Eye. na-sa.
       Green. na-sa.
         . **Near Eye.** na-sa.
       Near Eye. na-sa.
       Yellow. na-sa.
          Near Eye. na-sa.
    Yellow. na-sa.
Sight Impaired. na-sa.
Eyeball, Pressing. na-sa.
    Undefined. na-sa.
Orbit Inferiorly, Pressing. na-sa.
    Sensitive. na-sa.
    Shooting. na-sa.
    Softness, Feeling of. na-sa.
Backwards. Orbit Inferiorly, Shooting. na-sa.
Changing. Objects Imaginary, Mist, then Star Bright Green Yellow Near Eye. na-sa.
Objects Imaginary then Eyeball, Star Bright Green Yellow Near Eye, then Pressing. na-sa.
Sight Impaired then Objects Imaginary, [Star Bright Green Yellow Near Eye. na-sa.
LEFT. dt. frm.
Objects Imaginary, Blue. dt.
    Bright. dt.
    Spot Blue. dt.
       Bright. dt.
    Vibrations, Bright. dt.
Orbit Superiorly, Undefined. frm.

AFTER MIDNIGHT. (**Midnight to Sunrise.**)

cph. dt. frm.
OBJECTS IMAGINARY, dt.
Bright. (dt).
Spots. (dt).
    Bright. (dt).

EYEBALL. cph.
Undefined. cph. (frm).
ORBIT. frm.
ORBIT SUPERIORLY. frm.
LEFT. dt.
Objects Imaginary, Bright. dt.
                    Spot Bright. dt.
Orbit Superiorly, Undefined. frm.

In BED.

amb. ca-ca. ca-s. cr-o. dig. dl-s. dt. (ery). hg. hur. k-ca.
mg-ca. mgs-ar. mgs-au. na-ca. rn-b. si-x. spo. str.
OBJECTS, FALSE APPEARANCE **of.** dl-s.
Moving. dl-s.
    Circularly. dl-s.
OBJECTS IMAGINARY. ca-s. dt. (ery).
Blue. dt.
Bright. ca-s. dt.
Green. dt.
Flames. ca-s.
Moving with Eye. dt.
Spirits. ca-s.
Spots. dt.
        Blue. dt.
        Bright. dt.
Stripes. dt.
    Blue. dt.
        Moving with Eye. dt.
        Vertical. dt.
    Green. dt.
            Moving with Eye. dt.
            Vertical. dt.
    Moving with Eye. dt.
    Vertical. dt.
Threads. (ery).
Vertical. dt.
EYEBALL. ca-ca. cr-o. hg.
        Cutting. (cr-o). hg.
        Itching. (ca-ca). (hur). ·
        Lachrymation. cr-o.
Movements. (dt). (spo).
    Convulsions, Feeling of. dt.

Smarting. (hur).
EYELIDS. dt. hur. spo.
Movements, Closing. (spo).
      Spasmodically. (spo).
UPPER EYELID. dt.
PUNCTA LACHRYMALIA. hur.
Itching. hur.
Smarting. hur.
LENGTHWAYS. cr-o.
RIGHT. dt.
Upper Eyelid, Movements, Convulsions, Feeling of. dt.
LEFT. ca-ca. cr-o. dt. spo.
Objects Imaginary, Blue. dt.
     Bright. dt.
    Spots Blue. dt.
     Bright. dt.
Eyeball, Cutting. cr-o.
   Itching. ca-ca.
Eyelids, Movements, Closing Spasmodically. spo.
Lengthways. Eyeball, Cutting. cr-o.

COLD.

al-o. amm-cl. anth. ca-ca. cl-hx. cle. co. dig. elaps. hg-s.
k-ca. k-i. k-na. men. ni-ca. p-x. pul. rs. sb-t. sep. so-d. zn.
PHOTOPHOBIA. k-na.
SIGHT IMPAIRED. k-na.
EYEBALL. amm-cl. anth. cl-hx. cle. co. elaps. hg-s.
k-na. men. ni-ca. sb-t. sep. zn.
Color Red. ni-ca. sb-t. sep. zn.
False Sensations. sb-t.
    Sand. sb-t.
Heat. amm-cl. cl-hx. k-na. (rs). zn.
Itching. (rs).
Lachrymation. anth. co. dig. k-na.
Movements. (so-d).
 Convulsions. (so-d).
Shooting. (rs).
Smarting. zn.
Undefined. cle. co. elaps. hg-s. (men).

EYELIDS. rs. so-d.
Movements, Convulsions. so-d.
UPPER EYELID. rs.
RIGHT. rs.
Upper Eyelid, Heat. rs.
   Itching. rs.
    Shooting. rs.
LEFT. men.
Eyeball, Undefined. men.

HEAT.

ag-na. alli. bry. cmc. (dt). glo. hg. hg-s. na-sa. pul. rn-b.
s. se.
PHOTOPHOBIA. s.
SIGHT IMPAIRED. pul.
EYEBALL. ag-na. alli. bry. cmc. (dt). glo. hg. hg-s.
na-sa. s. se.
  Appearance Glassy. glo.
      Staring. glo.
, **Cutting.** hg. (hg-s).
  Heat. na-sa.
  Itching. (alli).
  Lacrymation. alli. cmc.
  Pressing. (dt). (hg-s).
  Shooting. s. se.
  Smarting. (hg-s).
  Swelling, Feeling of. (hg-s).
  Undefined. ag-na. bry. cmc.
  IRIS. glo.
  Pupils Contracted. glo.
  ORBIT. hg-s.
  ORBIT SUPERIORLY. hg-s.
  Cutting. hg-s.
  ORBIT INFERIORLY. hg-s.
  EYELIDS. alli.
  UPPER EYELID. alli.
  BACKWARDS. hg-s.
  Eyeball, Pressing. hg-s.
  FORWARDS. (dt).
  OUTWARDS. hg-s.
  Orbit Superiorly, Cutting. hg-s
  LEFT. alli. (dt). hg-s.

Orbit Inferiorly, Smarting. hg-s.
   Swelling, Feeling of. hg-s.
Upper Eyelid, Itching. alli.
Forwards. Eyeball, Pressing. (dt).

OPEN AIR.

acon. æth. aga. al-o. alli. amm-ca. amm-cl. anan. as-o.
asr. atp. bry. bz-x. ca-ca. ca-o. cb-v. cch. chd. cl-hx. cle.
cmc. co. cof. con. cth. cub. dig. dl-s. dt. ery. euphr. glo.
grp. hg. hg-s. hll. k-bicr. k-ca. k-i. k-o. klm. lau-c. led.
lpd. lyc. men. mgs-au. mll. mrl. n-x. na-cl. na-sa. ner. ol-a.
ol-t. p. pet. pol. pru-l. pul. pul-n. rhe. rho. rs. rut. s. s-x.
sb-t. sep. si-x. smc. snc. so-d. srr. str. te. teu. thu. trg.
trm. tx-b. vr-s. zn.
 OBJECTS, APPEARANCE of. cl-hx. ery. glo. k-ca.
k-o. ner.
 Confused. ner.
 Large. k-o.
 Moving. cl-hx. ery. k-ca. k-o.
   Circularly. cl-hx. ery. k-ca. k-o.
 Strange. glo.
OBJECTS IMAGINARY. amm-cl. cth. dl-s. dt. ery.
euphr. k-o. mrl. na-cl. ner. ol-a. pol.
 Black. ol-a.
 Blue. dt.
 Bright. dl-s. ery. na-cl. ner.
 Flashes Bright. dl-s.
 Mist. amm-cl. cth. euphr. k-o. mrl.
 Serpentine Bodies. ery.
    Bright. ery.
 Spots. dt. ery. na-cl. ner. ol-a.
  Black. ol-a.
  Blue. dt.
  Bright. na-cl. ner.
  White. ery.
 Threads. pol.
 White. ery.
SIGHT DAZZLED. ner.
SIGHT IMPAIRED. aga. al-o. amm-cl. con. cth.
euphr. k-o. men. mll. mrl. n-x. na-cl. thu.
 EYEBALL. acon. al-o. anan. bry. ca-ca. ca-o. cb-v. cch.
chd. cle. cmc. co. cof. con. cth. cub. dig. euphr. glo. grp.

hg. hg-s. k-bicr. k-ca. k-o. klm. lpd. n-x. na-cl. na-sa. ol-a. p. pet. pol. pul. pul-n. rhe. rho. rs. rut. s. s-x. sb-t. sep. si-x. snc. te. teu. thu. trm. tx-b. vr-s. zn.

Coldness. acon. al-o. con.

Color Red. hg. na-cl. sb-t. zn.

Contractive. euphr.

Cutting. rs.

Discharge. anan.

Drawing. klm.

Dryness. k-ca.

False Sensations. co. (s-x). sb-t.

         Sand. co. s-x). sb-t.

Heat. (co). con. grp. hg. k-ca. (na-sa). ol-a. (rs). s-x. zn.

Itching. (dl-s). (rs).

Lachrymation. al-o. anan. bry. ca-ca. ca-o. cch. chd. cmc. co. cof. cth. cub. dig. euphr. grp. hg. k-bicr. k-o. lpd. lyc. (n-x). na-cl. (na-sa). p. pet. pol. pul. rhc. rho. (rut). s. sb-t. sep. si-x. snc. srr. te. (teu). thu. trm. tx-b. vr-s. zn.

  Hot. euphr. (na-sa). teu.

Movements. (grp). (mrl). (so-d).

  Convulsions. (so-d).

Paralysis. (rs).

Pressing. (cb-v). euphr. (glo). (rs). (rut). s. s-x.

Shooting. (p). (rs). (sep). thu.

Smarting. euphr. hg. k-bicr. (rs). zn.

Undefined. acon. cle. co. euphr. hg-s. na-cl. pul-n.

EYEBALL SUPERIORLY. cb-v.

Pressing. cb-v.

EYEBALL ANTERIORLY. s-x.

Heat. s-x.

Pressing. s-x.

EYELIDS. co. dl-s. grp. mrl. rs. so-d. thu.

Adhesion of. .thu.

Heat. co.

Movements, Closing. grp.

  Convulsions. so-d.

  Winking. mrl.

Paralysis. rs.

Smarting. rs.

UPPER EYELID. dl-s. rs.

UPPER TARSAL EDGES. dl-s.

Itching. dl-s.
CANTHI. dl-s. p. s-x.
EXTERNAL CANTHUS. s-x.
False Sensations, Sand. s-x.
INTERNAL CANTHUS. dl-s. p.
Itching. dl-s.
Shooting. p.
RIGHT. glo. n-x. na-sa. rs.
Eyeball, Heat. na-sa.
   Lachrymation. n-x.
         Hot. na-sa.
   Pressing. glo. (rs).
Upper Eyelid, Heat. rs.
  Itching. rs.
  Shooting. rs.
LEFT. rut. sep. teu.
Eyeball, Lachrymation. rut. tcu.
      Pressing. rut.

ROOM, In.

æth. ag-na. alli. alm. amm-ca. anth. cl-hx. cro. dig. dro.
dt. ery. hg. hg-s. jnp-s. k-bicr. k-o. led. na-ca. na-sa. p.
pet. pt. pul. rn-b. s. se. sep. si-x. so-d. trg. tx-b. vtx.
OBJECTS, APPEARANCE of. dro. pt. si-x.
Moving. dro. si-x.
  Circularly. si-x.
  Vibrating. dro.
Small. pt.
Strange. pt.
OBJECTS IMAGINARY. dt. ery. na-sa. sep. so-d. trg.
Blue. dt. trg.
Bright. dt. ery. na-sa. so-d.
Flames. so-d.
Flashes, Bright. ery.
Green. dt.
Halo. trg.
  Blue. trg.
  Red. trg.
Mist. (na-sa). sep.
Moving with Eye. dt.
Near Eye. (na-sa).

Red. trg.
Spots. dt.
  Blue. dt.
  Bright. dt.
Stars. (na-sa).
  Bright. (na-sa).
      Near Eye. (na-sa).
  Green. (na-sa).
      Near Eye. (na-sa).
  Near Eye. (na-sa).
  Yellow. (na-sa).
      Near Eye. (na-sa).
Stripes. dt.
  Blue. dt.
    Moving with Eye. dt.
    Vertical. dt.
  Green. dt.
    Moving with Eye. dt.
    Vertical. dt.
  Moving with Eye. dt.
  Vertical. dt.
Vertical. dt.
Yellow. (na-sa).
PHOTOPHOBIA. dt.
SIGHT IMPAIRED. alm. dro. hg. na-ca. (na-sa). pul.
sep.
  EYEBALL. æth. ag-na. alli. anth. cro. dig. hg-s. k-bicr.
k-o. p. pt. s. se. tx-b. vtx.
Coldness. hg-s.
Dryness. s.
False Sensations. k-bicr.
        Sand. k-bicr.
Heat. æth. dig. k-bicr. pt.
Itching. (alli).
Lachrymation. alli. anth. cro. djg. k-o. p. pt. tx-b.
vtx.
  Hot. dig.
Pressing. k-bicr. (na-sa). (rn-b).
Sensitive. (na-sa).
Shooting. (na-sa). se.
Smarting. (hg-s).
Softness, Feeling of. (na-sa).

Swelling, Feeling of. (hg-s).
Undefined. ag-na.
EYEBALL EXTERNALLY. rn-b.
Pressing. rn-b.
ORBIT. hg-s. na-sa.
ORBIT INFERIORLY. hg-s. na-sa.
EYELIDS. alli. dig.
Movements, Closing. (dig).
UPPER EYELID. alli.
BACKWARDS. na-sa.
CHANGING CHARACTER or PLACE. na-sa.
**Objects Imaginary, Mist, then Star Bright Green
Yellow Near Eye.** na-sa.
  Eyeball, Sensitive then Pressing. (na-sa).
    ,,   **Shooting, then** ,,   (na-sa).
    ,,   **Softness, Feeling of, then** ,, (na-sa).
OBJECTS IMAGINARY then EYEBALL. na-sa.
SIGHT IMPAIRED then OBJECTS IMAGINARY.
na-sa.
  RIGHT. dig. na-sa.
  Objects Imaginary, Bright. na-sa.
        Green. na-sa.
        Mist. na-sa.
        Near Eye. na-sa.
        Star. na-sa.
           Bright. na-sa.
               Near Eye. na-sa.
           Green. na-sa.
               Near Eye. na-sa.
           Near Eye. na-sa.
           Yellow. na-sa.
               Near Eye. na-sa.
        Yellow. na-sa.
Sight Impaired. na-sa.
Eyeball, Pressing. na-sa.
Orbit Inferiorly, Pressing. na-sa.
  Sensitive. na-sa.
  Shooting. na-sa.
  Softness, Feeling of. na-sa.
Eyelids, Movements, Closing. dig.
Backwards. Orbit Inferiorly, Shooting. na-sa.

Changing. Objects Imaginary, Mist, then Star Bright Green Yellow Near Eye. na-sa.

Orbit Inferiorly, Sensitive then Pressing. na-sa.

„ **Shooting, then** „ na-sa.

„ **Softness, Feeling of, then** „ na-sa.

Objects Imaginary then Eyeball, Star Bright Green Yellow Near Eye, then Pressing. na-sa.

Sight Impaired, then Object Imaginary, Star Bright Green Yellow Near Eye. na-sa.

LEFT. alli. dt. hg-s.

Objects Imaginary, Blue. dt.

Bright. dt.

Spots Blue. dt.

Bright. dt.

Orbit Inferiorly, Smarting. hg-s.

Swelling. hg-s.

Upper Eyelid, Itching. alli.

UNCOVERING.

thu.

EYEBALL. thu.

Coldness. thu.

Undefined. thu.

WASHING.

al-o. amm-cl. cl-hx. elaps. k-ca. k-na. men. ni-ca. p-x. sa-l. sep.

PHOTOPHOBIA. k-na.

SIGHT IMPAIRED. k-ca.

EYEBALL. amm-cl. cl-hx. elaps. k-na. men. ni-ca. sa-l. sep.

Color Red. ni-ca. sep.

Heat. amm-cl. cl-hx. k-na.

Lacrymation. k-na.

Shooting. sa-l.

Smarting. sa-l.

Tensive. ni-ca.

Undefined. elaps. (men). ni-ca. sep.

LEFT. men.

Eyeball, Undefined. men.

WEATHER DAMP.

crt.
SIGHT IMPAIRED. crt.
EYEBALL. crt.
Lachrymation. crt.

WEATHER DULL.

aga.

WEATHER HOT.

s.
PHOTOPHOBIA. s.
EYEBALL. s.
Shooting. s.

WIND.

anan. asr. chd. euphr. k-bicr. lyc. na-cl. p. pul. sa-l. srr. thu.
EYEBALL. anan. asr. chd. euphr. k-bicr. lyc. na-cl. p. pul. sa-l. srr. thu.
Coldness. sa-l.
Discharge. anan.
Lachrymation. anan. chd. euphr. k-bicr. lyc. na-cl. p. pul. srr. thu.
  Hot. euphr.
Shooting. (sa-l). thu.
  Cold. sa-l.
Undefined. euphr. na-cl.

KNEELING.

mg-ca.
OBJECTS, FALSE APPEARANCE of. mg-ca.
Moving. mg-ca.
    Circularly. mg-ca.

LYING.

ag-na. cb-v. cld. cln. dt. f-hx. k-o. led. men. mgs. mtr. sep. zn.

OBJECTS, FALSE APPEARANCE **of.** sep.
Moving. sep.
    Circularly. sep.
OBJECTS, IMAGINARY. ag-na. dt. f-hx.
Black. k-o.
Blue. dt.
Bright. dt. f-hx.
Figures. ag-na.
Flashes Bright. f-hx.
Spots. dt. k-o.
   Black. k-o.
   Blue. dt.
   Bright. dt.
SIGHT IMPAIRED. mtr.
EYEBALL. cb-v. cld. cln. f-hx. men. zn.
Color Red. cln.
Lachrymation. zn.
    Hot. zn.
Pressing. cb-v. (f-hx).
Shooting. cld.
Tearing. led.
Undefined. (men). zn.
ORBIT. zn.
ORBIT SUPERIORLY. zn.
Undefined. zn.
RIGHT. cld. f-hx.
Eyeball, Pressing. f-hx.
    Shooting. cld.
    Undefined. f-hx.
LEFT. dt. men.
Objects Imaginary, Blue. dt.
    Bright. dt.
    Spot Blue. dt.
      Bright. dt.
Eyeball, Undefined. men.

LYING on LEFT SIDE.

hg-i.
OBJECTS, IMAGINARY. hg-i.

Black. hg-i.
Mist. hg-i.
    Black. hg-i.

LYING on RIGHT SIDE.

dt.
OBJECTS, IMAGINARY. dt.
Blue. (dt).
Bright. dt.
Spots. dt.
    Blue. (dt).
    Bright. dt.
LEFT. dt.
Objects, Imaginary, Blue. dt.
               Bright. dt.
               Spots, Blue. dt.
                  Bright. dt.

REST.

cl-hx. dro.
EYEBALL. cl-hx. dro.
Cutting. (cl-hx).
Itching. (cl-hx).
Shooting. (cl-hx). (dro).
CANTHI. cl-hx.
EXTERNAL CANTHUS. cl-hx.
RIGHT. cl-hx.
Eyeball, Cutting. cl-hx.
        Shooting. cl-hx.
External Canthus, Itching. cl-hx.
LEFT. dro.
Eyeball, Shooting. dro.

SITTING.

alm. cic. dt. eug. hg-s. hur. na-ca. na-sa. p. p-x. rut.
s-x. sep. smi.
OBJECTS, FALSE APPEARANCE **of.** cic. eug. rut.
s-x. sep.
  Inverted. eug.
  Moving. cic. rut. s-x. sep.
      Circularly. cic. rut. s-x. sep.

OBJECTS IMAGINARY. dt. hur. p-x. smi.
Bright. dt.
Cyphers. p-x.
Far off. dt.
Mist. smi.
Spots. dt.
    Bright. dt.
        Far off. dt.
    Far off. dt.
Zigzags. hur.
SIGHT IMPAIRED. alm.
EYEBALL. na-ca. na-sa. p.
Heat. (hg-s).
Lachrymation. (na-sa).
Shooting. (na-ca). p.
Tearing. p.
Undefined. na-ca.
ORBITAL INTEGUMENTS. hg-s.
ORBITAL INTEGUMENTS INFERIORLY. hg-s.
RIGHT. na-sa.
Eyeball, Lachrymation. na-sa.
      Shooting. na-sa.
LEFT. dt. hg-s.
Objects, Imaginary, Bright. dt.
  Far off. dt.
  Spots. dt.
    Bright. dt.
      Far off. dt.
    Far off. dt.
Orbital Integuments Inferiorly, Heat. hg-s.

STANDING.

bry. ca-ca. dt. euph. hg-s. k-o. mg-ca. pnx. pul.
OBJECTS, FALSE APPEARANCE **of.** bry. ca-ca.
euph. mg-ca. pnx.
  Moving. bry. ca-ca. euph. mg-ca. pnx.
      Circularly. bry. ca-ca. euph. mg-ca.
OBJECTS, IMAGINARY. dt. k-o.
Bright. dt.
Spots. dt.
    Bright. dt.

Veil. k-o.
EYEBALL.
Heat. (hg-s).
ORBITAL INTEGUMENTS. hg-s.
ORBITAL INTEGUMENTS INFERIORLY. hg-s.
LEFT. hg-s.
Orbital Integuments Inferiorly, Heat. hg-s.

PRESSURE.

alm. amm-cl. anth. art-v. ba-ca. bry. cit-c. dro. eryn. evo.
lac-cg. na-cl. p-x. pet. rs. s. si-x. smi. snp-n. vr-a.
SIGHT IMPAIRED. ba-ca.
EYEBALL. anth. cit-c. eryn. evo. na-cl. pet. rs. s. si-x.
smi. snp-n.
Bruised. (alm). s. (smi).
Eruptions. (bry).
  Undefined Pain. (bry).
Pressing. (art-v). evo. (p-x).
Shooting. pet. snp-n.
Smarting. (dro).
Tearing. (amm-cl).
Undefined. anth. (bry). (eryn). (lac-cg). (na-cl). rs. si-x.
  smi.
EYEBALL CENTRE OF. lac-cg.
Undefined. lac-cg.
CORNEA. lac-cg.
Undefined. lac-cg.
ORBIT. alm. amm-cl. art-v. smi.
ORBIT SUPERIORLY. amm-cl.
ORBIT INFERIORLY. alm. art-v. smi.
Bruised. smi.
Pressing. art-v.
EYELIDS. bry. dro. p-x.
UPPER EYELID. dro.
LOWER EYELID. bry. p-x.
Eruptions, Undefined Pain. bry.
BACKWARDS. cit-c.
DOWNWARDS. cit-c.
RIGHT. amm-cl. cit-c. na-cl.
Eyeball, Undefined. na-cl.
Orbit Superiorly, Tearing. amm-cl.

Backwards. Eyeball, Pressing. cit-c.
Downwards. Eyeball, Pressing. cit-c.
LEFT. alm. dro. eryn. p-x.
Eyeball, Undefined. eryn.
Orbit Inferiorly, Bruised. alm.
Upper Eyelid, Smarting. dro.
Lower Eyelid, Pressing. p-x.

RUBBING. (Scratching, Wiping).

aga. anan. cb-a. chd. chi. cit-c. con. frm-s. grc. (k-bicr).
k-o. klm. kre. lct. na-ca. nic. p-x. pol. pul. rn-b. rs. rut. sep.
smi. spi. sr-ca. trn. zn.
OBJECTS IMAGINARY. k-o. nic. pol. spi. sr-ca.
Blue. sr-ca.
Feathers. spi.
Halo. sr-ca.
    Blue. sr-ca.
    Red. sr-ca.
Mist. k-o. nic. pol.
Red. sr-ca.
Vibrations. pol.
SIGHT IMPAIRED. k-o. nic. pol. spi.
EYEBALL. aga. anan. chd. cit-c. frm-s. grc. (k-bicr).
klm. na-ca. p-x. rn-b. rs. sep. spi. sr-ca. zn.
Color Red. kre.
Eruptions. (smi).
  Hot. (smi).
False Sensations. kre. (rs). (sep). (spi). (sr-ca).
  Sand. kre. (rs). (sep). (spi). (sr-ca).
Heat. chd. frm-s. (smi).
Itching. (k-o). kre. rn-b. (rut). (sep). (trn). (zn).
Lachrymation. grc. (kre). na-ca. p-x.
  Hot. grc. kre.
  Salt. kre.
Pressing. aga. (pul). (sep). sr-ca.
Shooting. klm. (pul).
Smarting. anan. (k-o). kre. (rut). (sep). (zn).
Undefined. (k-bicr).
Wrinkled Feeling. anan.
EYEBALL SUPERIORLY. spi.
EYELIDS. kre. smi. trn.

Color Red. kre.
Eruption, Hot. smi.
Itching. kre.
Smarting. kre.
TARSAL EDGES. kre. trn.
Color Red. kre.
Itching. kre.
Smarting. kre.
CANTHI. cb-a. k-o. lct. pul. rs. rut. sep. zn.
EXTERNAL CANTHUS. lct. rs. sep.
Smarting. lct.
INTERNAL CANTHUS. cb-a. k-o. pul. rut. sep. zn.
Itching. rut.
Pressing. pul.
Shooting. pul.
Smarting. rut. sep.
FORWARDS. cit-c.
UPWARDS. cit-c.
RIGHT. cit-c. k-o. sep. spi. sr-ca.
Eyeball, False Sensations, Sand. sep. sr-ca.
   Pressing. sep.
Eyeball Superiorly, False Sensations, Sand. spi.
Internal Canthus, Itching. k-o.
   Smarting. k-o. zn.
Forwards. Eyeball, Pressing. cit-c.
Upwards. Eyeball, Pressing. cit-c.
LEFT. cb-a. rs. sep. zn.
Eyeball, False Sensations, Sand. rs.
   Itching. zn.
   Smarting. sep. zn.
External Canthus, Itching. sep.
   Smarting. sep.
Internal Canthus, Smarting. cb-a.

TOUCH.

acon. ag-na. aga. alo. atp. atrop. au. ba-ca. bry. buf.
buf-s. ca-s. cb-a. cch. chd. chi. chio. chlor. cit-c. cld. cle.
cof. cu. cu-asi. dig. dro. elaps. eryn. fe-mgs. gn-l. hg. hg-i.
hg-s. hll. hur. k-bicr. k-ca. k-o. lac-cg. ly-b. lyc. mg-cl.
mgs-ar. mn-ca. n-x. na-ca. na-cl. na-sa. ni-ca. ner. p. par.

pet. phy. pol. qu-sa. rs-r. rs-v. s. sang. sb-s. sb-t. sep. si-x.
sn. spi. spo. spo-f. str. str-i. thu. trn. trx. vtx.

EYEBALL. acon. ag-na. atp. atrop. au. bry. buf-s. ca-s.
cch. chi. chio. cit-c. cld. cle. cof. cu-asi. dig. elaps. eryn.
gn-l. hg. hg-s. hll. k-bicr. k-ca. ly-b. mg-cl. mgs-ar. na-ca.
na-cl. ni-ca. phy. pol. qu-sa. rs-v. sang. sb-s. sb-t. si-x.
spi. str-i. thu. trn. vtx.

Bruised. ca-s. (na-cl). sb-t. vtx.

Eruptions. (hg-s). (hur). (sb-s). (sn). (spo).

   Undefined Pain. (hg-s). (hur). (sb-s). (sn). (spo).

False Sensations. hg.

       Sand. hg.

Heat. (aga). (k-o). (thu).

Itching. (k-o).

Pressing. (au). ca-s.(chd).(chi). (cu).(na-cl).(thu).(trx).

Shooting. (ba-ca). (ni-ca).

Smarting. atrop. (chd). (dro). (hg-s). (ner). (spi). (str).

Softness, Feeling of. (na-sa).

Undefined. (sensitive). acon. ag-na. (aga). (alo). atp.
bry. buf-s. ca-s. (cb-a). cch. chi. chio. (chlor). cit-c. cld.
cle. cof. cu-asi. dig. elaps. (eryn). (fe-mgs). gn-l. hg. (hg-i).
hg-s. hll. (hur). k-bicr. k-ca. (lac-cg). ly-b. (lyc). mg-cl.
mgs-ar. (mn-ca). (n-x). na-ca. na-cl. (na-sa). ni-ca. (p).
(pet). phy. pol. qu-sa. (rs-r). rs-v. (sang). sb-s. sb-t. si-x.
(sn). spi. (spo). spo-f. (str). str-i. (thu). (trn).

EYEBALL SUPERIORLY. acon. thu.

Undefined. acon. .

EYEBALL CENTRE OF. lac-cg.

Undefined. lac-cg.

CORNEA. lac-cg.

Undefined. lac-cg.

ORBIT. alo. au. cu-asi. hg. hg-i. hg-s. ly-b. na-cl.
na-sa. p. pet. sep. spi. thu.

Undefined. alo. ly-b.

ORBIT CIRCUMFERENCE. ly-b. na-cl. p.

Undefined. ly-b. p.

ORBIT SUPERIORLY. cu-asi. hg. hg-i. hg-s. na-cl.
pet. sep.

Smarting. hg-s.

Undefined. hg. sep.

ORBIT INFERIORLY. au. hg-s. na-sa. thu.

ORBIT EXTERNALLY. spi.

Smarting. spi.

ORBITAL INTEGUMENTS. aga. ba-ca. chi. hll. hur.
n-x. ner. sb-s. sn. spo. str. thu. trx.
Undefined. n-x.
ORBITAL INTEGUMENTS SUPERIORLY. aga.
ba-ca. chi. hll. hur. ner. sb-s. sn. spo. str. thu. trx.
Eruptions, Undefined Pain. hur. sb-s. sn.
Pressing. chi.
Shooting. ba-ca.
Undefined. aga. str.
EYELIDS. atp. atrop. ca-s. cb-a. chd. chlor. cu. dro.
hg. k-bicr. k-o. lyc. mgs-ar. mn-ca. ni-ca. spo-f. str.
Eruptions, Undefined Pain. hg-s.
Pressing. cu.
Smarting. atrop. chd.
Undefined. ca-s. cb-a. chlor. hg. k-bicr. lyc. mgs-ar.
mn-ca. spo-f.
UPPER EYELID. atp. chd. mn-ca.
Undefined. mn-ca.
LOWER EYELID. dro. k-o.
Heat. k-o.
Itching. k-o.
TARSAL EDGES. ni-ca. str.
Shooting. ni-ca.
Smarting. str.
EYELIDS, INNER SURFACE. s.
Tensive. s.
CANTHI. aga. atp. fe-mgs. rs-r.
EXTERNAL CANTHUS. fe-mgs. rs-r.
Undefined. fe-mgs. rs-r.
INTERNAL CANTHUS. aga. atp.
Heat. aga.
LACHRYMAL GLAND. fe-mgs.
Undefined. fe-mgs.
RIGHT. au. dro. hg-s. na-cl. na-sa. ner. pet. sang. str.
thu. trn.
Eyeball, Pressing. au.
  Undefined. sang. thu. trn.
Orbit Superiorly Smarting. hg-s.
  Undefined. na-cl. pet.
Orbit Inferiorly, Softness, Feeling of. na-sa.
  Undefined. au. na-sa. thu.
Orbital Integuments Superiorly, Smarting. ner.
  Undefined. str.

Lower Eyelid, Smarting. dro.
LEFT. atp. chd. cu-asi. eryn. hg-i. hg-s. hll. na-cl. spo.
thu. trx.
Eyeball, Undefined. eryn.
Eyeball Superiorly, Heat. thu.
   Pressing. thu.
Orbit Circumference, Bruised. na-cl.
   Pressing. na-cl.
Orbit Superiorly, Undefined. cu-asi. hg-i.
Orbit Inferiorly, Undefined. hg-s.
**Orbital Integuments Superiorly, Eruption, Un-
defined Pain.** spo.
   Pressing. trx.
   Tensive. hll.
   Undefined. thu.
Upper Eyelid, Eruption, Undefined Pain. hg-s.
   Pressing. chd.
   Undefined. atp.
Internal Canthus, Undefined. atp.

ASCENDING.

cmf. ery. hg-s.
SIGHT IMPAIRED. ery.
EYEBALL. cmf.
Smarting. (hg-s).
Swelling, Feeling of. (hg-s).
Undefined. cmf.
ORBIT. hg-s.
ORBIT SUPERIORLY. hg-s.
Smarting. hg-s.
Swelling, Feeling of. hg-s.

DRIVING.

li-ca. na-cl.
EYEBALL. na-cl.
Dryness. na-cl.
Undefined. (li-ca).
ORBIT. li-ca.
Undefined. li-ca.

ORBITAL INTEGUMENTS. li-ca.
ORBITAL INTEGUMENTS SUPERIORLY. li-ca.
RIGHT. li-ca.
Orbital Integuments Superiorly, Undefined. li-ca.

LIFTING.

ol-a. sb-t.
OBJECTS IMAGINARY. sb-t.
Bright. sb-t.
Spots. sb-t.
   Bright. sb-t.
Vibrations. sb-t.

MOVING.

ca-ca. chi. led. na-cl. nic. pb. rn-b. spi.
OBJECTS IMAGINARY. ca-ca.
Black. ca-ca.
Spots. ca-ca.
   Black. ca-ca.
EYEBALL. nic. spi.
Boring. nic.
Drawing. nic.
Undefined. spi.

RISING. (Generally, including Varieties).

acon. amb. amm-cl. arn. art-v. as-o. bry. ca-ca. cb-a. cb-v.
cmc. cmf. dl-s. dt. glo. hg-i. hg-s. k-bicr. lct. ly-b. lyc. mg-ca.
myris. na-cl. ox-x. par. pru-l. pul. rn-b. rs. rs-r. sb-s. sb-t.
thr. thu. val. vr-a. vr-s. ziz. zn.
OBJECTS, FALSE APPEARANCE of. acon. arn.
bry. ca-s. cb-a. k-bicr. ly-b. mg-ca. zn.
Moving. acon. arn. bry. cb-a. k-bicr. ly-b. mg-ca. zn.
    Circularly. acon. arn. bry. cb-a. k-bicr. ly-b.
mg-ca. zn.
OBJECTS IMAGINARY. mg-cl. sb-t. vr-a.
Black. vr-a.
Bright. sb-t. vr-a.
Flames. vr-a.

High up. mg-cl.
Mist. mg-cl. sb-t.
Rocks. mg-cl.
   High up. mg-cl.
Spots. sb-t. vr-a.
   Black. vr-a.
   Bright. sb-t.
Vibrations. sb-t.
SIGHT IMPAIRED. amb. art-v. ca-s. cmc. dt. glo. myris. na-cl. pul. vr-s.
   EYEBALL. hg-s. lyc. ox-x. pul. rn-b. thr. thu. val.
Color Red. pul.
Heat. thu.
Pressing. (lct). (ox-x). rn-b. val.
Smarting. hg-s.
Tearing. lyc.
Throbbing. (thr).
Undefined. (hg-i).
EYEBALL SUPERIORLY. ox-x.
Pressing. ox-x.
ORBIT. hg-i. lct.
Pressing. lct.
ORBIT SUPERIORLY. hg-i.
EYELIDS. (dt).
Movements, Closing. (dt).
RIGHT. hg-i. thr.
Eyeball, Throbbing. thr.
Orbit, Undefined. hg-i.
Orbit Superiorly, Undefined. hg-i.

RISING from LYING.

amb. amm-cl. art-v. cb-a. cb-v. cmc. cmf. dt. hg-i. hg-s. lct. ly-b. mg-ca. par. pul. rn-b. rs. rs-r. sb-s. thr. thu. val. zn.

OBJECTS, FALSE APPEARANCE. of. cb-a. ly-b. mg-ca.
   Moving. cb-a. ly-b. mg-sa.
      Circularly. ly-b. mg-sa.
SIGHT IMPAIRED. amb. art-v. cmc. dt.
EYEBALL. hg-s. rn-b. thr. thu. val.
Heat. thu.
Pressing. (lct). rn-b. val.

Smarting. hg-s.
Throbbing. (thr).
Undefined. (hg-i).
ORBIT. hg-i. lct.
Pressing. lct.
ORBIT SUPERIORLY. hg-i.
RIGHT. hg-i. thr.
Eyeball, Throbbing. thr.
Orbit, Undefined. hg-i.
Orbit Superiorly, Undefined. hg-i.

RISING from SITTING.

acon. bry. k-bicr. mg-cl. sb-t. vr-a. vr-s.
OBJECTS, FALSE APPEARANCE **of.** acon. bry.
k-bicr.
Moving. acon. bry. k-bicr.
    Circularly. acon. bry. k-bicr.
OBJECTS IMAGINARY. mg-cl. sb-t. vr-a.
Bright. sb-t. vr-a.
Flames. vr-a.
High up. mg-cl.
Mist. mg-cl. sb-t.
Rocks. mg-cl.
    High up. mg-cl.
Spots. sb-t.
    Bright. sb-t.
SIGHT IMPAIRED. vr-s.

RISING from STOOPING. (Raising Head).

arn. as-o. ca-s. cb-a. na-cl. pul. zn.
OBJECTS, FALSE APPEARANCE **of.** arn. cb-a. zn.
Moving. arn. cb-a. zn.
    Circularly. arn. cb-a. zn.
SIGHT IMPAIRED. ca-s. na-cl.
EYEBALL. pul.
Color Red. pul.

STOOPING. (Bending Head Down).

anth. au. br. bry. ca-ca. cch. chi. cit-c. cmc. cof. cph. dl-s. dro. f-hx. grp. hg-i. hg-s. kre. lct. mll. mn-ca. mrl. msc. na-cl. p. pet. pol. s. stach. val. vin. ziz.

OBJECTS, FALSE APPEARANCE of. au. dl-s. val.
Moving. au. dl-s. val.
         Circularly. au. dl-s. val.
OBJECTS, IMAGINARY. lct. msc. vin.
Black. lct.
Mist. vin.
Moving Circularly. msc.
Spots. lct.
     Black. lct.
SIGHT IMPAIRED. cof. hg-s. na-cl. p.
EYEBALL. br. cit-c. cmc. dro. f-hx. kre. mrl. pol. s. stach.
Bursting. stach.
Cutting. (chi). (hg-s).
Drawing. (mn-ca). (val).
Lachrymation. cmc.
Looseness, Feeling of. br.
Pressing. (anth). (bry). cit-c. f-hx. (hg-s). kre. mrl. pol.
Shooting. dro. (s).
Smarting. cit-c.
Swelling, Feeling of. cph.
Throbbing. pol.
Undefined. cmc. (hg-i). mll. (pet). (ziz).
EYEBALL POSTERIORLY. anth.
Pressing. anth.
ORBIT. chi. hg-i. mn-ca. pet. val. ziz.
Cutting. chi.
Drawing. mn-ca.
ORBIT CIRCUMFERENCE. val.
Drawing. val.
ORBIT SUPERIORLY. hg-i. hg-s. pet.
Cutting. hg-s.
FORWARDS. br.
Eyeball, Pressing. br.
BACKWARDS. hg-s.
Eyeball, Pressing. hg-s.

OUTWARDS. hg-s.
Orbit Superiorly, Cutting. hg-s.
TO HEAD. kre.
TO VERTEX. kre.
Eyeball, Pressing. kre.
RIGHT. f-hx. hg-i. ziz.
Eyeball, Pressing. f-hx.
Orbit, Undefined. ziz.
Orbit Superiorly, Undefined. hg-i. pet.
LEFT. bry. s.
Eyeball, Shooting. s.
    Downwards Pressing. bry.

TURNING ROUND.

hg.
OBJECTS, FALSE APPEARANCE of. hg.
Moving. hg.
    Circularly. hg.

WALKING.

acon. aga. arn. as-o. atp. bry. ca-ça. ca-s. can-i. cb-v.
chi. cof. con. dl-s. dt. elaps. ery. euphr. fe-a. glo. grp. hg.
hur. itu. k-bicr. k-o. led. mgs-ar. na-cl. ner. nic. ol-t. ox-x.
p. pb. pet. phy. pul. pul-n. rn-b. s. s-x. sb-t. sep. smc. so-d.
spi. spo. str. te. thu. trg. vr-s. vr-v. ziz. zn.
OBJECTS, FALSE APPEARANCE of. arn. ery. glo.
na-cl. ner. p. sep. spi.
Confused. ner.
Moving. arn. ery. na-cl. p. sep. spi.
    Circularly. arn. ery. na-cl. p. sep. spi.
Strange. glo.
OBJECTS, IMAGINARY. acon. atp. can-i. dt. elaps.
ery. euphr. hur. k-o. na-cl. ner. nic. ol-t. sb-t. so-d.
Black. (atp). ca-ca. elaps. ol-t.
Blue. dt.
Bright. ery. hur. na-cl. ner. nic. sb-t. so-d.
Circles. elaps.
    Black. elaps.
Figures. can-i.
Flames. so-d.
Mist. euphr. k-o.

K

Serpentine Bodies. ery.
Bright. ery.
Spots. (atp). ca-ca. dt. ery. hur. na-cl. ner. nic. ol-t. sb-t.
    Black. (atp). ca-ca. ol-t.
    Blue. dt.
    Bright. hur. na-cl. ner. nic. sb-t.
    White. ery.
Vibrations. acon. sb-t.
White. ery.
Zigzags. hur.
SIGHT DAZZLED. ner.
SIGHT IMPAIRED. aga. euphr. fe-a. k-bicr. k-o. na-cl. pul. sep. so-d. vr-v.
EYEBALL. ca-s. cb-v. cof. con. euphr. glo. grp. hur. itu. nic. ox-x. phy. pul-n. s. smc. spi. spo. te. thu. vr-s.
Boring. nic.
Coldness. con.
Contractive. euphr.
Cutting. (chi).
Drawing. nic.
False Sensations. (s-x).
    Sand. (s-x).
Heaviness. itu.
Lachrymation. cof. grp. spo. te. (thu). vr-s.
Movements. (grp). (spo).
Pressing. (cb-v). euphr. (glo). (led). (ox-x). phy. s. (spi).
Shooting. smc.
Swelling, Feeling of. spi.
Tearing. smc.
Throbbing. (trg).
Undefined. ca-s. (chi). hur. (pd). (pet). phy. pul-n. spi. ziz.
EYEBALL SUPERIORLY. cb-v. ox-x.
Pressing. cb-v. ox-x.
ORBIT. chi. hur. led. pet. ziz.
Cutting. chi.
Undefined. hur.
ORBIT SUPERIORLY. chi. pet.
Undefined. chi.
ORBIT EXTERNALLY. led.
Pressing. led.

EYELIDS. cb-v. grp. spo.
Movements, Closing. grp. (spo).
                Spasmodically. spo.
UPPER EYELID. cb-v.
Pressing. cb-v.
CANTHI. s-x.
EXTERNAL CANTHUS. s-x.
RIGHT. glo. s-x. spi. trg. ziz.
Eyeball, Pressing. glo. spi.
        Throbbing. trg.
Orbit, Undefined. ziz.
Orbit Superiorly, Undefined. pet.
External Canthus, False Sensations, Sand. s-x.
LEFT. atp. pd. thu.
Objects Imaginary, Black. atp.
      Spots. atp.
           Black. atp.
Eyeball, Lachrymation. thu.
      Undefined. pd.

ANGER.

sep.
SIGHT IMPAIRED. sep.

ANXIETY.

chd.
OBJECTS IMAGINARY. chd.
Bright. chd.
Spots. chd.
    Bright. chd.

EMOTIONS.

dt.
EYEBALL. dt.
Movements. dt.
    Squinting. dt.

FRIGHT.

dt.
EYEBALL. dt.
Movements. dt.
    Squinting. dt.

MENTAL EXERTION

ag-na. art-v. au. eryn. lct. men. rn-b. s. stach. str. str-i.
OBJECTS IMAGINARY. au.
Bright. au.
Spots. au.
    Bright. au.
EYEBALL. art-v. eryn. lct. s. stach.
Bursting. stach.
Pressing. lct. (rn-b).
Tensive. s.
Undefined. art-v. eryn.
ORBIT. rn-b.
ORBIT SUPERIORLY. rn-b.
Pressing. rn-b.

Being ROUSED.

myris.
EYEBALL.
Movements. (myris).
EYELIDS. myris.
Movements, Winking. myris.

When SCOLDED.

dt.
IRIS. dt.
Pupils, Dilated. dt.

When OTHERS TALK about it.

ca-pa.
EYEBALL. ca-pa.
False Sensations. ca-pa.
    Sand. ca-pa.

MOVING HEAD.

acon. amm-ca. arn. cmc. dl-s. lac-cg. lch. lyc. msc. mtr. na-cl. pul. spi.
OBJECTS, FALSE APPEARANCE of. amm-ca. arn. dl-s.
Moving. amm-ca. arn. dl-s.
    Circularly. amm-ca. arn. dl-s.
OBJECTS IMAGINARY. msc.
Moving Up and Down. msc.
SIGHT IMPAIRED. acon. lch. na-cl.
EYEBALL. cmc. lac-cg. lyc. pul. stach.
Bursting. lac-cg. stach.
Pressing. cmc. (mtr).
Shooting. (pul).
Smarting. cmc.
Undefined. (cmc). lyc.
EYELIDS. mtr.
UPPER EYELID. mtr.
Pressing. mtr.
FORWARDS. cmc.
Eyeball, Pressing. cmc.
DOWNWARDS. cmc.
Eyeball Pressing. cmc.
To HEAD. cmc.
To OCCIPUT, cmc.
Eyeball Posteriorly, Undefined. cmc.
LEFT. lyc. pul.
Eyeball, Shooting. pul.
    Undefined. lyc.

· MOVING HEAD to SHOULDER.

gel.
OBJECTS, FALSE APPEARANCE of. gel.
Multiplied. gel.

MOVING HEAD ROUND.

dl-s.
OBJECTS, FALSE APPEARANCE of. dl-s.
Moving. dl-s.
    Circularly. dl-s.

MOVING HEAD ROUND to LEFT.

dt.
OBJECTS, IMAGINARY. dt.
Bright. dt.
Far off. (dt).
Spots. dt.
  Bright. dt.
      Far off. (dt).
  Far off. (dt).
LEFT. dt.
Bright. dt.
Far off. dt.
Spots. dt.
  Bright. dt.
      Far off. dt.
  Far off. dt.

RESTING HEAD on ARM.

na-cl.
EYEBALL. na-cl.
Pressing. na-cl.

MOVING SCALP.

chi.
EYEBALL.
Pressing. (chi).
ORBITAL INTEGUMENTS. chi.
ORBITAL INTEGUMENTS SUPERIORLY. chi.
Pressing. chi.

Before HEAD **Symptoms.**

acon. anm. ba-ca. cch. cic. con. cot. cth. dt. ery. hur. hyo.
k-bicr. lac-d. na-cl. pod. pso. rhe. sang. (sep). smi. thr. trg.
  OBJECTS, FALSE APPEARANCE of. ery. pod. pso.
thr.
  Confused. ery. pod.
  Far too. thr.
  Moving. pso.
  Multiplied. ery.

OBJECTS IMAGINARY. con. ery. hyo. na-cl. pod. pso. smi. thr. trg.

Black. pso.

Bright. ery. hyo. na-cl. pso. smi. trg.

Circles. pso.

Mist. pod.

    Moving. pod.

Moving. pod.

Spots. ery. hyo. pso.

    Black. pso.

    Bright. ery. hyo.

Veil. thr.

Vibrations. con. ery. pso. smi. thr. trg.

    Bright. con. ery.

Zigzags. na-cl. trg.

    Bright. na-cl.

SIGHT DAZZLED. na-cl.

SIGHT IMPAIRED. acon. con. cth. dt. (ery). k-bicr. lac-d. na-cl. pod. pso. (sep). smi. thr.

EYEBALL. acon. anm. ba-ca. cch. cic. cot. mrl. rhe. trg.

Appearance Glassy. anm.

    Staring. anm. cic.

Drawing. (cch).

Pressing. (trg).

Projecting. anm.

Smarting. cot.

Swelling. rhe.

Tearing. (cch).

Tensive. mrl.

Undefined. acon. (ba-ca). (hur). (k-bicr). (sang).

Same Symptom. (cch). mrl.

ORBIT. hur. k-bicr.

Undefined. hur.

ORBIT SUPERIORLY. k-bicr.

CANTHI. sang.

INTERNAL CANTHUS. sang.

RIGHT. k-bicr. sang. trg.

Eyeball Pressing. trg.

Orbit Superiorly, Undefined. k-bicr.

Internal Canthus, Undefined. sang.

LEFT. ba-ca. cch.
Eyeball, Drawing. cch.
   Tearing. cch.
   Undefined. ba-ca.
   Same Symptoms. cch.

With HEAD Symptoms.

ach. acon. æsc. æsc-g. æth. ag. ag-na. aga. al-o. alli. alm.
alo. amb. amm-ca. amm-cl. anag. anan. anm. apo. apo-a.
aps. ara. arn. art-v. as-o. asc. asr. ast. astac. atp. au. ba-a.
ba-ca. ba-cl. bap. bar. ber. bi-na. br. bru. bry. buf. ca-a.
ca-ca. ca-o. ca-s. can. cap. cast. cau. cb-a. cb-v. cch. ccs.
chd. cic. cis. cit-c. cl-hx. cld. cln. clv. cmc. cmf. cn-sa. co.
cof. con. cor. cot. cph. crb-x. cro. crot. crt. cth. cu. cu-ca.
cund. cy-hx. cyc. dig. dl-s. dol. dph. dph-i. drm. drò. dt.
elaps. erig. ery. eryn. eug. eupat. (eupat-p). euph. euph-c.
euphr. evo. f-hx. fe. fe-a. fe-mgs. frm. gel. glo. glp. gn-l.
grp. grt. gss. gua. gym. hg. hg-bicl. hg-bini. hg-cl. hg-i.
hg-s. hll. hpm. hpp. hum. hur. hydr. hyo. hyp. i. ind. irs.
itu. jat. jcr. jnc. jnp-s. jug. k-bicr. k-ca. k-i. k-na. k-o.
kd-o. kis. klm. kre. lac-cg. lac-d. lau-c. lch. lct. led. li-ca.
lpd. ly-b. lyc. men. menth. mg-ca. mg-cl. mg-sa. mgs.
mgs-ar. mgs-au. morph-a. mph. mrl. msc. mtr. myr. myris.
n-x. na-ba. ña-ca. na-cl. na-sa. narth. ner. ni-ca. nic. ol-t.
os. ox-x. p. p-x. pan. par. pb. ped. pet. phl. phy. physo.
pip. plb. pnc. pnx. pod. pol. ppv. pru-l. pso. pt. ptv. pul.
qu-sa. rhe. rho. rn-b. rs. rs-r. rut. s. s-x. sa-mgs. sang.
sb-t. scu. se. sep. si-x. smb. smc. smi. smr. sn. snc. so-d.
spi. spo. spo-f. sr-ca. srr. stach. str. str-i. tep. thr. thu. til.
trg. trn. tx-b. urt. val. vi-o. vin. vr-a. vr-s. vr-v. vtx. wis.
woo. zn. zng.

OBJECTS, FALSE APPEARANCE **of.** acon. ag-na.
al-o. (alm). amm-ca. anan. anm. arn. atp. au. ba-ca. ba-cl.
ber. bry. ca-a. ca-ca. ca-o. ca-s. can. cb-a. cb-v. chd. cic.
cl-hx. con. cy-hx. dl-s. dro. dt. ery. eug. euph. euph-c. fe.
frm. gel. glo. grt. gua. hg. hyo. jnc. k-bicr. k-ca. k-o. kis.
kre. lct. li-ca. lpd. ly-b. lyc. mg-ca. mg-cl. mrl. msc. mtr.
myris. na-cl. ner. nic. p. p-x. par. pb. pnx. ppv. pru-l.
pso. rho. rn-b. rs. rut. s. s-x. se. sep. si-x. smc. su. spi.
spo. str. tep. thr. thu. til. val. vin. vr-a. vr-s. vr-v. vtx.
wis. zn.

   Black. acon. al-o. hg. (na-cl). s-x. vin.

Blue. atp.

Bright. atp.

Confused. anan. ery. lct. ner. pnx.

Far. myris. smc. sn. thr.

Green. dt. hg. mg-cl. tep.

Grey. atp.

Inverted. eug. glo.

Large. ber. dt. k-o.

Moving. acon. ag-na. al-o. amm-ca. anm. arn. atp. au. ba-ca. ba-cl. ber. bry. ca-ca. ca-o. ca-s. can. cb-a. chd. cic. cl-hx. con. cy-hx. dl-s. dro. dt. ery. eug. cuph. euph-c. fe. frm. grt. gua. hg. jnc. k-bicr. k-ca. k-o. kre. lct. lpd. ly-b. lyc. mg-ca. mrl. msc. mtr. na-cl. ner. nic. p. p-x. par. pnx. ppv. pru-l. pso. rho. rn-b. rs. rut. s. s-x. se. sep. si-x. smc. spi. spo. str. tep. thu. til. val. vin. vr-a. vr-s. vtx. wis. zn.

    Backwards and Forwards. frm.

    Circularly. acon. ag-na. al-o. amm-ca. anm. arn. atp. au. ba-ca. ba-cl. ber. bry. ca-ca. ca-o. ca-s. can. cb-a. chd. cic. cl-hx. con. cy-hx. dl-s. dro. ery. euph. euph-c. fe. grt. gua. hg. jnc. k-bicr. k-ca. k-o. kre. lct. lpd. ly-b. lyc. mg-ca. mrl. msc. mtr. na-cl. ner. nic. p. p-x. par. ppv. pru-l. pso. rho. rn-b. rs. rut. s. s-x. se. sep. si-x. spi. str. tep. thu. val. vin. vr-a. vr-s. vtx. zn.

    Vertically. dt. msc. spo.

      Downward. dt.

      Up and Down. msc. spo.

    Vibrating. atp. cic. eug. grt. msc. pnx. s-x. smc. til. wis. zn.

Multiplied. (alm). atp. cic. ery. gel. hyo. kis. ner. nic. pb. spo. vr-v.

    Part Visible. li-ca. p. vr-v.

      Left half Visible. li-ca.

Red. atp. mg-cl.

Small. cb-v. dt.

Strange. ca-a. dt.

White. atp.

Yellow. k-bicr. tep.

OBJECTS, IMAGINARY. acon. ag. ag-na. al-o. amb. amm-ca. ara. arn. as-o. atp. au. ba-cl. bi-na. bry. ca-ca. ca-s. can. cb-a. cb-v. cch. chd. cmf. con. crb-x. cro. cth. cu. cyc. dig. dph. dt. elaps. ery. glo. hg. hyo. k-bicr. k-ca. k-o. kre. mg-ca. mg-cl. mgs-au. msc. myris. na-ca. na-cl. ner. nic. ol-t. p. pet. pnx. ppv. pru-l. pso. pt. pul. qu-sa.

rhe. s. sb-t. sep. si-x. smc.,smi. so-d. spo. sr-ca. srr. str. tep. thr. thu. trg. tx-b. vi-o. vin. vr-v. zn.

Black. acon. dt. elaps. (ery). glo. ol-t. str. thu.

Blue. (dt). pso.

Bright. acon. amm-ca. atp. au. ba-cl. ca-ca. ca-s. chd. con. dig. dph. dt. elaps. ery. hyo. k-ca. msc. ner. nic. p. ppv. qu-sa. s. sb-t. sep. spo. sr-ca. srr. str. tep. thr. trg. tx-b. vi-o. vin.

  Circles. p. tx-b. vr-v.

    Bright. tx-b.

      Moving. tx-b.

    Green. vr-v.

    Moving. tx-b.

    Red. vr-v.

Corpses. as-o. atp. ca-s. cth. na-ca. ppv. smc. str.

Figures. ag-na. amb. as-o. atp. bry. ca-ca. cb-a. cch. cmf. (cu). dt. hg. hyo. k-o. mg-ca. mg-cl. mgs-au. myris. na-ca. ppv. pul. rhe. s. sep. si-x. zn.

  Flames. atp. ca-ca. ca-s. s. spo. vin.

  Flashes, Bright. elaps. ery. hyo.

      Moving from Left to Right. elaps.

  Green. vr-v. (zn).

  Grey. atp. pnx.

  Halo. (zn).

  Light. qu-sa.

Mist. acon. ag. atp. bi-na. can. cb-a. cro. cyc. (ery). k-ca. k-o. pet. pru-l. pso. (s). sb-t. smi.

  Black. (ery).

  Grey. atp.

  Red. (ery).

Moving. tx-b.

Moving Circularly. ba-cl. msc.

Moving Downwards. ery.

Moving from Left to Right. elaps.

Red. elaps. (ery). vr-v.

Semicircle. vi-o.

  Bright. vi-o.

Spirits. as-o. atp. (cu). dt. hyo. ppv. pt. s. so-d. trg.

Spots. acon. atp. au. chd. dig. dt. elaps. ery. glo. k-ca. ner. nic. ol-t. ppv. qu-sa. sb-t. sep. sr-ca. srr. str. tep. thu. trg.

  Black. acon. dt. elaps. glo. ol-t. str. thu.

  Bright. acon. atp. au. chd. dig. dt. ery. k-ca. ner. nic. ppv. qu-sa. sb-t. sep. sr-ca. srr. str. tep. trg.

Moving Downwards. ery.
Grey. pnx.
Moving Downwards. ery.
Red. elaps.
White. elaps.
Stars. al-o. na-ca. pso.
Blue. pso.
White. al-o. na-ca.
Veil. as-o. cu. dt. k-bicr. kre. mrl. na-cl. pru-l. thr. vin.
Crooked. (na-cl).
Yellow. k-bicr.
Vibrations. acon. amm-ca. ara. arn. atp. ba-cl. chd.
con. crb-x. dph. dt. msc. ner. p. pt. sb-t. sep. thr. trg. vin.
Bright. acon. amm-ca. atp. ba-cl. chd. con. dph.
msc. ner. p. sb-t. sep. thr. trg.
Visions. ag-na. as-o. atp. cb-v. dt. ppv. pul. spo. str.
Beautiful. ppv.
Horrible. atp. cb-v. (dt). ppv. pul.
Water. ca-s. hg. sb-t.
Waves. ca-ca.
Light of. ca-ca.
White. al-o. elaps. na-ca.
Yellow. k-bicr.
Zigzags. p. trg.
Bright. p.
PHOTOMANIA. acon. amm-ca. atp. ca-a. ca-ca. dt.
PHOTOPHOBIA. acon. amm-ca. aps. arn. as-o. atp.
ba-ca. ca-ca. ca-s. chd. chi. cic. con. crb-x. cro. dig. (dt).
euphr. glo. grp. hg. hll. hyo. k-bicr. k-ca. lac-d. lau-c. lyc.
mgs-ar. mtr. na-ba. na-ca. p. p-x. pul. qu-sa. rs. s. scu.
sep. si-x. str. str-i. thu. trn. zn. zng.
Artificial Light, to. lac-d.
SIGHT DAZZLED. buf. cic. dig. euphr. (na-cl).
SIGHT IMPAIRED. acon. æsc-g. æth. ag. ag-na. aga.
al-o. alm. apo. apo-a. art-v. as-o. asc. ast. atp. bi-na. bry.
buf. ca-ca. ca-s. can. cap. cau. cb-a. cb-v. chd. chi. cic.
cit-c. cl-hx. clv. cof. con. cot. cro. crot. crt. cth. cu. cy-hx.
cyc. dig. dl-s. dph. drm. dt. (ery). eryn. evo. fe. fe-a. gel.
glo. grp. grt. gym. hg. hg-s. hydr. hyo. ind. irs. jnp-s.
k-bicr. k-ca. k-na. k-o. kre. lct. ly-b. lyc. mg-cl. mph. mrl.
msc. mtr. myris. n-x. na-ca. na-cl. na-sa. narth. ner. nic.
ol-a. ol-t. ox-x. p. p-x. par. pb. pet. phl. phy. pip. pnc.
pnx. pol. ppv. pru-l. pt. pul. qu-sa. rph. rs. rs-r. s. s-x.

sa-ıngs. sang. sb-t. se. sep. si-x. smc. smi. sn. so-d. spo.
srr. str. str-i. tep. til. thr. thu. trg. trn. trx. tx-b. urg.
vin. (vr-a). vr-s. vr-v. zn.

Hemeralopia (Night-blindness). vr-a.

Myopia (Short-sightedness). ca-ca. chi. na-cl.

EYEBALL. acon. æsc. æth. ag. ag-na. aga. al-o. alli-
(alm). alo. amb. amm-ca. anag. anau. anm. aps. ara. arn-
art-v. as-o. asr. ast. atp. ba-a. ba-ca. bap. ber. bi-na. br.
bru. bry. buf. c-bis. ca-a. ca-ca. ca-s. cast. cb-a. cb-v. cch.
ccs. chi. cic. cis. cit-c. cld. cln. clv. cmc. cmf. cn-sa. co.
cof. con. cot. cph. cro. crot. crt. cth. cu. cu-ca. cund. dig.
dol. dph. dph-i. dt. elaps. erig. ery. eug. eupat. eupat-p.
euph. euphr. evo. f-hx. fe-mgs. gel. glo. gn-l. gss. gym.
hg. hg-bicl. hg-bini. hg-i. hg-s. hll. hpm. hum. hur. hyo.
hyp. irs. itu. jat. jcr. jnp-s. jug. k-bicr. k-ca. k-i. k-na.
k-o. kd-o. kre. lac-cg. lac-d. lau-c. lch. lct. led. li-ca. ly-b.
lyc. mcn. menth. mg-ca. mg-cl. mgs-ar. morph-a. mrl.
msc. mtr. myr. myris. n-x. na-ba. na-ca. na-cl. nic. os. ox-x.
p. p-x. pan. pb: phy. physo. pnc. pnx. pod. pol. ppv. pru-l.
pso. pt. ptv. pul. rhe. rho. rn-b. rs. rs-r. s. s-x. sa-l. sang.
scu. se. sep. si-x. smb. sn. snc. spi. spo. spo-f. sr-ca. stach.
str. str-i. thr. thu. trg. trn. tx-b. val. vi-o. vp-t. vr-a. vr-s.
woo. zn.

Appearance Astonished. lau-c.

Bright. acon. (ag-na). (alm). atp. bry. cch. cth. dt.
eupat. hyo. jat. lch. lyc. morph-a. ppv. trg. trn.

Dim. ara. as-o. bry. buf. (cu). dt. ery. gym. k-ca.
ppv. trg.

Glassy. anm. atp. bry. (dt). glo. ppv. rs.

Impudent. (dt).

Spiteful. (dt).

Staring. acon. æth. al-o. amm-ca. anm. arn. as-o.
atp. ca-s. chi. cic. cit-c. clv. cof. con. cth. cu. dol. dt. ery.
glo. hg. hg-bicl. hyo. hyp. k-ca. k-o. lau-c. lyc. mgs. mgs-ar.
msc. mtr. p-x. ppv. pru-l. rs. s. sep. si-x. spi. (spo). str.
str-i. vr-a. zn.

Downwards. dt. ery.

Sideways. (dt).

Suspicious. dt.

Upward-looking. jat.

Wild. (alm). cu. cu-ca. dt. hyo. hyp. pb. vp-t.

Boring. bi-na. ca-ca. nic. s.

Bruised. (crt). (cu). (ly-b).

Bursting. acon. hg-s. lac-cg. sep. si-x. stach.

Coldness. (cro). s.

Color Dark. (anm). (as-o). (ca-s). (chi). (clv). (cu). (dl-s). (dt). (ery). (grp). (hg). (k-ca). (lyc). (mtr). (myris). (p). (p-x). (rs). (s). (s-x). (sep). (smc). (sn). (str). (str-i). (trg). (vr-a).

Red. acon. ag. (ag-na). al-o. arn. as-o. atp. bi-na. bry. buf. ca-ca. ca-s. cch. chi. cln. clv. cmf. (con). crot cu. cu-ca. dt. (eupat). (eupat-p). euphr. glo. gym. hg. hg-bini. hg-s. hum. hyo. (ind). k-bicr. kre. led. morph-a. myris. n-x. na-cl. p. (par). pnx. pol. ppv. pul. s. sep. si-x. (spi). (spo-f). str. str-i. trg. vr-a. (vr-s). (zn).

Contractive. (ag). ag-na. (anan). atp. bi-na. elaps. evo. (jnp-s). k-na. na-ba. physo. trg.

Crampy. buf. na-ca. sr-ca.

Creeping. crot.

Cutting. (cund). s.

Discharge. ag-na. (cch). (hg-bicl). (k-i). led. (na-cl).

　Fetid. led.

　Mucus. ag-na.

　Pus. (cch). (hg-bicl). (na-cl).

　Thin. (k-i).

Drawing. (acon). aga. (as-o). (atp). (cch). (ccs). (crt). (dph). k-o. kre. (ly-b). nic. p. pod. rho. (s). sr-ca. tx-b (val). (vr-s).

Dryness. myris. ppv.

Eruptions. (ca-ca). euphr. (hg-bicl). (rs). (zn).

　Pimples. (rs).

　Pterygium. (ca-ca). zn.

　Rhagades. (zn).

　Ulcers. (ca-ca). euphr. (hg-bicl).

　Vesicles. (rs).

False Sensations. ca-s. cmf. (cro). k-na.

　Sand. ca-s. cmf.

　Stones. k-na.

　Wind Cold. (cro).

Gnawing. ox-x. s.

Hæmorrhage. cb-v. (ery).

Hairs, Inverted. (zn).

Heat. (acon). æsc. (alm). amb. ara. asr. bi-na. br. c-bis. ca-ca. (cit-c). cro. crot. ery. eug. gym. hg-bini. hg-s. (hpm). jug. k-bicr. k-ca. k-na. (lau-c). lct. ly-b. mg-cl.

myris. n-x. na-ba. na-ca. (na-cl). (par). ppv. rho. s. s-x. sep. sn. spi. str-i. thu. trn. vr-a. zn.

Heaviness. alli. alo. anan. ast. chi. (cit-c). cmf. cph. (crot). ery. (euph). (frm). hg-s. (hur). jcr. k-bicr. (lac-d). lyc. (physo). pol. ptv. rs-r. s. str-i. thu. (trn). woo.

Itching. ca-ca. cot. (cu). (ly-b). s. sep. trg. (trn). vtx. zn.

Lachrymation. ag-na. alli. aps. asr. atp. ber. br. bru. bry. ca-ca. cb-a. cb-v. ccs. (chi). (con). cro. dt. eug. euph. euphr. fe-mgs. hg. k-bicr. k-ca. k-i. kd-o. kre. lac-d. lct. ly-b. (menth). myris. na-cl. os. p. pnx. ppv. pt. pul. rs-r. s. (sep). si-x. (smi). (spi). spo. str. str-i. trg. trn. tx-b. vr-a. zn.

Hot. bry. euphr. kre. (pul). (spi).

Feeling of. cro. (na-cl).

Movements. (ach). (acon). æth. (ag). (aga). (alm). (alo). (amm-ca). anm. aps. as-o. atp. (bar). (br). bry. buf. (ca-a). ca-ca. (ca-s). (can). (cb-a). (cb-v). (chd). (chi). cic. (cit-c). (cmf). (cof). (cor). (crb-x). cth. cu. (cyc). dig. (dol). dt. (dt-t). (euph). gel. glo. (glp). (hg-bicl). (hg-s). hll. hyo. (hyp). (jnp-s). (k-na). (k-o). kre. (lac-cg). lau-c. (li-ca). (ly-b). (lyc). (mg-ca). (mg-cl). (mg-sa). (msc). (mtr). (myris). (n-x). (na-cl). (na-sa). (ox-x). (p). (p-x). pb. (pet). (phl). (plb). (pnx). (pod). (ppv). (pru-l). (pt). (ptv). (qu-sa). (rs-r). s. (sb-t). (sep). si-x. (smr). (spi). (spo). (srr). (str). (thu). trg. vi-o. (vr-a). (vr-s).

Convulsions. (ach). æth. anm. as-o. atp. (br). bry. buf. (chi). cic. (cit-c). (cmf). cth. cu. dt. (hyo). kre. lau-c. (sep). si-x. trg. vi-o.

Feeling of. ara. glo. trn.

Squinting. æth. (alm). aps. atp. (ca-ca). dig. dt. gel. hll. hyo. (pb). s.

Feeling, of. ca-ca. pod.

Downwards. æth. cb-a.

Upwards. aps. buf. cic. cu. glo. hll.

Inwards. (alm). (ca-ca). (pb).

To the Left. buf.

Motion, in. eug.

Rolling. eug.

Numbness. hur.

Paralysis. (bap). (dt). (gel). (k-o). mg-ca. msc. (ped). (ptv). spi. (trg). (trn).

Pressing. acon. (æth). ag-na. aga. amb. anag. (as-o). asr. ast. atp. bap. ber. br. bry. buf. ca-a. ca-ca. cb-v. (ccs).

cis. (cit-c). cld. cmc. cmf. cu-sa. (con). cph. cro. crot. (crt).
ery. (f-hx). glo. gn-l. gym. hg-bini. (hg-s). itu. jcr. (jnp-s).
k-bicr. k-ca. (k-na). (k-o). kre. (lch). lct. (ly-b). lyc. men.
menth. mg-ca. mgs-ar. mrl. msc. (mtr). (myris). n-x. na-ba.
na-ca. na-cl. nic. (p). p-x. (pan). (ped). phy. pol. (pru-l). ppv.
(pso). ptv. (pul). (qu-sa). rn-b. rs. s. s-x. (sang). (scu). se.
sep. si-x. smb. (smc). spi. (spo). (spo-f). (sr-ca). (str). str-i.
thu. trg. val. (zn). (zng).

Like a Plug. asr. (smc).

Projecting. æth. anm. atp. (chi). glo. hyo. myris. ppv.
spi. (spo). str-i.

Sensitive. atp. (lac-cg). na-ba. (na-cl). (sep).

Shooting. (acon) anag. (anan). (as-o). (ba-ca). buf.
ca-ca. (chd). (cis). cit-c. (cld). cmf. gss. (hg-bini). hpp.
(k-bicr). k-ca. (lau-c). na-ca. ox-x. (pan). pnx. (pso). s. (sa-l).
se. sep. si-x. snc. (spi). trg. zn.

Cold. sa-l.

Hot. as-o.

Small Feeling. (kre) s.

Smarting. (acon). art-v. (as-o). asr. bap. bry. cast. cit-c.
cmc. (co). cro. hg-s. k-bicr. (lac-cg). li-ca. mg-cl. na-ba. ox-x.
pso. trn. zn.

Sticky Feeling. elaps.

Strained. dph.

Sunken. as-o. clv. (cu). dt. ery. k-ca. morph-a. rs. spo.
vp-t.

Feeling. amb. hg-s. lyc.

Swelling. anm. as-o. (bry). (cch). (clv). (dt). (eupat-p).
(hg-bicl). (hyo). (k-ca). (k-i). led. mg-ca. pb. rhe. sep. str-i.
trg. (u-na).

Chemosis. euphr.

Œdematous. (bry). (u-na).

Feeling of. ag-na. (cit-c). cro. mg-ca. p-x. pru-l.

Tearing. (ag-na). (anm). (as-o). bi-na. ca-ca. (cb-a).
cb-v. (cch). (chd). (con). (cro). (k-ca). (kd-o). led. lyc. na-ba.
na-ca. (ni-ca). (os). p. (pnc). pul. (s). sep. smb. (smc). str. zn.

Tensive. ba-a. ba-ca. ber. jnp-s. k-ca. (k-o). mrl. n-x.
ox-x. par. s. sep. si-x. trg.

Throbbing. (atp). (ba-a). bry. (cb-a). crb-x. (glo).
(myris). (na-cl). p. se. (sn). (thr). (thu). trg.

Tingling. crot.

Undefined. (alo). art-v. atp. (br). bry. cb-v. cit-c. cmf.
(co). con. cro. (cu). dph-i. dt. (erig). f-hx. fe-mgs. (frn).
(gym). hg-bini. hg-i. hpp. hur. irs. jug. k-i. lac-cg. lac-d.

(li-ca). (men). mg-ca. mgs-ar. myr. n-x. ox-x. pb. pod. (ppv).
pul. rs. (s). (sang). sep. si-x. (spi). spo-f. str-i. thr. thu. trg.
zn.

Wrinkled. (zn).

Same Symptom. (ach). acon. æsc. ag. ag-na. aga. alli.
alo. anag. ara. (as-o). asr. (atp). (ba-a). ba-ca. (ber). bi-na.
br. bry. buf. (ca-a). ca-ca. ca-o. cb-a. cb-v. (cch). (ccs). (chd).
(cic). cis. cit-c. (cld). cmf. (co). con. crb-x. cro. (crt). (cu).
(cund). dt. elaps. eug. fe-mgs. (glo). gn-l. gym. hg-bini. hg-s.
hur. irs. itu. jcr. jnp-s. jug. k-bicr. k-ca. k-na. (k-o). kre.
lac-d. (lau-c). lct. led. (ly-b). lyc. (men). mg-ca. mrl. msc.
myr. n-x. na-ba. na-ca. na-cl. (ni-ca). nic. ox-x. p. phy. physo.
(pnc). pnx. pod. ppv. (pso). (pul). (qu-sa). rn-b. s. s-x.
(sang). se. sep. si-x. (smc). snc. (spi). sr-ca. stach. str. (str-i).
thu. trg. urt. val. (vr-s). woo. zn. (zng).

EYEBALL SUPERIORLY. phy.

Pressing. phy.

EYEBALL EXTERNALLY. rn-b. spo.

Pressing. rn-b.

EYEBALL INTERNALLY. zn.

Color, Red. zn.

EYEBALL POSTERIORLY. co. menth. spo-f.

Pressing. menth. spo-f.

Undefined. co.

Same Symptom. co.

SCLEROTIC. as-o. eupat.

Color, Red. eupat.

    Yellow. as-o. eupat.

CORNEA. ca-ca. hg-bicl. lac-cg. rs. s.

Color, Red. s.

    White. hg-bicl. s.

Eruptions, Pimples. rs.

    Ulcers. ca-ca. hg-bicl.

    Vesicles. rs.

Sensitive. lac-cg.

Smarting. lac-cg.

CHAMBERS of EYE. hg-bicl.

Discharge, Pus. hg-bicl.

IRIS. æth. (alm). anm. aps. arn. ast. astac. atp. ba-ca.
(br). (buf). ca-ca. cap. chi. cic. clv. cmf. crb-x. cro. crt. cu.
cy-hx. dph. dt. ery. glo. hll. hyo. hyp. lau-c. lyc. morph.
morph-a. msc. mtr. myris. n-x. na-cl. nic. p. pb. phx.
ppv. pru-l. pul. rhe. s. sep. si-x. smc. str. str-i. thu. trg.
vr-v. zn.

Color, Discoloured. na-cl.

Pupils Contracted. anm. arn. ast. atp. cap. chi. cic. crb-x. cu. dph. dt. glo. lau-c. morph. msc. mtr. na-cl. p. pul. rhe. s. sep. si-x. smc. str-i. thu. zn.

Dilated. æth. (alm). anm. aps. astac. atp. br. buf. ca-ca. chi. cic. clv. cmf. cro. crt. cy-hx. dt. ery. hll. hyo. hyp. lyc. mgs. morph-a. myris. nic. pb. pnx. ppv. pru-l. rhe. str. vr-v.

Insensible. atp. ba-ca. buf. (cu). dt. hyo. mtr. myris. n-x. ppv. pru-l. trg.

Mobile. atp. mtr.

ORBIT. acon. alo. atp. ba-a. ba-ca. cb-a. cis. cit-c. con. crot. crt. cu. frm. glo. hg-i. hur. kd-o. lau-c. li-ca. lyc. msc. myris. na-cl. nic. os. ped. pol. ppv. pru-l. pul. qu-sa. sep. smc. sn. sr-ca. trg. val. zn.

Bruised. crt. cu.

Drawing. val.

Heaviness. crot. hur.

Pressing. acon. cit-c. crt. msc. na-cl. nic. ped. pol. pru-l. qu-sa. sr-ca.

Shooting. lau-c.

Tearing. cb-a. con. lyc.

Throbbing. cb-a.

Undefined. alo. con. hur. li-ca. trg.

Same Symptom. acon. alo. con. cu. hur. qu-sa. sr-ca.

ORBIT SUPERIORLY. cis. frm. hg-i. kd-o. myris. na-cl. os. sep. smc.

Tearing. kd-o. os.

Pressing. na-cl.

Sensitive. sep.

ORBITAL INTEGUMENTS. anm. as-o. ca-s. cb-a. chi. clv. cu. dl-s. dt. ery. grp. hg. lyc. mtr. myris. ox-x. p. p-x. par. rs. s. s-x. sep. smc. sn. spi. str. str-i. trg. vr-a. vtx.

Color Dark. anm. arn. ca-s. chi. clv. cu. dl-s. dt. ery. grp. hg. lyc. mtr. p. p-x. rs. s. sep. smc. sn. str. str-i. trg. vr-a.

Red. par.

Yellow. spi.

Shooting. as-o.

Hot. as-o.

Smarting. as-o.

Same Symptom. as-o.

ORBITAL, INTEGUMENTS SUPERIORLY. cb-a. ox-x. par. sep. vtx.

Gnawing. ox-x.

Itching. vtx.

L

Movements, Convulsions. sep.
   Downwards-Pressing. cb-a.
Smarting. ox-x.
Tensive. ox-x. par.
ORBITAL INTEGUMENTS INFERIORLY. dt.
myris. s-x.
Color, Dark. dt. myris.
EYELIDS. ach. acon. æth. ag. ag-na. alm. alo. amm-ca.
anm. aps. atp. bap. bar. br. bry. buf. ca-a. ca-ca. ca-s. can. cb-v.
cch. chd. chi. cit-c. clv. cmf. cof. con. cor. cph. crb-x. crot. cu.
cyc. dig. dol. dt. dt-t. ery. euph. euphr. frm. glo. glp.'grp.
hg-bicl. hg-s. hll. hpm. hyo. hyp. ind. jnp-s. k-bicr. k-ca.
k-na. k-o. kre. lac-cg. lac-d. lau-c. led. li-ca. ly-b. lyc. mg-ca.
mg-cl. mg-sa. msc. mtr. myris. n-x. na-cl. na-sa. ox-x. p. p-x.
par. pb. pet. phl. physo. plb. pnx. pod. ppv. pru-l. pt. ptv.
qu-sa. rs-r. s. sb-t. sep. smr. spi. spo. srr. str. thu. trg. trn.
u-na. vr-a. vr-s. zn.
   Adhesion. ca-ca. (con). k-ca. led.
   Color, Dark. clv. k-ca.
      Red. par.
   Discharge Fetid. led.
   Drawing. acon.
   Hæmorrhage. (ery).
   Hairs, Inverted. zn.
   Heat. lau-c. par.
   Itching. (cu). trn.
   Movements, Closing. acon. æth. ag. aga. alm. alo.
amm-ca. anm. aps. atp. bar. (br). bry. (buf). ca-a. (ca-ca).
ca-s. can. cb-v. chd. cor. crb-x. cu. cyc. (dig). (dt). euph. glo.
glp. (hg-bicl). hg-s. hll. hyo. (hyp). jnp-s. k-na. k-o. kre.
lac-cg. lau-c. li-ca. ly-b. lyc. mg-ca. mg-cl. mg-sa. msc. myris.
n-x. na-cl. (na-sa). ox-x. p. p-x. pb. pet. phl. plb. pnx. pod.
ppv. pt. ptv. qu-sa. rs-r. s. sb-t. sep. smr. spi. spo. srr. str.
thu. vr-a. vr-s.
      Spasmodically. br. ca-ca. cyc. hg-bicl. (hyp).
myris. spo.
   Convulsions. ach. (chi). cmf. cu. hyo. krc.
   Opening Wide. (alm). buf. cit-c. cof. dol. dt. dt-t.
lyc. mtr. pb. ppv. pru-l. vr-a.
   Upwards Drawn. acon. lyc.
   Winking. aga. myris.
   Paralysis. Opening Difficult. bap. gel. mg-ca. ped.
ptv. trg. trn.
   Pressing. æth. msc.
   Shooting. acon. k-bicr.

Small Feeling. kre.
Smarting. acon. trn.
Swelling. clv. hg-bicl. hyo. k-i.
Tensive. n-x.
Same Symptom. ach.
UPPER EYELID. cit-c. cph. crot. ery. euph. frm. hg-s. jnp-s. k-ca. lac-d. p. ptv. trn. zn.
Heaviness. cit-c. cph. crot. ery. euph. frm. hg-s. lac-d. ptv. trn.
Pressing. p.
Swelling. k-ca.
LOWER EYELID. bry. cch. grp. u-na.
Swelling. bry. u-na.
Œdematous. bry.
TARSAL EDGES. euphr. hpm. vr-s.
Color Red. euphr. vr-s.
Eruptions, Ulcers. euphr.
Heat. hpm.
EYELIDS, INNER SURFACE. cch. ind. k-bicr. zn.
Color Red. ind. k-bicr.
Wrinkled. zn.
CANTHI. anan. co. k-i. na-cl. ppv. zn.
Discharge. na-cl.
Pus. na-cl.
EXTERNAL CANTHUS. co. zn.
Eruptions, Rhagades. zn.
Smarting. zn.
INTERNAL CANTHUS. anan. k-i. ppv.
Contractive. anan.
Discharge. k-i.
Thin. k-i.
Shooting. anan.
Swelling. k-i.
Undefined. k-i.
CARUNCULA LACHRYMALIS. ca-ca.
LEFT then RIGHT. zn.
Eyeball, Eruption, Pterygium. zn.
FORWARDS. acon. anm. atp. br. cb-v. glo. gym. k-na. lch. mgs-ar. mtr. na-ca. na-cl. p. pan. pso. pul. rn-b. rs. sang. scu. sep. si-x. snc. str. str-i. val. zng.
Eyeball, Pressing. acon. atp. br. glo. gym. k-na. lch. mgs-ar. mtr. na-cl. p. pso. pul. rn-b. rs. sang. scu. sep. si-x. str. val.

Like a Plug. asr.

Shooting. na-ca. snc.

Tearing. anm. cb-v.

Orbit Superiorly, Pressing. na-cl.

BACKWARDS. acon. dph. hg-s. ly-b. s.

Eyeball, Drawing. dph. ly-b. s.

     Pressing. acon. hg-s.

UPWARDS, vr-s.

DOWNWARDS. atp. s.

Eyeball, Pressing. s.

To BACK. trg.

To NAPE. trg.

Eyeball, Tensive like a Thread. trg.

RIGHT. (alm). as-o. atp. ber. buf. ca-a. ca-ca. ccs. cis. cit-c. cld. cmf. con. cro. crt. dig. dt. erig. f-hx. hyp. k-bicr. k-o. ly-b. menth. mg-cl. na-cl. ner. pb. pnc. ppv. pso. pul. s-x. smc. sn. spi. spo-f. str-i. thr. thu. trg. vr-s. zn. zng.

Objects Imaginary, Veil Crooked. na-cl.

Photophobia. str-i.

Sight Impaired. cro. k-bicr. ner.

Eyeball Bruised. ly-b.

  Coldness. cro.

  Color Red. as-o. con. spo-f.

  Drawing. as-o. ccs. crt. vr-s.

  False Sensations, Wind Cold. cro.

  Heat. ly-b. thu.

  Itching. ly-b. trg.

  Lachrymation. con. menth.

    Hot. pul.

    Feeling of. na-cl.

  Movements, Squinting. (alm). pb.

    Inwards. (alm). pb.

  Paralysis. (k-o).

  Pressing. as-o. atp. ber. ca-a. ccs. cmf. con. f-hx. k-o. pul. spi. str-i. thu. trg. zn.

  Shooting. ca-ca. cld. pso.

  Tearing. as-o. cro. pnc.

  Tensive. k-o.

  Throbbing. atp. thr. thu. trg.

  Undefined. erig. f-hx. str-i.

  Same Symptom. as-o. atp. ber. ca-a. ca-ca. ccs. cld. cro. k-o. ly-b. pnc. pso. pul. spi. str-i. vr-s.

Eyeball Internally, Color Red. zn.
Swelling. zn.
Eyeball Posteriorly, Undefined. spo-f.
Orbit, Drawing. atp.
Pressing. pul.
Tearing. zn.
Throbbing. sn. trg.
Same Symptom. atp. ppv. trg.
Orbit Superiorly, Heat. na-cl.
Pressing like a Plug. smc.
Sensitive. na-cl.
Shooting. cis.
Throbbing. na-cl.
Orbital Integuments, Color Red. dt.
Swelling. dt.
Orbital Integuments Inferiorly, Color Dark. s-x.
Eyelids, Adhesion of. con.
Movements, Closing. ca-a. dig. mg-cl.
Spasmodically. hyp.
Open Wide. buf.
Upper Eyelid, Heat. na-cl.
Movements, Convulsions. cit-c.
Hangs Down. na-cl.
Tearing. zn.
Internal Canthus, Pressing. ppv.
Same Symptom. ppv.
Caruncula Lachymalis, Swelling. ca-ca.
Forwards. Eyeball, Pressing. str-i. zng.
Upwards. Eyeball, Drawing. vr-s.
Downwards. Orbit, Drawing. atp.
LEFT. acon. ag-na. ba-a. ba-ca. br. buf. ca-ca. cch. ccs.
chd. cit-c. co. cund. euph. frm. glo. grp. gym. hg-bini. hg-i.
jnp-s. k-ca. lac-cg. ly-b. men. myris. na-cl. na-sa. ni-ca. nic.
pan. ppv. s. sang. sep. smc. spi. spo. str-i. thu. trg. zn. zng.
Objects, False Appearance of, Dark. na-cl.
Objects Imaginary, Green. zn.
Halo. zn.
Green. zn.
Mist. s.
Sight Dazzled. na-cl.
Sight Impaired. ca-ca. ly-b. na-cl.
Eyeball Appears Bright. ag-na.
Boring. s.

Color Red. ag-na. glo. spi.
Contractive. ag. jnp-s.
Cutting. cund. s.
Drawing. cch. nic.
Eruptions, Pterygium. ca-ca.
Gnawing. s.
Heat. acon. k-ca. s.
Lachrymation. ag-na. euph. k-ca. ly-b. (sep). spi. trg.
     Hot. spi.
Movements, Convulsions. trg.
     Squinting. ca-ca.
     Inwards. ca-ca.
Pressing. acon. ccs. cit-c. hg-bini. ly-b. pan. s. spi. str-i. zng.
     Shooting. hg-bini. s. spi.
     Tearing. ag-na. cch. chd. k-ca. ni-ca. s. smc.
     Throbbing. na-cl.
     Undefined. br. cit-c. hg-bini. gym. lac-cg. men. ppv. sang. spi.
     Same Symptom. acon. ag-na. ba-a. br. cch. ccs. chd. cit-c. cund. glo. gym. hg-bini. ly-b. men. na-cl. ni-ca. nic. ppv. s. sang. smc. spi. str-i. zng.
Eyeball Externally, Pressing. spo.
Orbit, Heat. cit-c.
     Pressing. cit-c.
     Shooting. ba-ca.
     Swelling, Feeling of. cit-c.
     Throbbing. ba-a. glo.
     Same Symptom. ba-ca. glo.
Orbit Superiorly, Pressing. myris.
     Throbbing. myris.
     Undefined. frm. hg-i.
Eyelids, Movements, Closing. buf. euph. na-sa. thu.
     Convulsions. trg.
Upper Eyelid, Pressing. jnp-s.
Lower Eyelid, Movements, Hangs Down. grp.
     Swelling. cch.
Eyelids Inner Surface, Discharge. cch.
         Pus. cch.
External Canthus, Smarting. co.
Forwards. Eyeball, Shooting. pan.

After HEAD Symptoms.

anag. anm. ba-ca. ber. bry. cb-v. con. (cu). dt. frm-s, gel.
hyp. k-bicr. k-o. mg-ca. p. rhe. si-x. str-i. thu. trg.
OBJECTS IMAGINARY. p. trg.
Vibrations. p. trg.
Zigzags. trg.
PHOTOMANIA. gel.
SIGHT IMPAIRED. con. dt. frm-s. gel. k-bicr. k-o.
p. si-x.
EYEBALL. anag. anm. ba-ca. ber. bry. cb-v. con. hyp.
str-i.
Appearance Staring. hyp.
     Wild, hyp.
Heat. str-i.
Heaviness. str-i.
Itching. (p).
Lacrymation. (ba-ca). cb-v.
Movements. (ba-ca). cb-v.
Paralysis. (cu).
Pressing. anag. (ba-ca). ber. bry.
Shooting. anag.
Swelling. anm.
Tensive. ber.
Throbbing. (thu).
Undefined. con.
LENS. mg-ca.
Cataract. mg-ca.
IRIS. dt. hyp. rhe.
Pupils Dilated. dt. hyp. rhe.
EYELIDS. ba-ca. cb-v. (cu). hyp. p.
Itching. p.
Movements Closing. (ba-ca). cb-v. (hyp.)
    Spasmodically. (hyp).
Paralysis. (cu).
RIGHT. hyp. thu.
Eyeball, Throbbing. thu.
Eyelids, Movements, Closing Spasmodically. hyp.
LEFT. ba-ca.
Eyeball, Lacrymation. ba-ca.
  Pressing. ba-ca.
Eyelids, Movements, Closing. ba-ca.

DARKNESS or DUSK.

acon. ag-na. al-o. amm-cl. atp. ba-ca. ca-ca. cb-v. cd-sa. chd. cund. dig. dl-s. dt. ery. fe-mgs. hg. hyo. lyc. myris. na-cl. p. pul. rut. s-x. sr-ca. thu. val. vr-a.

OBJECTS, FALSE APPEARANCE of. myris.

Closer Together. myris.

Far, Too. myris.

Oblique. myris.

OBJECTS IMAGINARY. acon. ag-na. al-o. ba-ca. ca-ca. cb-v. cund. dig. dl-s. dt. ery. fe-mgs. lyc. p. sr-ca. thu. val.

Blue. (cund). dt. fe-mgs.

Bright. ag-na. al-o. ba-ca. ca-ca. dl-s. dt. ery. fe-mgs. lyc. p. thu. val.

Circles. fe-mgs.
> **Blue.** fe-mgs.
> **Bright.** fe-mgs.
> **Red.** fe-mgs.
> **Zigzags.** fe-mgs.

Flames. ag-na. dl-s.

Flashes, Bright. ag-na. dt. ery. thu.

Green. dt. sr-ca.

Light. al-o. val.

Mist. (ag-na).

Moving with Eye. dt.

Pyriform Body. (cund).
> **Blue.** (cund).

Red. fe-mgs.

Spots. ba-ca. ca-ca. dt. lyc. p. sr-ca. thu.
> **Blue.** dt.
> **Bright.** ba-ca. ca-ca. dt. lyc. p. thu.
> **Green.** sr-ca.
> **White.** sr-ca.

Stripes. dt.
> **Blue.** dt.
>> **Moving with Eye.** dt.
>> **Vertical.** dt.
> **Green.** dt.
>> **Moving with Eye.** dt.
>> **Vertical.** dt.

Moving with Eye. dt.

Vertical. dt.

Vertical. dt.
Vibrations. dig.
    Bright. dig.
Visions. cb-v. p.
    Horrible. cb-v.
White. sr-ca.
Zigzags. fe-mgs.
SIGHT IMPAIRED. ag-na. amm-cl. atp. cd-sa. chd.
dig. (dt). fe-mgs. grp. hg. hyo. rut. srr. vr-a.
EYEBALL. al-o. amm-cl. na-cl. s-x.
Heat. amm-cl. s-x.
Lachrymation. s-x.
Movements. (ba-ca). (na-cl). •
Paralysis. (na-cl).
Pressing. al-o. na-cl.
Smarting. (lyc).
EYELIDS. ba-ca. na-cl.
Closing. ba-ca. na-cl.
    Spasmodically. ba-ca. na-cl.
Paralysis. na-cl.
CANTHI. lyc.
EXTERNAL CANTHUS. lyc.
Smarting. lyc.
RIGHT. cund.
Objects Imaginary, Blue. cund.
        Pyriform Body. cund.
           Blue. cund.
LEFT. ag-na. dt.
Objects Imaginary, Blue. dt.
      Bright. dt.
      Mist. ag-na.
      Spots. dt.
        Blue. dt.
        Bright. dt.

LIGHT, Artificial.

(alm) alo. amph. art-v. as-o. asc. ber. ca-ca. ca-o. ca-pa. ca-s.
cb-v. chd. chi. cmc. con. cor. cph. cro. dl-s. dph. dro. dt. ele.
gel. grp. hg. i. k-ca. krm. lac-d. lo-c. lyc. mg-cl. mg-sa.
mn-ca. mrl. myris. n-x. na-ba. na-sa. ni-ca. ol-a. p. p-x. pb.
pet. phy. pol. pru-l. pt. pul. rs-r. rut. s. sb-t. sep. si-x. smi.
srr. stach. str-i. thu. til. trg.

OBJECTS, FALSE APPEARANCE of. ele. hg. lyc.
mrl. smi. til.
  Confused. ele. hg. mrl. til.
  Moving. lyc.
          Vibrating. lyc.
  Red. smi.
OBJECTS, IMAGINARY. ber. cb-a. chi. cro. dt. krm.
mn-ca. n-x. na-sa. p-x. sep. srr. til.
  Black. cb-a. dt. mn-ca.
  Blue. dt.
  Bright. chi. dt. (na-sa). p-x. srr. til.
  Circles. mn-ca.
          Black. mn-ca.
  Cobwebs. n-x.
  Light. chi.
          Red. chi.
          Yellow. chi.
  Mist. (na-sa). sep.
  Moving with Eye. dt.
  Near Eye. (na-sa).
  Red. chi.
  Spots. cb-a. dt. krm. srr.
          Black. cb-a. dt.
                  Moving with Eye. dt.
                  Symmetrical, Lines in. cb-a.
          Blue. dt.
          Bright. dt. srr.
          Moving with Eye. dt.
          Symmetrical Lines in. cb-a.
          White. krm.
          Yellow. cb-a.
                  Symmetrical Lines in. cb-a.
  Stars. (na-sa).
          Bright. (na-sa).
                  Near Eye. (na-sa).
          Green. (na-sa).
                  Near Eye. (na-sa).
          Near Eye. (na-sa).
          Yellow. (na-sa).
                  Near Eye. (na-sa).
  Veil. ber. cro.
  Vibrations. (dt). p-x. til.
    Bright. (dt). p-x. til.

White. krm.
Yellow. cb-a.
SIGHT DAZZLED. cph. hg. p.
SIGHT IMPAIRED. ber. cro. myris. na-sa. rs-r. sep.
EYEBALL. alo. amph. art-v. asc. ca-ca. ca-o. ca-pa.
cb-a. chd. cmc. con. cor. cph. cro. dro. dt. gel. grp. hg. i.
lac-d. lo-c. lyc. mg-cl. mg-sa. mn-ca. mrl. na-ba. na-sa.
ni-ca. ol-a. p. p-x. pet. pol. pru-l. pt. pul. rut. s. sb-t. sep.
smi. stach. str-i. thu.
Appearance Dim. lyc.
Bursting. pol. stach.
Color Red. sb-t.
Contractive. sep.
Cutting. ca-ca.
Dryness. (art-v). cro. mg-cl. pru-l.
Eruptions. sb-t.
    Blisters. sb-t.
False Sensations. art-v.
    Sand. art-v.
Heat. (art-v). ca-o. cor. cro. grp. mg-cl. mg-sa. ni-ca.
ol-a. p-x. pru-l. rut. thu.
Heaviness. (na-sa).
Lachrymation. cmc.
Movements. (ber). (cro). (mrl).
    Convulsions. (ber).
Pressing. (alo). (art-v). cb-a. cro. mn-ca. na-sa. pet.
pol. smi. str-i.
Sensitive. (na-sa).
Shooting. amph. ca-ca. lyc. (na-sa). pul. s. sep.
Smarting. (cro). lyc. p-x. (phy).
Softness, Feeling of. (na-sa).
Undefined. amph. art-v. asc. ca-ca. ca-pa. chd. cmc.
con. cph. dro. dt. gel. hg. i. lac-d. lo-c. lyc. mrl. na-ba.
p. pt. s.
IRIS. (alm). pb.
Pupils Dilated. (alm). pb.
ORBIT. na-sa.
ORBIT INFERIORLY. na-sa.
ORBITAL INTEGUMENTS. chd.
EYELIDS. art-v. as-o. ber. ca-ca. cro. mrl. na-sa. p-x. srr.
Cutting. ca-ca.
Dryness. art-v. as-o.
Heat. art-v. p-x.

Movements, Closing. srr.
     Convulsions. ber.
     Winking. cro. mrl.
Pressing. art-v.
Smarting. cro.
UPPER EYELID. na-sa.
Heaviness. na-sa.
CANTHI. art-v. p-x. phy.
Heat. p-x.
INTERNAL CANTHUS. art-v. phy.
Heat. art-v.
Smarting. phy.
FORWARDS. cmc. pol.
Eyeball, Pressing. cmc. pol.
BACKWARDS. na-sa.
DOWNWARDS. cmc.
Eyeball, Pressing. cmc.
To HEAD. cmc.
To OCCIPUT. cmc.
Eyeball Posteriorly, Undefined. cmc.
CHANGING CHARACTER or PLACE. na-sa.
**Objects Imaginary, Mist, then Star Bright Green
Yellow Near Eye.** (na-sa).
     Eyeball, Sensitive then Pressing. (na-sa).
     ,,   **Shooting then**   ,,   (na-sa).
     ,,   **Softness, Feeling of, then**   ,, (na-sa).
OBJECTS IMAGINARY, then EYEBALL. na-sa.
SIGHT IMPAIRED then OBJECTS IMAGINARY.
na-sa.
    RIGHT. alo. chd. na-sa.
    Objects Imaginary, Bright. na-sa.
        Green. na-sa.
        Mist. na-sa.
        Near Eye. na-sa.
        Star. na-sa.
           Bright. na-sa.
              Near Eye. na-sa.
           Green. na-sa.
              Near Eye. na-sa.
           Near Eye. na-sa.
           Yellow. na-sa.
              Near Eye. na-sa.
        Yellow. na-sa.

Sight Impaired. na-sa.
Eyeball, Pressing. alo. na-sa.
Orbit Inferiorly, Pressing. na-sa.
    Sensitive. na-sa.
    Shooting. na-sa.
    Softness, Feeling of. na-sa.
Backwards. Orbit Inferiorly, Shooting. na-sa.
Changing. Objects Imaginary, Mist, then Star Bright Green Yellow Near Eye. na-sa.
    Orbit Inferiorly, Sensitive then Pressing. na-sa.
       „   **Shooting then**   „ na-sa.
       „   **Softness, Feeling of then**   „ na-sa.
    Objects Imaginary then Eyeball, Star Bright Green Yellow Near Eye then Pressing. na-sa.
    Sight Impaired then Objects Imaginary, Star Bright Green Yellow Near Eye. na-sa.
LEFT. dt.
Objects Imaginary, Blue. dt.
    Bright. dt.
    Spots. dt.
        Blue. dt.
    Vibrations. dt.
        Bright. dt.

LIGHT, Natural.

acon. æth. ag-na. aga. al-o. alli. ale. amm-ca. amm-cl. amph.
anan. aps. arn. art-v. arum-t. as-o. ast. atp. ba-ca. ber. br.
bry. buf. ca-ca. (ca-i). ca-o. ca-pa. ca-s. cast. cb-a. cch. chd.
chi. chio. cic. cl-hx. cle. cmc. co. cof. con. cop. crb-x. cro.
crv. cu-a. cund. dig. dl-s. drm. dro. dt. elaps. ery. eryn.
eug. eupat. euphr. fe-mgs. gel. grc. grp. hg. hg-bicl. hg-bini.
hll. hyo. irs-f. k-bicr. k-ca. k-i. k-na. k-o. kre. lac-d. lac-f.
lau-c. lct. li-ca. lo-c. lyc. mg-ca. mg-cl. mg-sa. mgs-ar.
mgs-au. mn-ca. mrl. mtr. myris. n-x. na-ba. na-ca. na-cl.
na-sa. nic. ol-a. p. p-x. pb. pet. phl. phy. pnx. pol. pru-l.
pso. pul. qu-sa. rho. rs. rs-r. rs-v. s. s-x. sa-l. sb-s. sb-t.
scu. sep. si-x. smb. smc. smi. sn. so-d. spi. srr. str. str-i.
thr. thu. trn. trx. u-na. vr-a. vr-s. vtx. woo. ziz. zn. zng.
  OBJECTS, FALSE APPEARANCE of. thr.
Multiplied. thr.
  OBJECTS IMAGINARY. alo. con. cund. dt. (ery).
fe-mgs. k-ca. qu-sa. s. sb-t. sep. so-d. thr. thu.

Black. dt. k-ca. (s). thu.
Blue. dt. fe-mgs.
Bright. dt. fe-mgs. (qu-sa). sb-t. sep. so-d. thr.
Circle. fe-mgs.
    Blue. fe-mgs.
    Bright. fe-mgs.
    Red. fe-mgs.
    Zigzags. fe-mgs.
Flames. so-d.
Flashes Bright. sb-t.
Halo. con.
    Variegated. con.
High up. dt.
Pyriform Body. (cund).
    Red. (cund).
Rain. thu.
Red. (cund). fe-mgs.
Semicircle. dt.
    Bright. dt.
        High Up. dt.
    High Up. dt.
Spots. amm-cl. dt. k-ca. (qn-sa). s. thu.
  Black. dt. k-ca. (s). thu.   :
  Blue. dt.
  Bright. dt. (qu-sa).
  White. s. thu.
  Yellow. amm-cl.
Stripes. dt.
  Bright. dt.
      Upwards to Right. dt.
      Vertical. dt.
  Upwards to Right. dt.
  Vertical. dt.
Threads. (ery).
Upwards to Right. dt.
Variegated. con.
Vertical. dt.
Veil. k-ca.
Vibrations. alo. (dt). sep. thr.
  Bright. (dt). sep. thr.
White. s. thu.
Yellow. amm-cl.
Zigzags. fe-mgs.
SIGHT DAZZLED. dt. cuph. mrl. p. sa-l. sep.

SIGHT IMPAIRED. atp. con. dt. eug. fe-mgs. grp. k-ca. k-o. myris. p. s. sb-s. si-x. trn. vr-a.

EYEBALL. acon. æth. ag-na. aga. al-o. (alli). amm-ca. amm-cl. anan. aps. arn. art-v. arum-t. as-o. ast. atp. au. ba-ca. ber. br. bry. buf. ca-ca. (ca-i). ca-o. ca-pa. ca-s. cast. cb-a. cch. (chd). chi. chio. cic. cl-hx. cle. clv. cmc. co. cof. con. cop. cro. crv. cu-a. dig. dl-s. drm. dro. dt. elaps. ery. eryn. eug. eupat. euphr. gel. grc. grp. hg. hg-bicl. hg-bini. hll. hyo. irs-f. k-bicr. k-ca. k-i. k-na. k-o. kre. lac-d. lac-f. lau-c. (led). li-ca. lo-c. lyc. mg-ca. mg-cl. mg-sa. mgs-ar. mgs-au. mn-ca. mrl. mtr. myris. n-x. na-ba. na-ca. na-cl. na-sa. nic. ol-a. p. p-x. pb. pet. phl. phy. pnx. pol. pru-l. pso. pul. qu-sa. rho. rs. rs-r. rs-v. s. s-x. sa-l. sb-s. sb-t. scu. sep. si-x. smc. smi. spi. srr. str. str-i. thr. thu. trn. trx. (u-na). vr-s. vtx. woo. ziz. zn. zng.

Color Red. eryn. sb-t.
Dryness. (mn-ca). rho.
Eruptions. sb-t.
  Blisters. sb-t.
Heat. (chd). dl-s. eryn. (k-bicr). kre. mg-ca. mg-cl. rho.
Heaviness. (lyc).
Itching. anan.
Lachrymation. al-o. bry. dig. dl-s. dt. eug. grp. k-bicr. kre. lyc. mg-cl. qu-sa. s-x. (str-i). vr-s. zn.
  Hot. al-o. dig. dl-s. str-i.
Movements. (as-o). eryn. (k-bicr). (mrl).
  Convulsions. (k-bicr).
  Squinting. eryn.
Paralysis. ast. lyc.
Pressing. mg-cl. phy. (pul). s. sep. (str).
Shooting. co. euphr. grp. pul. s. thu.
Smarting. as-o. (chd). co. dl-s. eryn. grp.
Undefined. (Photophobia). as-o. æth. ag-na. aga. al-o. (alli). amm-ca. amm-cl. anan. aps. arn. art-v. arum-t. as-o. ast. atp. au. ba-ca. ber. br. bry. buf. ca-ca. (ca-i). ca-o. ca-pa. ca-s. cast. cb-a. cch. chi. chio. cic. cl-hx. cle. clv. cmc. co. cof. con. cop. cro. crv. cu-a. dig. dl-s. drm. dro. dt. elaps. ery. eupat. euphr. gel. grc. grp. hg. hg-bicl. hg-bini. hll. hyo. irs-f. k-bicr. k-ca. k-i. k-na. k-o. kre. lac-d. lac-f. lau-c. (led). li-ca. lo-c. lyc. mg-ca. mg-cl. mg-sa. mgs-ar. mgs-au. mn-ca. mrl. mtr. myris. n-x. na-ba. na-ca. na-cl. na-sa. nic. ol-a. p. p-x. pb. pet. phl. phy. pnx. pol. pru-l. pso. pul. rs. rs-r. rs-v. s. s-x. sa-l. sb-s. scu. sep. si-x. smc. smi. spi. srr. str. str-i. thr. thu. trn. trx. (u-na). vtx. woo. ziz. zn. zng.

EYELIDS. as-o. k-bicr. lyc. mn-ca. mrl. (myris). s. sa-l.
Dryness. mn-ca.
Heat. k-bicr.
Movements, Closing. (as-o). sa-l.
              Spasmodically. as-o.
   Convulsions. k-bicr.
    Winking. mrl. (myris).
Pressing. s.
UPPER EYELID. lyc.
Heaviness. lyc.
RIGHT. aps. atp. cund. (hg-bini). lac-f. str-i.
Objects Imaginary, Pyriform Body. cund.
                  Red. cund.
            Red. cund.
Eyeball Undefined. aps. atp. (hg-bini). lac-f. str-i.
LEFT. al-o. alli. as-o. atp. dt. led. s. u-na.
Objects Imaginary, Black. s.
           Blue. dt.
           Bright. dt.
           Spots. dt. s.
              Black. s.
              Blue. dt.
              Bright. dt.
          Vibrations. dt.
              Bright. dt.
Sight Impaired. atp.
Eyeball, Lacrymation. alo.
       Undefined. alli. as-o. led. u-na.

CHANGE of LIGHT.

dt.
EYEBALL. dt.
Pressing. (dt).
EYEBALL INTERIORLY. dt.
Pressing. dt.

During LIGHTNING Flash.

rn-b.
OBJECTS IMAGINARY. rn-b.
Rope across Sky. rn-b.

READING.

ach. ag-na. aga. al-o. amm-ca. anan. anm. aps. ara. art-v. as. as-o. asr. atp. atrop. bar. ber. br. bry. c-bis. ca-ca. ca-o. ca-pa. ca-s. cb-v. cd-sa. chd. chi. cic. cmc. co. cof. con. cot. cro. crt. cth. cund. cyc. dl-s. dph. drm. dro. dt. ery. glo. glp. gn-c. grp. grt. hæm. hg. hrc. hur. hyo. i. jnp-s. k-ca. k-i. k-o. klm. kre. lac-c. lac-d. lac-f. lch. li-ca. lpd. lyc. men. mg-ca. mg-cl. mgs-ar. mn-ca. mph. mrl. myris. n-x. na-ca. na-cl. na-sa. narth. ner. nic. p. p-x. pet. phy. pnx. pol. pul. rho. rmx. rs-v. rut. s. s-x. sb-t. sep. si-x. smi. so-d. sr-ca. stach. str-i. thu. trg. val. vi-o. vin. vtx. zn.

OBJECTS, FALSE APPEARANCE of. aga. anm. atp. atrop. bry. chd. chi. co. cro. cund. dro. dt. ery. glo. gn-c. grp. hg. hyo. jnp-s. lac-c. li-ca. lyc. na-cl. pb. pnx. pol. sb-t. si-x. smi. thu. trg. vi-o.

Black. hg. thu.

Blue. atp.

Confused. anm. atp. atrop. bry. chd. chi. co. (cund). dro. dt. ery. glo. grp. hæm. hg. hyo. jnp-s. k-o. lyc. na-cl. pnx. pol. si-x. trg. vi-o.

Green. lac-c.

Grey. dt.

Large. atp.

Moving. aga. atp. cic. con. dt. hg. hyo. k-o.

Vertically. con.

Vibrating. atp. k-o.

Multiplied. dt. sb-t.

Horizontally. sb-t.

Part Visible. lac-c. li-ca. pb.

Vertical. ph.

Red. cro. lac-c. smi.

Small. glo.

Variegated. atp. cic. lac-c.

White. chi. dro. ery. si-x.

Yellow. atp. lac-c.

OBJECTS, IMAGINARY. ag-na. ca-ca. ca-pa. cd-sa. chi. cic. cot. cro. dl-s. dro. dt. ery. gn-c. grt. hæm. k-ca. k-o. lac-c. lch. mg-cl. mph. n-x. na-ca. p-x. pet. pol. rmx. sb-t. sr-ca. trg. vin.

Black. ca-ca. ca-pa. ery. k-ca. sb-t. trg.

Bright. dl-s. dt. sb-t.

M

Circles. k-ca.
Cobweb. k-ca.
Figures. ca-pa.
  Moving from Right to Left. ca-pa.
Flashes, Bright. dl-s. sb-t.
Green. lac-c. n-x. sr-ca.
Grey. (ca-pa). lch.
Halo. chi. cic.
  Variegated. cic.
  White. chi.
High up. mg-cl.
Mist. (ag-na). cd-sa. cro. dro. gn-c. grt. hæm. k-ca. k-o. mg-cl. mph. na-ca. p-x. pet. pol. rmx. vin.
 Moving from Right to Left. ca-pa.
Red. cot. lac-c.
Rocks, High up. mg-cl.
Spots. ca-ca. ca-pa. cot. dt. ery. k-ca. lac-c. lch. n-x.
 Black. ca-ca. ca-pa. ery. k-ca.
 Bright. dt.
 Green. lac-c. n-x.
 Grey. ca-pa. (lch).
 Red. cot. lac-c.
 White. ery.
 Yellow. cot. lac-c. lch.
Variegated. cic.
Veil. dro. gn-c.
Vibrations. dt. p-x. pol. trg.
 Black. trg.
 Bright. dt.
Waves. sr-ca.
 Green. sr-ca.
White. chi. ery.
Yellow. cot. lac-c. lch.
PHOTOPHOBIA. (lac-f).
SIGHT DAZZLED. pol.
SIGHT IMPAIRED. ag-na. aga. art-v. asr. br. bry. ca-ca. ca-s. cd-sa. chd. cro. crt. dph. dro. dt. glo. gn-c. grt. hæm. hur. i. k-ca. k-i. k-o. lac-f. lch. li-ca. men. mg-ca. mph. myris. n-x. na-ca. na-cl. p. p-x. pet. pol. rho. rmx. rs-v. s. sep. smi. str-i. thu. vin.
 Myopia. p-x.
 Presbyopia. rmx.
EYEBALL. ach. aga. al-o. amm-ca. aps. ara. art-v. as.

asr. bar. c-bis. ca-ca. ca-o. cmc. con. cro. cyc. dph. ery.
grp. grt. hrc. k-ca. k-i. lac-c. lac-f. li-ca. lpd. mn-ca. mrl.
n-x. na-ca. na-sa. ner. nic. p. pet. phy. pol. pul. rho. rs-v.
rut. s. s-x. sep. smi. so-d. stach. thu. vtx.

Bursting. asr. stach.

Color, Red. (lac-f).

Contractive. sep.

Cutting. ca-ca. pet.

Drawing. art-v.

Dryness. art-v. (as-o). bar. (grp). li-ca. na-ca. p.

False Sensations. pul.

 Sand. pul.

Gnawing. (str-i).

Heat. bar. ca-ca. ca-o. cro. cyc. (grp). na-ca. ner. nic.
pol. rho. rut. s. s-x. thu. vtx. (zn).

Heaviness. (na-sa).

Lachrymation. amm-ca. c-bis. cro. grt. hrc. (lac-f).
lpd. n-x. ner. p. s-x..

Movements. (aga). (ber). (ca-ca). (cro). (lac-d). (mrl).

 Convulsions. (aga). (ber). (lac-d).

  Feeling of. ara.

Paralysis. asr. k-i.

Pressing. ach. (aga). (al-o). con. cro. mn-ca. na-sa.
pul. smi. zn.

Shooting. ach. aps. k-ca.

Smarting. (ca-ca). cro. (li-ca). p. (s-x). (sep). (str-i).

Stiffness. ca-ca.

Tensive. ca-ca. ner.

Throbbing. (lac-f).

Undefined. art-v. as-o. (chd). dph. ery. lac-c. (lac-d).
li-ca. phy. rs-v. rut.

ORBITAL INTEGUMENTS. chd.

EYELIDS. as-o. ber. ca-ca. cro. grp. mrl. na-sa. ner.
str-i. zn.

Cutting. ca-ca.

Dryness. as-o. grp.

Heat. ca-ca. grp.

Movements, Convulsions. ber.

  Winking. ca-ca. cro. mrl.

Smarting. ca-ca.

UPPER EYELID. na-sa. zn.

Heaviness. na-sa.

TARSAL EDGES. li-ca. str.

Gnawing. str-i.
Smarting. li-ca. str-i.
CANTHI. lac-d. sep.
INTERNAL CANTHUS. li-ca. sep.
Smarting. sep.
FORWARDS. cmc.
Eyeball, Pressing. cmc.
BACKWARDS. lac-f.
DOWNWARDS. cmc.
Eyeball, Pressing. cmc.
To HEAD. lac-f.
To FOREHEAD. lac-f.
To TEMPLE. lac-f.
RIGHT. al-o. lac-f. mg-ca. rho.
Photophobia. lac-f.
Sight Impaired. mg-ca.
Eyeball, Color Red. lac-f.
    Heat. rho.
    Lachrymation. lac-f.
    Pressing. al-o.
    Shooting. lac-f.
Backwards, Eyeball Shooting. lac-f.
To Forehead. Eyeball, Shooting. lac-f.
          Throbbing. lac-f.
To Temple. Eyeball, Shooting. lac-f.
          Throbbing. lac-f.
LEFT. ag-na. agà. cund. dt. lac-d. lch. ner. s-x. zn.
Objects, False Appearance of, Confused. cund.
Objects, Imaginary, Bright. dt.
      Grey. lch.
      Mist. ag-na.
      Spots, Bright. dt.
      Grey. lch.

Eyeball, Heat. s-x.
    Lachrymation. s-x.
    Movements, Convulsions. aga.
    Pressing. aga.
    Smarting. s-x.
Eyelids, Tensive. ner.
Upper Eyelid, Heat. zn.
      Pressing. zn.
Internal Canthus, Movements, Convulsions. lac-d.
      Undefined. lac-d.

READING WRITING.

con. dt. lch.
OBJECTS, FALSE APPEARANCE of. con. dt.
Moving. con.
      Vertically. con.
Multiplied. dt.
OBJECTS, IMAGINARY. lch.
Grey. (lch.)
Spots. (lch).
    Grey. (lch).
LEFT. lch.
Objects, Imaginary, Grey. lch.
           Spots. lch.
             Grey. lch.

SEWING.

ag-na. amm-ca. amm-cl. ca-ca. eupat. k-ca. lac-d. lct, mrl.
OBJECTS, FALSE APPEARANCE of. lct. mrl.
Confused. lct. mrl.
OBJECTS IMAGINARY. ag-na. amm-ca. amm-cl.
Black. amm-ca.
Mist. (ag-na).
Spots. amm-ca. amm-cl.
    Black. amm-ca.
    Yellow. amm-cl.
Yellow. amm-cl.
SIGHT IMPAIRED. ca-ca. eupat.
EYEBALL. k-ca. rmx.
Movements. (lac-d).
    Convulsions. (lac-d).
Shooting. k-ca.
Smarting. rmx.
Undefined. (lac-d).
CANTHI. lac-d.
INTERNAL CANTHUS. lac-d.
LEFT. ag-na. lac-d.
Objects Imaginary, Mist. ag-na.
Internal Canthus, Movements, Convulsions. lac-d.
        Undefined. lac-d.

SPINNING.

dt. mg-sa.
OBJECTS IMAGINARY. mg-sa.
Figures. mg-sa.
SIGHT IMPAIRED. dt.

WRITING.

ag-na. al-o. alo. ara. ca-ca. ca-s. cb-v. chd. cle. co. crb-x.
cth. dl-s. dph. ele. ery. fe. grp. grt. k-bicr. k-ca. lac-f. lch.
lct. lyc. mrl. na-ca. na-cl. narth. ol-a. p-x. pet. physo. pol.
ppv. rho. rs-v. sep. sr-ca. thu. val. vin. zn.
OBJECTS, FALSE APPEARANCE of. chd. cle.
crb-x. ery. grp. k-ca. lyc. ppv.
  Confused. chd. cle. crb-x. ery. k-ca. lyc. ppv.
  Moving. k-ca. thu.
      Circularly. k-ca.
      Vibrating. thu.
  Multiplied. cle. ery. grp.
OBJECTS IMAGINARY. cle. ery. grt. k-ca. na-ca.
ol-a. p-x. sr-ca. vin.
  Black. na-ca.
  Bright. cle. ery. ol-a.
  Green. sr-ca.
  Mist. vin.
  Spots. ery. na-ca. ol-a.
      Black. na-ca.
      Bright. ery. ol-a.
  Stars. k-ca.
  Veil. grt. ol-a. p-x.
  Vibrations. cle.
      Bright. cle.
  Waves. sr-ca.
      Green. sr-ca.
PHOTOPHOBIA. (lac-f).
SIGHT IMPAIRED. ag-na. alo. chd. co. cth. ele. grt.
k-ca. lct. na-cl. ol-a. p-x. physo. rho. sep. zn.
  Myopia. p-x.
EYEBALL. al-o. ara. ca-ca. co. dl-s. fe. lac-f. na-ca.
na-cl. ol-a. pol. rho. rs-v. sep. thu. zn.
  Color Red. (lac-f).

Contractive. sep.
Creeping. ol-a.
Dryness. na-ca. na-cl.
Heat. dl-s. (k-bicr). (lct). na-ca. na-cl. pol. rho. thu. zn.

Lachrymation. ca-ca. fe. (lac-f). ol-a. zn.
Movements. (ca-s). (dph). (ery).

Convulsions, Feeling of. ara.

Paralysis. (fe).
Pressing. co.
Shooting. co. (lac-f).
Smarting. co. dl-s.
Throbbing. (lac-f).
Undefined. rs-v.
IRIS. lct.
Pupils Dilated. lct.
EYELIDS. ca-s. dph. ery. fe. lct. pol.
Heat. lct. pol.
Movements, Closing. dph. ery.

Winking. ca-s.

Paralysis. fe.
CANTHI. k-bicr.
INTERNAL CANTHUS. k-bicr.
Heat. k-bicr.
BACKWARDS. lac-f.
To HEAD. lac-f.
To FOREHEAD. lac-f.
To TEMPLE. lac-f.
RIGHT. al-o. lac-f.
Photophobia. lac-f.
Eyeball, Color Red. lac-f.

Lachrymation. lac-f.

Pressing. al-o.

Shooting. lac-f.

Backwards. Eyeball Shooting. lac-f.
To Forehead. Eyeball, Shooting. lac-f.

Throbbing. lac-f.

To Temple. Eyeball, Shooting. lac-f.

Throbbing. lac-f.

LOOKING FIXEDLY. (Long, Exerting Eyes).

ac-s. aga. al-o. amm-ca. amm-cl. aps. art-v. au. ba-a. ba-ca. ca-ca. cast. cb-v. chd. cic. cl-hx. cmc. co. con. (cph). cro. cth. dl-s. dro. eug. gel. grp. hæm. hg. hg-s. k-bicr. (k-ca). k-o. kre. lac-c. lch. led. lyc. mg-ca. mn-ca. mtr. n-x. na-cl. na-sa. ni-ca. nic. p. p-x. pet. pnx. pol. pru-l. pt. qu-sa. rhe. rho. rn-b. rs. rs-v. rut. s. s-x. smc. smi. spi. spo. sr-ca. thu. trn. tx-b. val.

OBJECTS, FALSE APPEARANCE of. aga. amm-ca. cic. cl-hx. con. eug. k-o. lac-c. n-x. pnx. pol.

Black. n-x.

Confused. cic. cl-hx. eug. (k-bicr). k-o.

　　Outlines. k-bicr.

Moving. eug. k-o. pol.

　　Vibrating. eug. k-o. pol.

Multiplied. amm-ca. con. pnx.

Red. lac-c.

White. aga.

OBJECTS, IMAGINARY. ac-s. aga. al-o. amm-ca. amm-cl. art-v. ca-ca. lac-c. lch. na-sa. nic. p-x. pet. rut.

Black. ac-s. amm-ca.

Bright. (na-sa). nic. p-x.

Circles. lch.

　　Grey. lch.

Green. sr-ca.

Grey. lch.

Mist. (na-sa).

Near Eye (na-sa).

Red. lac-c.

Spots. ac-s. amm-ca. amm-cl. lac-c.

　　Black. ac-s. amm-ca.

　　Red. lac-c.

　　Yellow. amm-cl.

Stars. (na-sa).

　　Bright. (na-sa).

　　　　Near Eye. (na-sa).

　　Green. (na-sa).

　　　　Near Eye. (na-sa).

　　Near Eye. (na-sa).

　　Yellow. (na-sa).

　　　　Near Eye. (na-sa).

Veil. aga. al-o. art-v. ca-ca. lch. pet. rut.

Vibrations. nic. p-x.

    Bright. nic. p-x

Waves. sr-ca.

    Green. sr-ca.

Yellow. amm-cl.

SIGHT DAZZLED. s.

SIGHT IMPAIRED. aga. al-o. art-v. ca-ca. cast. cb-v. hæm. k-bicr. lch. mg-ca. mn-ca. n-x. (na-sa). nic. pet. qu-sa. rs-v. rut. spi. thu. trn.

Myopia. cb-v.

EYEBALL. aps. au. ba-ca. cb-v. cmc. dl-s. dro. hg. hg-s. k-bicr. kre. mn-ca. na-cl. na-sa. ni-ca. nic. p. pet. pol. pru-l. pt. rhe. rho. rs. s. s-x. smc. smi. spo. sr-ca. tx-b. val.

Color Red. au. sr-ca.

Drawing. (pru-l).

Dryness. rho.

False Sensations. hg.

    Sand. hg.

Heat. ba-ca. k-bicr. ni-ca. pet. rho. s-x. sr-ca.

Lachrymation. (cph). (hg-s). (k-ca). kre. nic. pol. (s). spo. sr-ca. tx-b.

    Hot. (k-ca).

Movements. (gel).

Pressing. ba-ca. cmc. mn-ca. na-cl. (na-sa). p. pet. rhe. rs. s-x. smc. val.

Shooting. dl-s.

Smarting. cmc. (co). dro.

Tensive. au.

Undefined. aps. (cb-v). (cmc). (co). nic. pt. rhe. (rut). smi.

EYEBALL SUPERIORLY. pru-l.

Drawing. pru-l.

EYEBALL ANTERIORLY. s-x.

Heat. s-x.

Pressing. s-x.

IRIS. p-x.

Pupils, Dilated. (p-x).

EYELIDS. co. gel. pru-l.

Movements, Closing. gel.

Smarting. co.

Undefined. co.

UPPER EYELID. co. pru-l.

Smarting. co.

TARSAL EDGES. pru-l.

UPPER TARSAL EDGE. pru-l.

Drawing. pru-l.

CANTHI. p-x.

INTERNAL CANTHUS. p-x.

Pressing. p-x.

CHANGING CHARACTER or PLACE in EYES. na-sa.

Objects Imaginary Mist, then Star Bright Green Yellow Near Eye. (na-sa).

OBJECTS IMAGINARY then EYEBALL. na-sa.

SIGHT IMPAIRED then OBJECTS IMAGINARY. na-sa.

RIGHT. hg-s. mg-ca. na-sa. p-x. s. trn.

Objects Imaginary, Bright. na-sa.

   Green. na-sa.

   Mist. na-sa.

   Near Eye. na-sa.

   Star. na-sa.

     Bright. na-sa.

        Near Eye. na-sa.

     Green. na-sa.

        Near Eye. na-sa.

     Near Eye. na-sa.

     Yellow. na-sa.

        Near Eye. na-sa.

   Yellow. na-sa.

Sight Impaired. mg-ca. na-sa. trn.

Eyeball, Lachrymation. hg-s. s.

     Pressing. na-sa.

Iris, Pupil Dilated. p-x.

Changing. Objects Imaginary Mist, then Star Bright Green Yellow Near Eye. na-sa.

       Objects Imaginary, then Eyeball, Star Bright Green Yellow Near Eye, then Pressing. na-sa.

       Sight Impaired, then Star Bright Green Yellow Near Eye. na-sa.

LEFT. cb-v.

Eyeball Undefined. cb-v.

LOOKING UP.

al-o. as-o. atp. ba-ca. cb-v. chd. crot. cu. dt. hg-s. jup-s.
k-ca. lac-c. mn-ca. p. pul. s. vr-s. zn.
OBJECTS IMAGINARY. atp. cu. dt. p. zu.
Black. p. (zn).
Bright. dt. zn.
High up. dt.
Mist. atp. p.
    Black. p.
    White. atp.
Semicircle. dt.
    Bright. dt.
        High up. dt.
    High up. dt.
Spots. dt. zn.
    Bright dt.
        High up. dt.
    High up. dt.
Stars. atp.
    White. atp.
Stripes. dt. (zn).
    Black. (zn).
        Upwards to Left. zn.
    Bright. dt.
        High up. dt.
        Upwards to Right. dt.
        Vertical. dt.
    High up. dt.
    Upwards to Right. dt.
    Upwards to Left. (zn).
    Vertical. dt.
Upwards to Right. dt.
Upwards to Left. (zn).
Veil. cu.
Vertical. dt.
White. atp.
SIGHT IMPAIRED. cu.
EYEBALL. al-o. as-o. atp. ba-ca. cb-v. chd. crot. hg-s.
k-ca. lac-c. mn-ca. p. s. vr-s.
Heat. al-o.
Movements. (al-o).
    Convulsions. (al-o).

Paralysis. (dt).
Pressing. (as-o). atp. ba-ca. crot. mn-ca. vr-s.
Shooting. (as-o).
Swelling, Feeling of. (hg-s).
Tensive. (hg-s). p. s. vr-a.
Undefined. (as-o). cb-v. chd. (k-ca). lac-c.
EYEBALL SUPERIORLY. as-o.
Pressing. as-o.
Undefined. as-o.
EYELIDS. as-o. hg-s.
Swelling, Feeling of. hg-s.
UPPER EYELID. as-o.
Undefined. as-o.
LEFT. al-o. as-o. k-ca. zn.
Objects Imaginary, Black. zn.
    Stripe. zn.
        Black. zn.
           Upwards to Left. zn.
      Upwards to Left. zn.
Eyeball, Movements, Convulsions. al-o.
    Undefined. k-ca.
Eyeball Superiorly, Shooting. as-o.

LOOKING DOWN.

acon. al-o. dt. klm. mll. ner. p. pnx. s. tep.
OBJECTS, FALSE APPEARANCE of. mll. ner. pnx.
tep.
Large. mll.
Moving. pnx. tep.
Multiplied. ner.
OBJECTS, IMAGINARY. dt. klm. p.
Black. p.
Blue. dt.
Bright. klm.
Mist. p.
    Black. p.
Spots. dt.
    Blue. dt.
Vibrations. klm.
    Bright. klm.
SIGHT IMPAIRED. klm.

EYEBALL. acon. al-o.
Heat. acon.
Movements. (al-o).
      Convulsions. (al-o).
Pressing. acon. (s).
EYELIDS. s.
UPPER EYELID. s.
Pressing. s.
LEFT. alo.
Eyeball, Movements, Convulsions. alo.

LOOKING SIDEWAYS. (Around).

acon. ba-a. gel. mg-ca. mg-sa. ner. pol. sr-ca.
OBJECTS, FALSE APPEARANCE of. ca-ca. gel.
Moving. ca-ca.
      Circularly. ca-ca.
Multiplied. gel.
OBJECTS IMAGINARY. pol. sr-ca.
Bright. pol.
Green. sr-ca.
Spots. pol. sr-ca.
      Bright. pol.
      Green. sr-ca.
SIGHT IMPAIRED. ner.
EYEBALL. acon. ba-a. mg-sa. si x.
Heat. acon.
Pressing. acon. ba-a. mg-sa.
Undefined. si-x.
FORWARDS. mg-sa.
Eyeball, Pressing. mg-sa.

LOOKING INWARDS.

mn-ca.
EYEBALL. mn-ca.
Pressing. mn-ca.

LOOKING to RIGHT.

dig. sep.
OBJECTS, FALSE APPEARANCE of. dig.
Multiplied. dig.
EYEBALL. dig. sep.
Pressing. sep.
Undefined. dig.

LOOKING to LEFT.

na-sa. smi.
OBJECTS, IMAGINARY. na-sa.
Bright. (na-sa).
Green. (na-sa).
Mist. (na-sa).
Near Eye. (na-sa).
Star. (na-sa).
    Bright. (na-sa).
        Near Eye. (na-sa).
    Green. (na-sa).
        Near Eye. (na-sa).
    Near Eye. (na-sa).
    Yellow. (na-sa).
        Near Eye. (na-sa).
Yellow. (na-sa).
SIGHT IMPAIRED. (na-sa).
EYEBALL. smi.
Bruised. (smi).
RIGHT. na-sa. smi.
Objects, Imaginary, Bright. na-sa.
    Green. na-sa.
    Mist. na-sa.
    Near Eye. na-sa.
    Star. na-sa.
        Bright. na-sa.
            Near Eye. na-sa.
        Green. na-sa.
            Near Eye. na-sa.
        Near Eye. na-sa.
        Yellow. na-sa.
            Near Eye. na-sa.
    Yellow. na-sa.
Sight Impaired. na-sa.
Eyeball, Bruised. smi.

LOOKING into the AIR.

amm-cl. dt. k-ca. s. thu.
OBJECTS, IMAGINARY. amm-cl. dt. k-ca. s. thu.
Black. k-ca.

Bright. dt.
Far off. dt.
Spots. amm-cl. dt. k-ca. s. thu.
    Black. k-ca.
    Bright. dt.
        Far off. dt.
   Far off. dt.
   White. s. thu.
   Yellow. amm-cl.
Veil. k-ca.
White. s. thu.
Yellow. amm-cl.
LEFT. dt.
Objects Imaginary, Bright. dt.
    Far off. dt.
    Spots. dt.
      Bright. dt.
        Far off. dt.
      Far off. dt.

LOOKING at NEAR Objects.

ag-na. al-o. amm-ca. atp. bry. buf. ca-a. ca-ca. cb-a. chd. con. cub. dph. dro. dt. f-hx. glp. grt. hyo. k-o. lyc. mg-cl. mn-ca. na-cl. p-x. pet. phy. pul. s. sep. si-x. spi. srr. str. trg. val.

OBJECTS, FALSE APPEARANCE of. amm-ca.
Multiplied. amm-ca.
OBJECTS, IMAGINARY. (dt).
Figures. (dt).
SIGHT DAZZLED. p-x.
SIGHT IMPAIRED. **(Presbyopia).** ag-na. al-o. amm-ca. atp. bry. buf. ca-a. ca-ca. cb-a. con. dph. dro. dt. f-hx. glp. grt. hyo. k-o. lyc. mg-cl. na-cl. p-x. pet. phy. pul. rmx. s. sep. si-x. spi. srr. str. trg. val.
EYEBALL. mn-ca. p-x.
Pressing. mn-ca. p-x.
LEFT. cb-a.
Sight Impaired. cb-a.

LOOKING at DISTANT Objects.

ach. aga. amm-ca. as-o. atp. ber. buf. ca-ca. ca-s. cac.
cb-v. chi. cmf. con. cyc. dig. dph. dt. eupat-p. euph. euphr.
gel. glp. grp. grt. hyo. i. krm. lyc. mn-ca. n-x. na-ca. na-cl.
ni-ca. nic. ol-a. p-x. pb. pet. physo. pul. rut. s. s-x. sb-t.
se. si-x. smc. spo. srr. thu. trg. val. vi-o. vi-t. vrb. woo.
OBJECTS, FALSE APPEARANCE of. atp. chi. gel.
i. n-x. ni-ca. nic.
Blue. i.
Confused. chi. gel.
Large. ni-ca.
Multiplied. amm-ca. atp. n-x. nic.
     Horizontally. n-x.
OBJECTS, IMAGINARY. dig.
Black. dig.
Spots. dig.
     Black. dig.
SIGHT IMPAIRED. (**Myopia**). ach. aga. amm-ca.
(as-o). ber. buf. ca-ca. ca-s. cac. cb-v. chi. cmf. con. cyc.
dph. dt. eupat-p. euph. gel. glp. grp. grt. hyo. krm. lyc.
mn-ca. n-x. na-ca. na-cl. ol-a. p. p-x. pb. pet. physo. pul.
rut. s. s-x. sb-t. se. si-x. smc. spo. srr. thu. trg. val. vi-o.
vi-t. vrb. woo.
LEFT. as-o. ca-ca.
Sight Impaired. as-o. ca-ca.

CHANGING AXIS of VISION.

lac-c.
SIGHT IMPAIRED. lac-c.

LOOKING at SMALL Objects.

atp. cd-sa. cof. cyc. dro. dt. clc. eupat. i. mph. na-ca.
pet. s.
OBJECTS, FALSE APPEARANCE of. dt.
Multiplied. dt.

OBJECTS, IMAGINARY. dro.
Bright. dro.
Vibrations. dro.
    Bright. dro.
SIGHT IMPAIRED. (atp). cd-sa. cyc. dt. ele. eupat.
mph. na-ca. pet. s.
Presbyopia. atp.

LOOKING at LINEAR **Objects.**

ox-x.
OBJECTS, FALSE APPEARANCE of. ox-x.
Far. ox-x.
Large. ox-x.

LOOKING at FIXED **Objects.**

pb.
OBJECTS, FALSE APPEARANCE of. pb.
White. pb.

LOOKING at DIFFERENT **Objects.**

lac-c.
EYEBALL. lac-c.
Pressing. lac-c.

LOOKING at FLOWING WATER.

fe.
OBJECTS, FALSE APPEARANCE of. fe.
Moving. fe.
    Circularly. fe.

LOOKING at BLACK **Objects.**

dt. (str). trn.
OBJECTS, FALSE APPEARANCE of. dt. (str).
Grey. dt. (str).
OBJECTS, IMAGINARY. trn.
Mist. trn.

N

LOOKING at BLUE Objects.

art-v. lpd. snt.
OBJECTS, FALSE APPEARANCE of. art-v.
Green. art-v.
Grey. lpd.

LOOKING at GREEN Objects.

trn.
OBJECTS, IMAGINARY. trn.
Mist. trn.

LOOKING at GREY Objects.

snt.
OBJECTS, FALSE APPEARANCE of. snt.
Blue. snt.
Yellow. snt.

LOOKING at RED Objects.

art-v. grp. trn.
OBJECTS, FALSE APPEARANCE of. art-v.
Yellow. art-v.
OBJECTS, IMAGINARY. trn.
Mist. trn.
EYEBALL. grp.
Shooting. grp.
INWARDS. grp.
Eyeball, Shooting. grp.

LOOKING at WHITE Objects.

acon. as-o. cro. dt. (ery). grp. hyo. k-ca. mtr. na-cl. nic.
(p). smi. sr-ca.
OBJECTS, FALSE APPEARANCE of. art-v. cro.
smi.
Red. cro. smi.
Yellow. art-v.
OBJECTS, IMAGINARY. acon. dt. (ery). hyo. k-ca.
(p). sr-ca.
Black. acon. (p).

Blue. dt.
Bright. acon. dt.
Figures. hyo. (p).
Green. sr-ca.
Grey. dt.
Halo. dt. hyo.
    Grey. dt.
    Red. dt.
    Yellow. hyo.
Red. dt.
Spots. acon. dt. k-ca. (p).
    Black. acon. (p).
    Blue. dt.
    Bright. acon. dt.
    White. k-ca.
Threads. (ery).
Waves. sr-ca.
    Green. sr-ca.
White. k-ca.
Yellow. hyo.
SIGHT DAZZLED. as-o. grp.
SIGHT IMPAIRED. mtr. nic.
EYEBALL. grp.
Lachrymation. grp.
Shooting. grp.
INWARDS. grp.
Eyeball, Shooting. grp.

LOOKING at YELLOW Objects.

snt. trn.
OBJECTS, FALSE APPEARANCE of. snt.
Red. snt.
OBJECTS, IMAGINARY. trn.
Mist. trn.

LOOKING at BRIGHT OBJECTS.

amm-cl. buf. cch. cmc. dt. grp. grt. mg-cl. p-x. sep. str-i.
vr-s.
SIGHT DAZZLED. p-x.
SIGHT IMPAIRED. dt. grt.
EYEBALL. buf. cmc. grp. p-x.
Pressing. cmc. p-x.

N 2

Shooting. grp.
Undefined. buf. (cmc).
EYEBALL POSTERIORLY. cmc.
FORWARDS. cmc.
Eyeball, Pressing. cmc.
DOWNWARDS. cmc.
Eyeball, Pressing. cmc.
INWARDS. grp.
Eyeball, Shooting. grp.
To HEAD. cmc.
To OCCIPUT. cmc.
Eyeball Posteriorly, Undefined. cmc.

LOOKING at ARTIFICIAL LIGHT.

acon. ag-na. al-o. anan. atp. ba-ca. ca-ca. (chd). cic. cmc.
cph. dig. dl-s. dt. euph. euphr. fe-mgs. hpp. i. k-ca. k-na. k-o.
kre. lyc. mg-cl. mim. mtr. n-x. ni-ca. os. os-x. p. p-x. pb. ptv.
pul. rut. s. sep. smc. smi. sn. sr-ca. srr. til. trg. vr-v. zn.

OBJECTS, FALSE APPEARANCE of. (**Appear-
ance of Flame**). acon. ag-na. anan. atp. ba-ca. (chd) dig.
euphr. fe-mgs. hpp. i. k-na. k-o. kre. lyc. n-x. ni-ca. os. pb.
ptv. smc. sn. til.
　Black. euphr. k-o. smc.
　Blue. dig. hpp. kre.
　Bright. dig.
　Confused. ag-na. euphr. i. n-x. os. os-x. til.
　Large. anan. dig. os. os-x.
　Moving. acon. euphr. lyc. smc.
　　　Vibrating. acon. euphr. lyc. smc.
　Multiplied. ni-ca. pb.
　Small. (chd).
　Variegated. ag-na. atp. ba-ca. fe-mgs. k-na. ni-ca. sn.
　Yellow. ptv.
OBJECTS IMAGINARY. al-o. atp. ba-ca. ca-ca. cic.
cmc. cph. dig. dl-s. dt. euph. k-ca. k-na. k-o. mg-cl. mim.
mtr. n-x. os. p. p-x. ptv. pul. rut. s. sep. smc. smi. sn. sr-ca.
srr. trg. vr-v. zn.
　Black. k-o. p.
　Blue. cph. trg.
　Bright. ca-ca. dt. pul. trg.
　Green. k-o. mg-cl. p. rut. sep. vr-v. zn.

Grey. p. sep.

Halo. al-o. atp. ba-ca. ca-ca. cic. cmc. cph. dig. dl-s. euph. k-ca. k-na. k-o. mg-cl. mim. n-x. os. p. p-x. ptv. pul. rut. s. sep. smc. smi. sn. sr-ca. trg. vr-v. zn.

    Black. k-o. p.
    Blue. cph. trg.
    Bright. ca-ca. dt. pul. trg.
    Green. k-o. mg-cl. p. rut. sep. vr-v. zn.
    Grey. p. sep.
    Red. atp. (cmc). cph. ptv. rut. s. trg. vr-v.
    Star-like. pul.
    Variegated. atp. ba-ca. cic. k-na. k-o. os.

Rays. atp. k-ca. mtr. srr. trg.

Red. atp. (cmc). cph. ptv. rut. s. trg. vr-v.

Spots. dt.

    Bright. dt.

Stars. pul.

Variegated. atp. ba-ca. cic. k-na. k-o. os.

RIGHT. cmc.

Objects Imaginary, Halo. cmc.
                    Red. cmc.
            Red. cmc.

LEFT. atp. zn.

Objects Imaginary. **Green**. zn.
                Halo. atp.
                    Green. zn.
                    Variegated. atp.
                Rays. atp.
                Variegated. atp.

LOOKING SUDDENLY in the DARK.

p-x.

EYEBALL. p-x.

Pressing. p-x.

LOOKING through SPECTACLES.

na-ba.

EYEBALL. na-ba.

Heat. . na-ba.

Movements. (na-ha).
EYELIDS. na-ba.
Movements, Closing. na-ba.
                    Spasmodically. na-ba.

LOOKING with RIGHT EYE.

lyc.
OBJECTS, FALSE APPEARANCE of. lyc.
Part Visible. lyc.
        Vertical. lyc.
                Left Side Visible. lyc.

LOOKING into IMAGINARY BRIGHT SPOT.

chd.
EYEBALL. chd.
Lachrymation. chd.

LACHRYMATION.

(ca-s). mgs.
EYEBALL. ca-s. mgs.
Eruptions. (ca-s).
        Blisters. (ca-s).
Undefined. mgs.
EYEBALL ROUND CORNEA. (ca-s).
Eruptions, Blisters. (ca-s).

MOVING EYES.

acon. ag-na. arn. as-o. atp. bry. ca-a. ca-ca. ca-o. ca-s. cb-v.
chd. chi. cit-c. cle. cmc. con. cor. cph. crt. cu. dig. eryn. gel.
hg. hpp. k-bicr. k-ca. k-o. klm. lau-c. lo-cœ. lyc. mg-ca.
mn-ca. mph. mtr. n-x. na-cl. nic. ox-x. p. pb. pul. rn-b. rn-s.
rs. s. sa-l. sep. si-x. sn. spi. spo. spo-f. sr-ca. stc. str-i. trg.
val. vi-t. vtx. ziz. zn.
OBJECTS, FALSE APPEARANCE of. gel.
Confused. gel.
OBJECTS IMAGINARY. atp. p.
Black. p.
Bright. atp.

Mist. p.
    Black. p.
Spots. atp.
    Bright. atp.
PHOTOPHOBIA. ca-s.
SIGHT IMPAIRED. con.
EYEBALL. acon. ag-na. as-o. atp. bry. ca-ca. ca-s. cb-v.
chd. chi. cmc. cor. cph. crt. eryn. hg. hpp. k-bicr. k-ca. klm.
lau-c. lo-cœ. lyc. mph. n-x. nic. ox-x. pb. pul. rn-b. rn-s. rs.
s. sa-l. sep. sn. spi. spo-f. sr-ca. stc. str-i. trg. val. vi-t. vtx.
    Bruised. (cu). (vtx).
    Bursting. acon. (lau-c).
    Drawing. pb.
    Dryness. (arn). (as-o). atp. crt.
    False Sensations. chi. hg. (rs).
        Sand. chi. hg. (rs).
    Heat. acon.
    Heaviness. chi. pb.
    Motion, in. (rs).
        Passing Round, like Something. (rs).
    Movements. gel.
        Convulsions. gel.
    Pressing. acon. atp. ca-s. cph. crt. hg. mn-ca. (mtr).
nic. sep. spi. trg. (val).
    Shooting. acon. (as-o). (sn). (spi). (spo). sr-ca. (vi-t).
    Smarting. (arn). (chd). (cmc). cor. lo-cœ. stc.
    Stiffness. atp. ca-ca.
    Swelling, Feeling of. spi.
    Tensive. ca-ca. n-x. s. (sn). (spo). (vi-t).
    Undefined. acon. ag-na. (as-o). bry. (ca-o). cb-v. chd.
eryn. hpp. k-bicr. k-ca. klm. lyc. mph. ox-x. pul. rn-b. rn-s.
rs. s. (sa-l). si-x. spi. spo-f. str-i. (ziz).
EYEBALL SUPERIORLY. acon.
    Bursting. acon.
    Undefined. acon.
EYEBALL EXTERNALLY. vtx.
    Bruised. vtx.
EYEBALL INTERIORLY. as-o.
ORBIT. chd. cu. ziz.
    Bruised. cu.
    Smarting. chd.
EYELIDS. arn. as-o. ca-a. ca-o. mtr.
    Adhesion of. ca-a.

UPPER EYELID. ca-o. mtr.
Pressing. mtr.
Undefined. ca-o.
TARSAL EDGES. arn. as-o.
Dryness. arn. as-o.
Smarting. arn.
Undefined. as-o.
CANTHI. spo.
EXTERNAL CANTHUS. spo.
FORWARDS. val.
Eyeball, Pressing. val.
To HEAD. spo-f.
To TEMPLE. spo-f.
Eyeball, Undefined. spo-f.
RIGHT. as-o. cmc. lau-c. rs. spi. vi-t. ziz.
Eyeball, Bursting. lau-c.
　　　　　　Motion in, Passing Round like Something. rs.
　　　　　　Shooting. as-o. spi. vi-t.
　　　　　　Smarting. cmc.
　　　　　　Tensive. vi-t.
Orbit, Undefined. ziz.
LEFT. as-o. sa-l. sn. spi. spo.
Eyeball, Pressing. spi.
　　　　　　Shooting. as-o. sn.
　　　　　　Tensive. sn.
　　　　　　Undefined. sa-l.
Eyeball Interiorly, Shooting. as-o.
External Canthus, Shooting. spo.
　　　　　　Tensive. spo.

MOVING EYELIDS.

alm. arn. as-o. atp. ber. c-bis. chd. chi. cor. euphr. k-bicr.
mgs-au. mn-ca. str-i. thu. trg.
OBJECTS, IMAGINARY. atp.
Bright. atp.
Spots. atp.
　　　　Bright. atp.
EYEBALL. arn. chd. chi. k-bicr. str-i. trg.
Bruised. (alm). trg.
Dryness. (as-o). chi.

False Sensations. chi. (thu).
    Sand. chi. (thu).
Heaviness. (ber).
Scraping. chd. k-bicr.
Smarting. arn. (c-bis).
Undefined. euphr. (mn-ca). str-i.
ORBIT. alm. trg.
Bruised. trg.
ORBIT INFERIORLY. alm.
EYELIDS. as-o. ber. c-bis. mn-ca.
Dryness. as-o.
Undefined. mn-ca.
UPPER EYELID. ber. c-bis.
Heaviness. ber.
CANTHI. thu.
INTERNAL CANTHUS. thu.
RIGHT. thu.
Internal Canthus, False Sensations, Sand. thu.
LEFT. alm. c-bis.
Orbit Inferiorly, Bruised. alm.
Upper Eyelid, Smarting. c-bis.

When EYELID is STILL.

asr.
EYEBALL. asr.
Movements. (asr).
    Convulsions. (asr).
EYELIDS. asr.
UPPER EYELID. asr.
LEFT. asr.
Upper Eyelid, Movements, Convulsions. asr.

OPENING EYELIDS.

acon. ag-na. al-o. asr. atp. au. (ca-i). chd. co. con. cph.
cro. cth. euph. grp. hg. k-bicr. mg-cl. na-ba. p. p-x. physo.
rs-r. s-x. spi. str. str-i. zn.
 OBJECTS, IMAGINARY. (spi).
Black. (spi).
Bright. (spi).

Spots. (spi).
    Black. (spi).
    Bright. (spi).
EYEBALL. acon. al-o. au. (ca-i). cph. grp. mg-cl. p-x. s-x. str-i. zn.
Bursting. acon.
Discharge. hg.
False Sensations. chd. s-x. str-i.
    Sand. chd. s-x. str-i.
Hæmorrhage. (atp).
Heat. al-o. mg-cl.
Lachrymation. au. (ca-i). con. cph. physo. (spi). zu.
    Hot. au. (ca-i). (spi).
Movements. (chd). (k-bicr).
    Convulsions. (k-bicr).
Pressing. acon. (na-ba). str-i.
Shooting. str-i.
Smarting. chd. (cth).
Undefined. al-o. (cth). grp. p-x.
EYELIDS. atp. chd. co. cth. k-bicr. na-ba.
Hæmorrhage. atp.
Movements, Closing. (chd).
    Spasmodically. chd.
    Convulsions. k-bicr.
As if connecting Strings Snapped. co.
UPPER EYELID. cth. na-ba.
Pressing. na-ba.
Undefined. cth.
TARSAL EDGES. cth.
Smarting. cth.
CANTHI. s-x.
EXTERNAL CANTHUS. s-x.
FORWARDS. acon.
Eyeball, Pressing. acon.
OUTWARDS. s-x.
RIGHT. s-x.
External Canthus, False Sensation, Sand. s-x.
Outwards. Eyeball, False Sensation, Sand. s-x.
LEFT. (spi).
Objects Imaginary, Black. (spi).
    Bright. (spi).
    Spots, Black. (spi).
    Bright. (spi).
Eyeball, Lachrymation. (spi).

CLOSING EYELIDS.

ag-na. aga. al-o. am-ni. as-o. atp. atrop. ba-ca. ber. ca-ca. ca-s. cb-v. chd. cle. cmf. con. cor. cro. cu. dig. dl-s. dt. elaps. f-hx. grt. hll. hpm. hur. jnp-s. k-o. lac-d. lau-c. lch. led. lo-c. lyc. mn-ca. na-ca. os. p. p-x. phy. pod. ptv. pul. rs-r. s. s-x. sep. si-x. smi. smr. spo. stc. str. thr. thu. vr-v.

OBJECTS, FALSE APPEARANCE of. ca-s. grt. si-x.

Moving. ca-s. grt. si-x.

  Circularly. ca-s. grt. si-x.

OBJECTS, IMAGINARY. ag-na. al-o. am-ni. as-o. atp. atrop. ba-ca. ca-ca. con. dig. dt. elaps. f-hx. k-o. lau-c. led. mn-ca. na-ca. p. pod. ptv. pul. s. sep. spo. thr. thu. vr-v.

Black. thu.

Bright. al-o. as-o. atp. dig. f-hx. k-o. mn-ca. na-ca. p. sep. spo. thr.

Circles. am-ni. elaps. f-hx. mn-ca.

  Bright. mn-ca.

  Red. elaps.

  Yellow. am-ni.

Figures. ag-na. k-o.

Flames. spo.

Flashes, Bright. as-o. atp. na-ca. sep.

Green. dt.

Halo. vr-v.

  Red. vr-v.

Increasing and Decreasing in Size. lau-c.

Light. al-o. p.

Low Down. dt.

Mist. ba-ca. pod.

  Moving. pod.

Moving. dt. pod.

Red. elaps. vr-v.

Spots. dig. dt. k-o. thu.

  Black. thu.

  Bright. dig. k-o.

  Green. dt.

    Low Down. dt.

    Moving. dt.

  Low Down. dt.

  Moving. dt.

Stars. p.
Vibrations. f-hx. thr.
   Bright. f-hx. thr.
Visions. atp. ca-ca. k-o. led. ptv. pul. s. sep. thu.
   Horrible. atp. ca-ca. k-o.
Waves. (p).
   Concentric. (p).
Yellow. am-ni.
Zigzags. con.
SIGHT IMPAIRED. ba-ca. (os).
Sensation as if Axis of Vision was Moved Backwards and Forwards. os.
EYEBALL. aga. al-o. atp. ber. ca-ca. cle. con. cor. cro. (cu). hll. k-o. lac-d. lo-c. lyc. p-x. s. sep. si-x. smi. smr. spo. stc.
 Broken. si-x.
 Bruised. s.
 Coldness. (hur). (p-x).
 Contractive. lac-d.
   Like a Band. lac-d.
 Dryness. (ber).
 False Sensations. (s-x). (sep).
   Sand. (s-x). (sep).
 Heat. (aga). ca-ca. (cb-v). cle. cor. cro. (hpm). lyc. (ptv). si-x.
 Lachrymation. ber. spo.
 Movements. (al-o). (cu). (lch). (na-cl).
   Convulsions. (al-o). (cu). (lch).
 Pressing. aga. atp. (chd). con. (dl-s). (hll). (jnp-s). lac-d. (sep).
 Shooting. hll. smi.
 Smarting. (dig). lo-c. smr. stc. (str-i).
 Stiffness. k-o.
 Undefined. (cmf). lac-d. lyc. (rs-r). si-x. (thu).
EYEBALL SUPERIORLY. aga.
Pressing. aga.
ORBIT. p-x. thu.
ORBIT INTERNALLY. p-x.
Coldness. p-x.
ORBIT INFERIORLY. thu.
EYELIDS. ber. cb-v. chd. cro. dig. dl-s. hpm. hur. jnp-s. lac-d. lch. na-cl. ptv.
 Coldness. hur.

Dryness. ber.
Heat. cb-v. cro.
Movements, Closing. na-cl.
        Spasmodically. na-cl.
UPPER EYELID. chd. cmf. dl-s. jnp-s. lch.
Movements, Convulsions. lch.
Pressing. dl-s.
TARSAL EDGES. dig. hpm. lac-d. p-x. ptv.
Coldness. p-x.
Heat. hpm. ptv.
Small Feeling. lac-d.   •
Smarting. dig.
CANTHI. aga. hll. rs-r. s-x. str-i.
EXTERNAL CANTHUS. rs-r. str-i.
Smarting. str-i.
Undefined. rs-r.
INTERNAL CANTHUS. aga. hll. s-x.
Heat. aga.
INWARDS. s-x.
RIGHT. cmf. hll. s-x. sep. thu.'
Eyeball, False Sensations, Sand. sep.
        Pressing. sep.
Orbit Inferiorly, Undefined. thu.
Upper Eyelid, Undefined. cmf.
Internal Canthus, False Sensations, Sand. s-x.
        Pressing. hll.
Inwards. Eyeball, False Sensations, Sand. s-x.
LEFT. al-o. chd. jnp-s.
Eyeball, Movements, Convulsions. al-o.
Upper Eyelid, Pressing. chd. jnp-s.

NOISE.

hg-i.
EYEBALL.
Undefined. (hg-i).
ORBIT. hg-i.
ORBIT SUPERIORLY. hg-i.
LEFT. hg-i.
Orbit Superiorly, Undefined. hg-i.

Before EAR Symptoms.

anag. ery. frm. pet.
OBJECTS, FALSE APPEARANCE of. ery.
Confused. ery.
Multiplied. ery.
OBJECTS, IMAGINARY. ery.
Bright. ery.
Spots. ery.
    Bright. ery.
Vibrations. ery.
EYEBALL. anag. pet.
Boring. (frm).
Pressing. anag.
Undefined. (pet).
ORBIT. frm.
RIGHT. frm.
Orbit, Boring. frm.
LEFT. pet.
Eyeball, Undefined. pet.

With EAR Symptoms.

acon. al-o. as-o. atp. ba-cl. buf. ca-ca. can. cb-v. chi. cic.
cle. clv. cmf. crot. cy-hx. dig. dro. dt. ery. fe-a. frm-s. glo.
ind. k-bicr. k-ca. k-i. kre. ly-b. men. mgs. mph. n-x. na-cl.
na-sa. ni-ca. p. pb. ppv. pul. qu-sa. s. sa-l. sep. si-x. spo. srr.
thu. trg. trn. vr-a.
OBJECTS, FALSE APPEARANCE of. al-o. cic.
ery. si-x.
Black. al-o.
Confused. ery.
Moving. si-x.
    Vertically. si-x.
        Up and Down. si-x.
Multiplied. cic. ery.
OBJECTS IMAGINARY. as-o. atp. can. (dt). ery.
k-ca. p. qu-sa. spo. trg. vr-a.
Bright. ery. k-ca. p. qu-sa. spo. vr-a.
Flames. spo. vr-a.
Light. qu-sa.
Mist. can.

Spots. ery. k-ca. qu-sa.
  Bright. ery. k-ca. qu-sa.
Vibrations. atp. ery. p. trg.
  Bright. p.
Visions. as-o. spo.
PHOTOPHOBIA. ca-ca. cle. k-na.
SIGHT IMPAIRED. acon. al-o. as-o. can. cb-v. chi. clv. cy-hx. dt. (ery). fe-a. k-bicr. mph. pb. ppv. pul. qu-sa. sep. srr. trn.
EYEBALL. ba-cl. bi-na. buf. ca-ca. cle. crot. dro. dt. frm-s. glo. k-ca. ly-b. men. n-x. na-sa. ppv. s. sa-l. thu. vr-a.
Appearance Bright. dt.
    Dim. k-ca. vr-a.
    Staring. k-ca.
Bursting. frm-s.
Coldness. (ni-ca). (sa-l).
Color Dark. (k-ca).
  Red. bi-na. (ca-ca). crot. glo. (ind). n-x. ppv. s.
Discharge. ba-cl.
Dryness. (thu).
Eruptions. ca-ca. (p).
    Pterygium. (ca-ca).
    Styes. (p).
    Ulcers. ca-ca.
False Sensations. (ni-ca). (thu).
    Sand. (thu).
    Water, Cold. (ni-ca).
Heat. crot. (dro). (k-ca). s. thu.
Itching. ly-b. na-sa. s.
Lachrymation. (dt). k-ca. vr-a.
Movements. (ca-ca). (dt). (kre). (ppv).
Pressing. k-ca. (na-cl).
Projecting. dt.
Shooting. ca-ca. k-ca. n-x. (sa-l). (thu).
  Cold. sa-l.
Swelling. (ca-ca). (k-i).
Tearing. (k-ca).
Undefined. buf. cle. (men).
Same Symptom. ba-cl. buf. cmf. crot. frm-s. ly-b. (men). na-sa. thu.
EYEBALL INTERNALLY. ca-ca.
CORNEA. ca-ca.
Eruptions, Ulcers. ca-ca.

IRIS. cic. dt. mgs. ppv.
Pupils Dilated. cic. dt. mgs. ppv.
   Insensible. dt. ppv.
ORBIT. na-cl.
Pressing. na-cl.
EYELIDS. ca-ca. dig. dt. ind. k-ca. k-i. kre. p. ppv. thu.
Color Dark. k-ca.
Movements, Closing. (ca-ca). (dig). dt. kre. p. ppv.
     Spasmodically. ca-ca.
Swelling. k-i.
UPPER EYELID. k-ca. thu.
Heaviness. thu.
Swelling. k-ca.
LOWER EYELID. p. thu.
TARSAL EDGES. thu.
LOWER TARSAL EDGE. thu.
EYELIDS, INNER SURFACE. ind.
Color Red. ind.
CANTHI. ca-ca. ni-ca. thu.
EXTERNAL CANTHUS. ni-ca. thu.
INTERNAL CANTHUS. ca-ca.
CARUNCULA. ca-ca.
RIGHT. ca-ca. dig. dro. na-sa. ni-ca. thu.
Eyeball, Dryness. thu.
   Heat. dro.
   Itching. na-sa.
   Same Symptom. na-sa.
Eyeball Internally, Color Red. ca-ca.
     Swelling. ca-ca.
Eyelids, Movements, Closing. dig.
Lower Tarsal Edge, Heat. thu.
External Canthus, Coldness. ni-ca.
    Dryness. thu.
    False Sensations, Sand. thu.
      Water Cold. ni-ca.
    Shooting. thu.
Caruncula, Swelling. ca-ca.
LEFT. ca-ca. cle. (dt). glo. k-ca. men. na-sa. p.
Eyeball, Color Red. glo.
   Eruptions Pterygium. ca-ca.
   Heat. k-ca.
   Itching. na-sa.

Lachrymation. (dt). k-ca.
Tearing. k-ca.
Undefined. cle. men.
Same Symptom. men. na-sa.
Lower Eyelid, Eruptions Stye. p.

After EAR Symptoms.

arn. hur. thu.
EYEBALL. arn. thu.
Drawing. arn.
Shooting. arn.
Tearing. thu.
Undefined. (hur).
Same Symptom. thu.
ORBIT. hur.
OUTWARDS. arn.
Eyeball, Drawing. arn.
LEFT. hur.
Orbit, Undefined. hur.

BLOWING NOSE.

al-o. k-o. n-x. na-cl. na-sa..
OBJECTS, IMAGINARY. al-o. na-sa.
Bright. na-sa.
Spots. na-sa.
    Bright. na-sa.
    Yellow. na-sa.
Stars. al-o.
Yellow. na-sa.
SIGHT IMPAIRED. k-o.
EYEBALL. k-o. n-x.
False Sensations. (k-o).
       Pellicle. (k-o).
Swelling. (na-cl).
Tensive. (k-o).
Undefined. n-x.
EYEBALL INTERNALLY. k-o.
False Sensations, Pellicle. k-o.
LACHRYMAL SAC. na-cl.
Swelling. na-cl.

o

RIGHT. k-o.
Sight Impaired. k-o.
Eyeball, False Sensations, Pellicle. k-o.
          Tensive. k-o.

HÆMORRHAGE from NOSE.

cb-v.
SIGHT IMPAIRED. cb-v.

SNEEZING.

amm-ca. (hydr). k-cla.
OBJECTS, IMAGINARY. amm-ca. (hydr). k-cla.
Bright. k-cla.
Spots. k-cla.
          Bright. k-cla.
Stars. amm-ca.
Vibrations. (hydr).
          Bright. (hydr).

Before NOSE Symptoms.

br. ca-ca. cic. k-bicr. k-i. mgs. sang.
SIGHT IMPAIRED. k-i.
EYEBALL. br. ca-ca. cic. k-bicr. k-i. sang.
Dryness. (mgs).
Heat. k-bicr. (sang).
Lachrymation. (sang).
Sensitive. (sang).
Shooting. ca-ca. cic.
Smarting. k-i.
Throbbing. ca-ca.
Undefined. br.
EYELIDS. mgs.
Dryness. mgs.
CANTHI. ca-ca.
INTERNAL CANTHUS. ca-ca.
Shooting. ca-ca.
To HEAD. cic.
To OCCIPUT. cic.

Eyeball, Shooting. cic.
RIGHT. sang.
Eyeball, Heat. sang.
    Lachrymation. sang.
    Sensitive. sang.

With NOSE Symptoms.

ag-na. aga. al-o. alli. amm-ca. anan. anm. arn. art-v. arum. as-o. atp. au. ba-cl. ber. bi-na. br. bru. bry. ca-ca. (ca-i). ca-pa. ca-s. cau. cb-v. ccs. chi. cit-c. clv. co. con. cr-o. crb-x. cro. crt. (cu). cu-asi. dl-s. dt. eug. (eupat-p). euphr. fe. fe-a. fe-mgs. frm. frm-o. gel. grc. hg. hg-bini. hg-s. hll. hydr. ind. jcr. k-bicr. k-ca. k-cla. k-i. k-o. lyc. mg-ca. mg-cl. mrl. na-ca. na-cl. ox-x. p. pb. pet. pnx. ppv. pt. qu-sa. rho. rn-b. rph. rs. rs-r. s. s-x. sep. smc. smi. so-d. spi. (spo). str. te. teu. thu. trg. trn. urg. vr-a. vr-s. vr-v. woo. ziz.

    OBJECTS, FALSE APPEARANCE of. gel.
Multiplied. gel.
    OBJECTS, IMAGINARY. amm-ca. atp. (hydr). k-cla. na-ca. smi.
    Bright. atp. (hydr). k-cla.
    Mist. smi.
    Spots. atp. k-cla.
        Bright. atp. k-cla.
    Stars. amm-ca. na-ca.
        White. na-ca.
    Vibrations. (hydr).
        Bright. (hydr).
    White. na-ca.
    PHOTOPHOBIA. alli. atp. ca-ca. con. euphr. k-bicr.
    SIGHT IMPAIRED. atp. br. dt. fe-a. gel. (grc). ind. ox-x. pb. qu-sa. sep. smi.
    EYEBALL. ag-na. aga. al-o. alli. anan. anm. arn. art-v. as-o. atp. au. ba-cl. ber. bi-na. br. bru. bry. ca-ca. ca-pa. ca-s. cb-v. ccs. chi. cit-c. clv. co. con. cr-o. crb-x. crot. dt. (eupat-p). euphr. fe-mgs. frm. frm-o. grc. hg. hg-s. hll. hydr. jcr. k-bicr. k-ca. k-i. lyc. mg-ca. mg-cl. mrl. na-cl. pnx. pt. rho. rn-b. rph. s. s-x. sep. smc. so-d. spi. str. te. teu. thu. trg. trn. urg. vr-a. vr-v. woo. ziz.
    Appearance, Bright. trg.
        Dim. alli. as-o. (con). (cu). k-ca. urg.
        Staring. (cu). (spo).

Boring. bi-na.

Bursting. (mg-ca).

Coldness. pnx.

Color, Dark. (art-v). (chi). (clv). (cu). (rs).

    Red. al-o. (alli). arn. atp. (ca-i). clv. con. (eupat-p). euphr. (hg-s). k-i. rn-b. teu. (vr-s). vr-v.

    Yellow. as-o.

Creeping. frm-o.

Discharge. ba-cl.

Drawing. ca-s.

Dryness. atp. (cr-o). grc. spi.

Eruptions. (ca-ca). (p).

    Styes. (p).

    Ulcers. (ca-ca).

False Sensations. ca-pa. (grc).

    Sand. ca-pa. (grc).

Heat. aga. al-o. as-o. (bry). (cit-c). hg. lyc. na-cl. rho. (s). thu. ziz.

Heaviness. jcr. thu. woo.

Itching. arum. eug. (hg-s). (s). sep. (smi).

Lachrymation. ag-na. aga. al-o. alli. anan. atp. au. ber. br. bru. bry. cb-v. ccs. chi. co. con. (crb-x). crot. dl-s. (eupat-p). euphr. hg. hg-bini. (hg-s). hydr. k-bicr. k-i. mg-ca. mg-cl. mrl. pt. rn-b. s. smc. so-d. spi. str. te. (teu). trg. urg. vr-a..

    Cold. (trg).

    Hot. atp. bry. euphr.

Movements. (aga). art-v. (ca-ca). dt. (k-o). (lyc). spi.

    Convulsions. (aga). art-v. dt.

    Squinting. art-v. hll. spi.

Paralysis. (ppv).

Pressing. al-o. (atp). br. (cit-c). (crt). (fe). (grc). (hg-s). lyc. (na-cl). (rs-r). thu.

Projecting. spi. (spo).

Sensitive. thu.

Shooting. (aga). ca-ca. cit-c. (hg-s). s. sep.

Smarting. alli. bry. ca-s. (cb-v). (cu-asi). k-bicr. rn-b. s-x. ziz.

Sunken. ag-na. as-o. chi. rph.

Swelling. anm. (clv). (con). (euphr). (hg). (k-i). (pet).

    Chemosis. euphr.

    Feeling of. cit-c.

Throbbing. (atp). trn.

Undefined. co. fe-mgs. scp.

Same Symptom. aga. al-o. anm. arum. as-o. ba-cl. br. ca-pa. ca-s. (cit-c). co. (cr-o). (cu-asi). eug. k-i. lyc. rn-b. (rs-r). s. sep. (smi). spi. ziz.

SCLEROTIC. con.

Color Red. con.

CORNEA. ca-ca. con.

Eruptions, Ulcers. ca-ca.

Opacity. con.

IRIS. art-v. as-o. atp. hll. spi.

Pupils, Dilated. art-v. as-o. atp. hll. spi.

   Insensible. as-o.

ORBIT. cit-c. crt. cu-asi. na-cl. trn.

Pressing. crt. na-cl.

Throbbing. trn.

ORBITAL INTEGUMENTS. art-v. bry. chi. (cu). fe. rs. s. smi.

Color Dark. art-v. chi. (cu).

Itching. smi.

Same Symptom. s. smi.

ORBITAL INTEGUMENTS SUPERIORLY. bry. fe. s.

Heat. bry.

Itching. s.

Pressing. fe.

ORBITAL INTEGUMENTS INFERIORLY. rs.

Color Dark. rs.

EYELIDS. aga. alli. clv. con. hg. hg-s. k-ca. k-i. k-o. lyc. p. ppv. vr-s.

Adhesion of. k-ca. k-o.

Color Dark. clv.

   Red. k-o. lyc.

Movements, Closing. (ca-ca). k-o. lyc.

       Spasmodically. ca-ca.

     Convulsions. aga.

Paralysis, Opening Difficult. ppv.

Swelling. clv. con. k-i.

Same Symptom. aga.

LOWER EYELID. aga. hg. hg-s. p.

Swelling. hg.

TARSAL EDGES. vr-s.

Color Red. vr-s.

CANTHI. cb-v. grc. hg-s. pet. rs-r.

Smarting. cb-v.
INTERNAL CANTHUS. grc. hg-s. pet.
Swelling. pet.
FORWARDS. mg-ca.
RIGHT. aga. atp. br. cr-o. frm. grc. hg-s. na-cl. s.
Sight Impaired. grc.
Eyeball, Color Red. hg-s.
       Dryness. cr-o.
       Heat. s.
       Lachrymation. br. hg-s. teu.
       Pressing. atp. na-cl.
       Shooting. aga. s.
       Throbbing. atp.
       Same Symptom. aga. cr-o. s.
Lower Eyelid, Itching. hg-s.
         Movements, Convulsions. aga.
         Pressing. hg-s.
         Shooting. hg-s.
Internal Canthus, False Sensations, Sand. grc.
         Itching. hg-s.
         Pressing. grc. hg-s.
         Shooting. hg-s.
LEFT. alli. cit-c. crb-x. cu-asi. mg-ca. p. rs-r. s. trg.
Photophobia. alli.
Eyeball, Bursting. mg-ca.
       Color Red. alli.
       Lachrymation. alli. crb-x.
           Cold. trg.
       Shooting. s.
       Same Symptom. s.
Orbit, Heat. cit-c.
       Pressing. cit-c.
       Smarting. cu-asi.
       Swelling, Feeling of. cit-c.
       Same Symptom. cit-c. cu-asi.
Lower Eyelid, Eruptions, Styes. p.
Internal Canthus, Pressing. rs-r.
         Same Symptom. rs-r.
Forwards. Eyeball Pressing. mg-ca.

After NOSE, Symptoms.

ca-s. cb-v. hg.
SIGHT IMPAIRED.   cb-v.
EYEBALL.   ca-s. hg.
Heat.   (hg).
Lachrymation.   hg.
Smarting.   ca-s.
Swelling.   (hg).
EYELIDS.   hg.
LOWER EYELID.   hg.
LEFT.   hg.
Lower Eyelid, Heat.   hg.
            Swelling.   hg.

Moving FACE Muscles.

pul. (spi).
EYEBALL.   (spi).
Drawing.   (pul).
Eruptions.   (pul).
            Styes.   (pul).
Tensive.   (pul).
Undefined.   (spi).
CANTHI.   pul.
Drawing.   pul.
Eruptions, Stye.   pul.
Tensive.   pul.

Moving JAWS.

ca-a.
EYEBALL.
Boring.   (ca-a).
Shooting.   (ca-a).
ORBITAL INTEGUMENTS.   ca-a.
ORBITAL INTEGUMENTS SUPERIORLY.   ca-a.
LEFT.   ca-a.
Orbital Integuments Superiorly, Boring.   ca-a.
                  Shooting.   ca-a.

YAWNING.

(arn). atp. ba-ca. ca-pa. dl-s. drm. fe. hg-bicl. k-ca. mph. p-x. sb-t. smi. str. str-i. vi-o. vr-s.
OBJECTS, FALSE APPEARANCE of. hg-bicl.
Far. hg-bicl.
Small. hg-bicl.
EYEBALL. (arn). atp. ba-ca. ca-pa. dl-s. drm. fe. hg-bicl. k-ca. mph. p-x. sb-t. smi. str. str-i. vi-o. vr-s.
Heat. hg-bicl.
Lachrymation. (arn). atp. ba-ca. ca-pa. dl-s. drm. fe k-ca. mph. p-x. sb-t. smi. vi-o. vr-s.

PRESSING on CHEEK.

atp.
OBJECTS, IMAGINARY. atp.
Flames. atp.
Mist. atp.

Before FACE Symptoms.

anm.
EYEBALL. anm.
Appearance, Glassy. anm.
      Staring. anm.
Projecting. anm.

With FACE Symptoms.

acon. æth. ag-na. al-o. alo. amb. anm. ara. (arn). art-v. as-o. ast. atp. au. ba-ca. ber. bi-na. bry. buf. ca-ca. ca-pa. cap. cast. chi. cic. cit-c. clv. cmf. cn-sa. con. cop. cph. cr-o. crb-x. cro. crot. crt. cth. cu. cu-ca. cub. cyc. dig. dl-s. dor. dph. drm. dt. ery. eupat. (eupat-p). f-hx. fe. glo. glp. grp. grt. gym. hg. hg-bicl. hg-bini. hg-i. hg-s. hll. hyo. hyp. jat. jup-s. k-bicr. k-ca. k-i. k-na. kre. lau-c. lch. lct. led. ly-b. lyc. men. mg-cl. mgs-ar. morph-a. mph. mrl. msc. mtr. myris. n-x. na-ba. na-ca. na-cl. na-sa. ner. (nic). ox-x. p. p-x. pb. pet. pnx. ppv. pso. pt. pul. qu-sa. rhe. rph. rs. rs-v. rut. s. s-x. sb-t. sep. si-x. smb. smi. sn. spi. spo. str. str-i. teu. trg. trn. urg. urt-u. val. vi-o. vp-r. vp-t. vr-a. vr-s. woo. zn.
OBJECTS, FALSE APPEARANCE of. atp. cic. hg-bicl. mg-cl. myris. s-x.
Black. s-x.

Blue. atp.
Bright. atp.
Far. hg-bicl. myris.
Green. mg-cl.
Grey. atp.
Moving. s-x.
    Vibrating. s-x.
Multiplied. atp. cic.
Red. atp. mg-cl.
Small. hg-bicl.
White. atp.
OBJECTS, IMAGINARY. alo. atp. au. dt. (ery). (hg).
k-ca. pet. pt. qu-sa. trg. (vr-a). zn.
  Black. (ery).
  Bright. au. k-ca. qu-sa. (vr-a).
  Circles. zn.
    Variegated. zn.
  Figures. dt.
  Green. (zn).
  Grey. atp.
  Halo. (zn).
    Green. (zn).
  Mist. atp. (ery).
    Black. (ery).
    Grey. atp.
    Red. (ery).
  Red. (ery).
  Spots. au. k-ca. qu-sa. (vr-a).
    Bright. au. k-ca. qu-sa. (vr-a).
  Veil. pet.
  Vibrations. alo. (hg). pt. trg.
  Visions. dt.
    Horrid. (dt).
PHOTOMANIA. dt.
PHOTOPHOBIA. acon. au. ca-ca. con. k-ca. str.
SIGHT IMPAIRED. ag-na. as-o. ast. atp. cap. chi.
cro. dt. grp. grt. msc. pet. pul. s-x. str-i. trn.
  Myopia. chi. grt.
EYEBALL. acon. æth. ag-na. al-o. amb. anm. ara. arn.
art-v. as-o. atp. au. ba-ca. ber. bry. buf. ca-ca. ca-pa. cap.
cast. chi. cit-c. clv. cmf. cn-sa. con. crot. crt. cth. cu. cu-ca.
cyc. dl-s. dor. dph. drm. dro. dt. ery. eupat. f-hx. fe. glo.
gym. hg. hg-bicl. hg-bini. hg-i. hg-s. hll. hyo. hyp. jnp-s.

k-bicr. k-ca. k-na. lau-c. lch. lct. led. ly-b. lyc. mg-cl. morph-a. mph. mrl. msc. mtr. myris. n-x. na-ba. na-ca. na-cl. na-sa. ox-x. p. p-x. pb. pet. pnx. ppv. pt. pul. qu-sa. rph. rs. rs-v. rut. s. sb-t. sep. si-x. smc. smi. sn. spi. spo. str. str-i. teu. trg. trn. urg. urt-u. vi-o. vp-r. vp-t. vr-a. vr-s. zn.

Appearance Bright. atp. crot. cth. dt. eupat. hg-bicl. hyo. jnp-s. lch. lyc. mtr. pb. trg. trn.

Dim. acon. ara. as-o. bry. buf. cit-c. (con). cu. dt. ery. hg. jnp-s. k-ca. lch. mtr. p-x. ppv. qu-sa. sep. trg. vr-a.

Glassy. anm. atp. (dt). glo. ppv.

Impudent. (dt).

Spiteful. (dt).

Staring. acon. æth. aum. atp. chi. crot. cth. cu. dor. dt. glo. hyp. k-ca. lau-c. lyc. msc. p-x. ppv. si-x. (spo). urg.

Wild. dt. hyp. ppv. .

Coldness. lch.

Color Dark. (art-v). (as-o). (ber). (bi-na). (buf). (chi). (clv). (cn-sa). (cph). (cu). (cub). (dig). (dl-s). (dt). (ery). (jat). (jnp-s). (lyc). (myris). (na-ca). (ner). (p). (p-x). (rs). (s-x). (sep). (str-i). (woo).

Red. acon. (as-o). atp. buf. (ca-ca). clv. cmf. con. crot. (cu). cu-ca. dt. (eupat). (eupat-p). hg-s. hyo. led. morph-a. myris. na-cl. (pet). pnx. ppv. qu-sa. rs-v. rut. s. sep. str. (zn).

White. (hg-bicl).

Yellow. as-o. cth. (eupat). mg-cl. (n-x). s. sep. (spi) (str). vr-a.

Contractive. k-na.

Cutting. au.

Discharge. lyc. s.

Drawing. (as-o). (dph). (f-hx). (nic). p. val.

Eruptions. (ca-ca). (hg-bicl). (kre). (rs). zn.

Dry. (kre).

Herpetic. (kre).

Dry. (kre).

Pimples. (rs).

Pterygium. (ca-ca). zn.

Rhagades. (zn).

Scales. (kre).

Dry. (kre).

Ulcers. (ca-ca). (hg-bicl).

Vesicles. (rs).

Gnawing. (s).

Heat. amb. (aps) ara. hg-bicl. k-bicr. lct. ly-b. lyc. mrl. mtr. n-x. na-ca. pet. pt. s. spi. trn. vr-a. zn.

Itching. (cr-o). pet. s. zn.

Lachrymation. ag-na. al-o. (arn). atp. (au). ba-ca. (br). bry. ca-pa. con. crt. dl-s. drm. dt. (eupat). (eupat-p). fe. gym. k-ca. lct. lyc. mph. (na-sa). p-x. pnx. ppv. pt. (pul). qu-sa. sb-t. smi. spi. (spo). str. str-i. (trg). vi-o. vr-a. vr-s. zn.

Hot. au. bry. (pul). spo.

Movements. acon. æth. anm. art-v. atp. (ba-ca). buf. (ca-ca). (chi). cth. cu. (dig). dt. (glp). (grp). hg-bicl. hll. lau-c. (lyc). (men). mtr. ppv. (rhe). si-x. (smb). spi. (spo). trg.

Convulsions. acon. anm. art-v. atp. buf. cth. cu. dt. hg-bicl. (hll). lau-c. (men). mtr. (rhe). si-x. trg.

Squinting. æth. art-v. atp. dt. hll. spi.

Downwards. æth. (grp).

Upwards. acon. buf. (cu). lau-c.

To Left. buf.

Paralysis. (ppv).

Pressing. (as-o). cit-c. dph. (dt). (hg-bini). k-ca. lyc. (myris). na-ba. (na-cl). (ner). p. (pul). s.

Projecting. æth. anm. atp. au. cap. cu. dt. myris. pb. ppv. qu-sa. spo. vp-r. vp-t.

Shooting. ca-ca. (hg-bini). k-ca. (mgs-ar). pnx. (spo).

Smarting. (aps). bry. cast. na-ba. zn.

Small Feeling. al-o.

Strained. dph.

Sunken. ag-na. as-o. ber. buf. ca-ca. chi. cit-c. clv. cn-sa. cu. cyc. dl-s. dro. (dt). ery. hg. k-bicr. k-ca. lyc. n-x. ox-x. p. p-x. pb. ppv. pul. qu-sa. rph. s. smc. sn. spo. teu. vp-t.

Swelling. (as-o). au. (bry). buf. (ca-ca). (con). (cu). dt. (hg-s). (k-i). na-ca. (p). (pb). (pso). rs. s. urt-u.

Feeling of. lch.

Tearing. ca-ca. lyc. p. pul. (spo).

Tensive. jnp-s. k-ca. (nic). spi.

Throbbing. (myris).

Undefined. hg-i. str. trg.

Wrinkled. (zn).

Same Symptom. ara. as-o. (bry). buf. cmf. (cr-o). crot. cth. (cu). (dig). dph. dt. (hg-bini). hg-i. (hg-s). k-bicr. lau-c. ly-b. lyc. mg-cl. (mgs-ar). morph-a. mtr. n-x. (na-cl). pet. ppv. (rhe). s. sep. si-x. sn. spi. (spo). trg. trn. vr-a.

EYEBALL INTERNALLY. zn.

Color Red. zn.

SCLEROTIC. con. eupat.

Color Red. eupat.

  Yellow. eupat.

CORNEA. au. ca-ca. con. hg-bicl. rs.

Color Red. au.

  White. hg-bicl.

Eruptions, Pimples. rs.

    Ulcers. ca-ca. hg-bicl.

    Vesicles. rs.

Opacity. con.

CHAMBERS of EYE. hg-bicl.

Discharge, Pus. hg-bicl.

IRIS. acon. æth. anm. art-v. as-o. ast. atp. buf. chi. cic. crb-x. crt. cu. dt. glo. hg-bicl. hll. hyo. hyp. lyc. msc. mtr. na-ca. pnx. ppv. spi. str. trg.

Pupils Contracted. acon. ast. atp. crb-x. dt. glo. hg-bicl. msc. pnx.

   Dilated. æth. anm. art-v. as-o. atp. buf. chi. cic. crt. cu. dt. hll. hyo. hyp. lyc. msc. mtr. na-ca. ppv. spi. str. trg.

   Insensible. acon. æth. as-o. buf. (crb-x.) cu. dt. ppv.

   Irregular. trg.

ORBIT. hg-i. lyc. myris. na-cl. pul. sn. val.

Drawing. sn. val.

Pressing. na-cl.

Tearing. lyc.

Same Symptom. na-cl. sn.

ORBIT SUPERIORLY. myris.

ORBITAL INTEGUMENTS. art-v. as-o. ber. bi-na. buf. chi. clv. cn-sa. cph. cr-o. crt. cu. cub. dl-s. dt. ery. hg-s. hll. jat. jnp-s. k-i. lyc. myris. n-x. na-ca. ner. p. p-x. pb. rs. sep. smc. spi. str. str-i. woo.

Color Dark. art-v. ber. bi-na. buf. chi. clv. cn-sa. cph. crt. cu. cub. dl-s. ery. jat. jnp-s. lyc. na-ca. ner. p. p-x. sep. smc. str-i. woo.

  Yellow. n-x. spi. str.

Itching. cr-o.
Swelling. as-o. hg-s. k-i. p. pb. rs.
Same Symptom. cr-o. hg-s.
ORBITAL INTEGUMENTS SUPERIORLY. hll.
Movements, Convulsions. hll.
ORBITAL INTEGUMENTS INFERIORLY. dt. jat.
myris. p. rs. s-x.
Color Dark. dt. jat. myris. p. rs.
Swelling. dt. p.
Same Symptom. dt.
EYELIDS. acon. anm. aps. as-o.˜atp. au. ba-ca. bry.
buf. ca-ca. chi. clv. con. cu. dig. dt. (ery). glp. grp. hg-bicl.
hll. k-ca. kre. lau-c. lyc. men. mtr. pnx. ppv. rhe. spo. zn.
Adhesion of. au. k-ca.
Color Dark. as-o. clv. dig.
     Red. con. cu.
Eruptions, Dry. kre.
       Herpes. kre.
           Dry. kre.
       Scales. kre.
           Dry. kre.
Hæmorrhage. (ery).
Hairs Inverted. zn.
Heat. aps.
Movements, Closing. acon. anm. (atp). ba-ca. (buf).
(ca-ca). chi. cu. dt. glp. (hg-bicl). lau-c. mtr. pnx. ppv.
smb. spo.
              Spasmodically. ca-ca. hg-bicl. spo.
        Convulsions. hll. men. rhe.
        Opening Wide. acon. (cu). lau-c. lyc. mtr.
ppv.
Paralysis, Opening Difficult. ppv.
Smarting. aps.
Swelling. bry. clv. con. cop. cu. hg-bicl. na-ca. pso.
Same Symptom. as-o. bry. cop. cu. dig. hll. men. rhe.
UPPER. EYELID. k-ca.
Swelling. k-ca.
LOWER EYELID. bry.
Swelling. bry.
EYELIDS, INNER SURFACE. zn.
Wrinkled. zn.
CANTHI. ca-ca. mgs-ar. zn.
EXTERNAL CANTHUS. zn.

Eruptions, Rhagades. zn.
Smarting. zn.
INTERNAL CANTHUS. ca-ca. mgs-ar.
Shooting. mgs-ar.
Same Symptom. mgs-ar.
CARUNCULA. ca-ca.
LACHRYMAL SAC. pet.
FORWARDS. (dt). p.
Eyeball, Pressing. p.
BACKWARDS. dph.
Eyeball, Drawing. dph.
DOWNWARDS. ner.
LEFT then RIGHT. zn.
Eyeball, Eruptions, Pterygium. zn.
RIGHT. as-o. br. ca-ca. cit-c. dig. grp. na-sa. pul. s-x.
Objects Imaginary, Vibrations. hg.
Eyeball, Color Red. as-o.
    Drawing. as-o.
    Lachrymation. br. na-sa.
        Hot. pul.
    Pressing. as-o. cit-c. pul.
    Same Symptom. cit-c.
Eyeball Internally, Color Red. ca-ca.
        Swelling. ca-ca.
Orbit, Pressing. pul.
Orbital Integuments Inferiorly, Color Dark. s-x.
Eyelids, Movements, Closing. dig.
        Opening Wide. grp.
Caruncula, Swelling. ca-ca.
LEFT. atp. buf. ca-ca. (dt). f-hx. grp. hg-bini. k-ca.
myris. ner. s. spo. trg. vr-a. zn.
    Objects Imaginary, Bright. vr-a.
        Green. zn.
        Halo Green. zn.
        Spots Bright. vr-a.
Eyeball, Drawing. f-hx.
    Eruptions, Pterygium. ca-ca.
    Gnawing. s.
    Heat. k-ca.
    Lachrymation. k-ca. trg.
    Movements, Convulsions. trg.
    Pressing. hg-bini. ner.
    Shooting. hg-bini. spo.

Tearing. k-ca. spo.
Undefined. s.
Same Symptom. hg-bini. ner. s. spo.
Orbit Superiorly, **Pressing.** myris.
Throbbing. myris.
Eyelids, Movements, Closing. atp. buf. grp.
Convulsions. trg.
Forwards. Eyeball, Pressing. (dt).
Downwards. Eyeball, Pressing. ner.

After FACE Symptoms.

rho.
EYEBALL. rho.
Pressing. rho.
LEFT. rho.
Eyeball, Pressing. rho.

Before TEETH Symptoms.

anm. hur.
EYEBALL. anm. hur.
Appearance Glassy. anm.
Staring. anm.
Projecting. anm.
Undefined. hur.

With TEETH Symptoms.

aps. art-v. as-o. atp. bry. ca-ca. cast. chi. cit-c. cle. cmc.
cro. cth. dt. hg. hur. ind. k-ca. k-i. k-o. lyc. mn-ca. myris.
na-ba. s. sep. spi. trg. trn.
OBJECTS, FALSE APPEARANCE **of.** dt.
Large. dt.
OBJECTS IMAGINARY. (hg).
Vibrations. (hg).
PHOTOPHOBIA. cle. k-ca.
SIGHT IMPAIRED. as-o. (cro). sep.
EYEBALL. aps. art-v. as-o. atp. bry. ca-ca. cast. chi.
cle. cmc. cro. cth. dt. hur. k-ca. k-o. lyc. myris. na-ba. s.
trg. trn.

Appearance Bright. cth. trg.

    Dim. dt.

    Staring. cth. k-o.

Boring. s.

Color Dark. (dt).

Coldness. (cro).

Drawing. (s).

Heat. atp. (cit-c). (myris).

Lachrymation. bry. chi. dt.

     Hot. bry.

Movements. aps. art-v. cth. dt. (k-o).

   Convulsions. cth. dt.

    Squinting. aps. art-v.

Numbness. hur.

Pressing. (cit-c). na-ba.

Shooting. ca-ca. (myris).

Smarting. bry. cast. cmc.

Tearing. (cro). lyc.

Throbbing. trn.

Undefined. cle. hur. s.

Same Symptom. (cro). hur. lyc. (myris).

IRIS. aps. dt. mn-ca.

Pupils Dilated. aps. dt. mn-ca.

ORBIT. cit-c. hg-i. hur. k-i. myris.

Pressing. cit-c.

Throbbing. trn.

ORBIT SUPERIORLY. hg-i.

ORBITAL INTEGUMENTS. dt. spi.

Color Yellow. spi.

ORBITAL INTEGUMENTS INFERIORLY. dt.

Color Dark. dt.

EYELIDS. ind. k-o.

Movements, Closing. k-o.

EYELIDS, INNER SURFACE. ind.

Color Red. ind.

RIGHT. as-o. cro. hg. k-i.

Objects Imaginary, Vibrations. hg.

Sight Impaired. cro.

Eyeball, Coldness. cro.

   Color Red. as-o.

   Drawing. as-o.

   Pressing. as-o.

Tearing. cro.
 Same Symptom. cro.
Orbit, Tearing. k-i.
 Same Symptom. k-i.
LEFT. cit-c. (dt). hg-i. hur. k-ca. myris. s.
Eyeball, Drawing. s.
  Heat. k-ca. myris.
  Lachrymation. (dt). k-ca.
  Shooting. hur. myris.
  Tearing. k-ca.
  Undefined. cle. s.
  Same Symptom. hur. myris. s.
Orbit, Heat. cit-c.
 Pressing. cit-c.
Orbit Superiorly, Undefined. hg-i.
   Same Symptom. hg-i.

After TEETH Symptoms.

ccs.
EYEBALL. ccs.
Pressing. (ccs).
LEFT. ccs.
Eyeball, Pressing. ccs.

PRESSING on THROAT.

trg.
EYEBALL. trg.
Pressing. trg.
FORWARDS. trg.
Eyeball, Pressing. trg.

Before THROAT Symptoms.

hyp. na-cl.
SIGHT DAZZLED. (na-cl).
SIGHT IMPAIRED. (na-cl).
EYEBALL. hyp.
Appearance, Staring. hyp.
 Wild. hyp.

P

IRIS. hyp.
Pupils, Dilated. hyp.
LEFT. na-cl.
Sight Dazzled. na-cl.
Sight Impaired. na-cl.

With THROAT Symptoms.

acon. æth. ag-na. (alm). anm. aps. as-o. atp. br. bru. bry. buf. ca-ca. cast. cb-v. ccs. cic. cld. clv. con. cop. cth. cu. dt. dt-t. ery. eug. eupat. (eupat-p). gel. glo. hg. hg-bini. hll. hyo. jnp-s. k-bicr. k-ca. k-i. k-na. k-o. klm. lau-c. lyc. mgs. morph-a. msc. myris. na-ba. na-cl. nic. p. par. pb. ppv. pru-l. pt. pul. rn-b. rs. s. sb-t. si-x. smb. spi. spo. str. thu. trg. trn. vr-a.

OBJECTS, FALSE APPEARANCE of. (alm). atp. cic. dt. gel. myris. pb.
　Blue. atp.
　Bright. atp.
　Far. gel. myris.
　Grey. atp.
　Inverted. gel.
　Large. dt.
　Multiplied. (alm). atp. cic. gel. pb.
　Red. atp.
　White. atp.
OBJECTS, IMAGINARY. atp. dt. pt.
　Black. dt.
　Bright. atp.
　Grey. atp.
　Mist. atp.
　　　Grey. atp.
　Spots. atp. dt.
　　　Black. dt.
　　　Bright. atp.
　Vibrations. pt.
PHOTOPHOBIA. acon. aps. con. hg. na-ba.
　SIGHT IMPAIRED. (alm). as-o. atp. cb-v. dt. gel. klm. par. pb. pru-l.
　EYEBALL. acon. æth. ag-na. (alm). anm. aps. as-o. atp. br. bru. bry. buf. ca-ca. cast. cb-v. ccs. cic. cld. clv. cth. cu. dt. ery. eug. eupat. (eupat-p). glo. hg. hg-bini. hll. hyo. jnp-s.

k-ca. k-na. klm. lau-c. lyc. mgs. msc. myris. na-ba. nic. p. pb. ppv. pul. rn-b. rs. s. sb-t. si-x. spi. spo. str. thu. trg. trn. vr-a.

Appearance, Bright. (alm). atp. bry. cth. dt. eupat. lyc. pb.

Dim. as-o. bry. buf. (cu). dt. ery. k-ca. trg. vr-a.

Glassy. anm. atp. bry. (dt). glo. rs.

Impudent. (dt).

Spiteful. (dt).

Staring. æth. anm. atp. cth. (cu). dt. glo. lyc. msc. si-x. spo.

Wild. dt.

Color Dark. (ery). (p).

Red. acon. atp. bry. cld. clv. cu. dt. (eupat). hg. myris. ppv. s. sb-t. str.

White. (s).

Yellow. as-o. (eupat). (eupat-p). s. str. vr-a.

Discharge. (str).

Hard. (str).

Yellow. (str).

Dryness. atp. (mgs). spi.

Eruptions. (k-bicr).

Granulations. (k-bicr).

Pustules. (k-bicr.)

Heat. as-o. eug. k-na. na-ba. myris. s.

Heaviness. ppv. thu.

Itching. s.

Lachrymation. ag-na. aps. br. bru. bry. cb-v. ccs. dt. nic. ppv. pt. rn-b. str. (trg). vr-a.

Movements. æth. (alm). buf. cic. cth. cu. dt. dt-t. hll. (k-o). lau-c. lyc. pb. ppv. pul. si-x. spi. trg.

Convulsions. buf. cic. cth. cu. dt. lau-c. ppv. pul. si-x. trg.

Squinting. æth. (alm). dt. hll. (pb). spi.

Upwards. buf. cic. cu. ppv.

Downwards. æth.

Inwards. (alm). (pb).

To Left. buf.

Paralysis. (trg).

Pressing. atp. (hg-bini). (myris). (na-cl). p. thu.

Projecting. acon. anm. atp. cu. hyo. myris. pb. (spo).

Shooting. (cth). (hg-bini). k-ca. klm. (myris). (trn).

Smarting. ca-ca. cast. rn-b.

Sunken. as-o. (cu). (dt). ery. k-ca. p. rs.

228

Swelling. (cu). dt. (k-i).
      Feeling of. cld.
Tearing. pul.
Tensive. jnp-s. k-ca.
Throbbing. (myris).
Undefined. (hg-bini). (s). trg.
Same Symptom. as-o. atp. buf. dt. (hg-bini). lau-c. pul. spi. trg.
EYEBALL ROUND CORNEA. k-bicr.
Color Red. k-bicr.
SCLEROTIC. eupat.
Color Red. eupat.
      Yellow. eupat.
CORNEA. k-bicr. s.
Color Red. s.
      White. s.
Eruptions, Pustules. k-bicr.
IRIS. æth. (alm). anm. as-o. atp. buf. cic. dt. glo. hll. lyc. morph-a. msc. pb. ppv. pul. spi. str. trg.
Pupils Contracted. atp. dt. glo.
      Dilated. æth. (alm). anm. as-o. atp. buf. cic. dt. hll. lyc. morph-a. msc. pb. ppv. pul. spi. str.
      Insensible. æth. as-o. buf. dt. ppv.
      Irregular. trg.
ORBIT. myris. na-cl.
Pressing. na-cl.
ORBIT SUPERIORLY. myris.
ORBITAL INTEGUMENTS. cth. cu. ery. p.
ORBITAL INTEGUMENTS SUPERIORLY. cth.
Color Dark. cu. ery. p.
EYELIDS. (alm). buf. clv. cop. cu. dt. dt-t. k-bicr. k-ca. k-i. k-o. lyc. mgs. p. pb. ppv. smb. trg.
Adhesion of. k-ca.
Color Dark. clv. k-ca.
      Red. cu.
Dryness. mgs.
Eruptions, Granulations. k-bicr.
Movements, Closing. (buf). cu. dt. k-o. ppv. smb.
      Convulsions. cu.
      Opening Wide. (alm). dt-t. lyc. pb. ppv.
Paralysis, Opening Difficult. trg.
Swelling. clv. cop. cu. k-i.
UPPER EYELID. k-o,

Heaviness. k-o.
CANTHI. str.
Discharge, Hard. str.
         Yellow. str.
FORWARDS. atp. p. trg.
Eyeball, Pressing. atp. p. trg.
To HEAD. cth.
To FOREHEAD. cth.
Orbital Integuments Superiorly, Shooting. cth.
RIGHT. (alm). as-o. pb.
Eyeball, Color Red. as-o.
      Drawing. as-o.
      Movements, Squinting. (alm). pb.
            Inwards. (alm). pb.
      Pressing. as-o.
LEFT. buf. hg-bini. k-ca. myris. s. trg. trn.
Eyeball, Heat. myris.
      Lachrymation. trg.˙
      Movements, Convulsions. trg.
      Pressing. hg-bini.
      Shooting. hg-bini. myris. trn.
      Undefined. hg-bini. s.
      Same Symptom. hg-bini. s.
Orbit Superiorly, Pressing. myris.
      Throbbing. myris.
Eyelids, Adhesion of. k-ca.
      Movements, Closing. buf.
            Convulsions. trg.

DRINKING.

crot.
SIGHT IMPAIRED. crot.

EATING.

aga. al-o. amb. arum. atp. ba-ca. ca-ca. cb-v. cro. dig. dph.
dt. ery. grt. hg. i. irs-f. k-bicr. k-o. lct. li-ca. lyc. mg-ca.
mg-cl. n-x. na-ca. na-sa. ner. ol-a. p. pb. phl. pol. ppv. ptv.
rut. s. si-x. str. str-i. thu. val. vr-a. zn.
OBJECTS, FALSE APPEARANCE of. dt. hg. p.
Black. hg.

Green. hg.
Moving. hg.
       Circularly. hg.
Multiplied. dt.
Part Visible. p.
OBJECTS, IMAGINARY. ba-ca. dig. dph. ery. lct. p. si-x. str-i. zn.
Black. lct. lyc. p.
Bright. dig. dph. ery. p.
Circles. p.
Mist. si-x.
Serpentine Bodies. ery. str-i.
       Bright. ery.
Spots. dig. ery. lct. lyc. p.
    Black. lct. lyc. p.
    Bright. dig.
    White. ery.
Veil. ba-ca. zn.
Vibrations. dph. p.
       Bright. dph. p.
White. ery.
Zigzags. p.
     Bright. p.
PHOTOPHOBIA. str.
SIGHT DAZZLED. dig. si-x.
SIGHT IMPAIRED. atp. ba-ca. ca-ca. cb-v. k-bicr. na-sa. (ner). p. ppv. ptv. str. zn.
EYEBALL. aga. al-o. amb. dph. k-o. lyc. mg-ca. mg-cl. na-ca. na-sa. ol-a. s. thu. zn.
Color Red. s.
Drawing. aga.
Dryness. (vr-a).
Heat. (cb-v). k-o. mg-cl. na-ca. thu. zn.
Heaviness. (cro).
Itching. (mg-ca).
Lachrymation. dph. (na-sa). (ol-a). zn.
Movements. (arum). (dph). (grt). (n-x).
       Convulsions. (dph). (grt). (n-x).
Presssing. aga. pol. s. (val).
Shooting. (irs-f). (na-ca). ol-a.
Small Feeling. al-o.
Smarting. mg-cl.
Swelling, Feeling of. (cro).

Tearing. amb. (ol-a). (phl).
Undefined. lyc.
IRIS. s. str.
PUPILS, **Dilated.** s. str.
ORBIT. pol.
Pressing. pol.
ORBITAL INTEGUMENTS. amb. n-x. phl.
Tearing. amb.
ORBITAL INTEGUMENTS SUPERIORLY. phl.
ORBITAL INTEGUMENTS INFERIORLY. n-x.
EYELIDS. arum. cb-v. cro. dig. dph. grt. irs-f. phl.
vr-a.
Heat. cb-v.
Movements, Closing. arum.
        Convulsions. dph. grt. •
Swelling, Feeling of. cro.
UPPER EYELID. cro. vr-a.
Dryness. vr-a.
Heaviness. cro.
LOWER EYELID. phl.
FORWARDS. val.
Eyeball, Pressing. val.
RIGHT. dig. irs-f. mg-ca. n-x. na-sa. ner. ol-a. phl.
Sight Impaired. ner. •
Eyeball, Itching. mg-ca.
        Lachrymation. na-sa. ol-a.
Orbital Integuments Superiorly, Tearing. phl.
**Orbital Integuments Inferiorly, Movements,
Convulsions.** n-x.
Eyelids, Movements, Closing. dig.
Upper Eyelid, Shooting. irs-f.
LEFT. lyc. ol-a. phl.
Eyeball, Shooting. ol-a.
        Tearing. ol-a.
        Undefined. lyc.
Lower Eyelid, Tearing. phl.

VOMITING.

aga. as-o. ca-ca. cu. eug. k-bicr. nic. sb-t. vr-v.
EYEBALL. aga. asr. ca-ca. cu. eug. k-bicr. sb-t. vr-v.
Appearance Dim. sb-t.

Color Red. (k-bicr).
Heat. eug. k-bicr.
Lachrymation. asr. ca-ca. cu. k-bicr. sb-t. vr-v.
Motion in. eug.
   Rolling. eug.
Swelling, Feeling of. (aga).
EYELIDS. k-bicr.
Color Red. k-bicr.
LEFT. aga.
Eyeball, Swelling Feeling of. aga.

During STOOL.

so-t. spi.
EYEBALL. so-t. spi.
Color Red. (so-t).
Lachrymation. so-t.
Pressing. (spi).
SCLEROTIC. so-t.
Color Red. so-t.
RIGHT. spi.
Eyeball, Pressing. spi.

After STOOL.

crot. na-ca.
SIGHT IMPAIRED. crot.
EYEBALL. na-ca.
Heat. na-ca.

Before ABDOMINAL Symptoms.

amb. anm. (ery). eug. hyp. na-cl. narth. rn-b. sep. trg.
vr-a.
OBJECTS, IMAGINARY. na-cl. vr-a.
Bright. (vr-a).
Spots. (vr-a).
  Bright. (vr-a).
Zigzags. na-cl.
  Bright. na-cl.
SIGHT IMPAIRED. amb. (ery). narth.

EYEBALL. anm. eug. hyp. rn-b. sep. trg.
Appearance Glassy. anm.
     Staring. anm. hyp.
     Wild. hyp.
Heat. eug.
Itching. rn-b.
Lachrymation. eug.
Motion in. eug.
     Rolling. eug.
Pressing. sep.
Projecting. anm.
IRIS. hyp.
Pupils Dilated. hyp.
LEFT. vr-a.
Objects Imaginary, Bright. vr-a.
     Spots, Bright. vr-a.

During ABDOMINAL Symptoms.

 acon. æsc. æth. aga. alli. alm. anan. aps. ara. arn. art-v.
as-o. asr. ast. atp. bi-na. br. bry. buf. ca-ca. cac. can. cast.
cb-a. cb-v. chd. chi. chio. cic. cit-c. cld. clv. cmf. con. cop.
cph. crn. cro. crot. cth. cu. cyc. dig. dor. drm. dt. dt-t.
ery. eupat. (eupat-p). glo. gn-l. grc. gym. hg. hg-bicl. hg-cl.
hg-s. jat. jnp-s. k-bicr. k-ca. k-i. k-na. k-o. klm. lac-f. lam.
lau-c. lct. li-ca. ly-b. lyc. mg-cl. msc. mtr. myris. n-x. na-ba.
na-ca. na-cl. na-sa. ner. ni-ca. nic. p. pb. pet. pip. pnc.
pnx. pod. ppv. pru-l. pso. pt. pul. qu-sa. rho. rph. rn-b.
s. sb-t. sep. spi. spo. srr. str. str-i. thr. thu. trg. trn. tx-b.
vr-a. vr-s. vr-v. zn. zng.
OBJECTS, FALSE APPEARANCE of. (alm). atp.
cic. hg. klm. mg-cl. nic. pb. s. spo. str. thr.
 Black. hg. klm.
 Blue. atp.
 Bright. atp.
 Green. mg-cl. nic.
 Grey. atp.
 Moving. spo. str.
   Vertically. spo. str.
     Up and Down. spo. str.
 Multiplied. (alm). atp. cic. pb. s. spo. thr.
 Red. atp. mg-cl.

White. atp.
Yellow. as-o. nic.
OBJECTS, IMAGINARY. atp. ca-ca. can. cyc. dt. cry. k-ca. klm. myris. na-cl. pso. pt. qu-sa. sep. str. thr. trg. tx-b.
Black. thr.
Blue. pso.
Bright. atp. cyc. ery. k-ca. klm. qu-sa. sep. thr.
Circles. tx-b.
Figures. dt. myris.
Grey. atp.
Light. qu-sa.
Mist. atp. can. k-o. pso.
  Grey. atp.
Spots. atp. cyc. ery. k-ca. qu-sa.
  Bright. atp. cyc. ery. k-ca. qu-sa.
Stars. pso.
  Blue. pso.
Veil. dt. (na-cl).
Vibrations. atp. klm. pt. sep. thr. trg.
  Black. thr.
  Bright. klm. sep. thr.
Visions. dt. str.
PHOTOMANIA. dt.
PHOTOPHOBIA. acon. aps. atp. ca-ca. con. hg. k-ca. (lac-f). na-ba. thr.
SIGHT DAZZLED. (na-cl).
SIGHT IMPAIRED. alm. as-o. ast. atp. bi-na. br. buf. ca-ca. can. cb-v. chi. crot. cyc. dt. (ery). glo. gym. hg. k-bicr. k-ca. klm. lac-f. lam. na-ca. na-cl. (ner). pet. pip. pnc. pru-l. pt. pul. qu-sa. rph. sep. spo. srr. trg. trn. (vr-a).
  Hemeralopia. vr-a.
EYEBALL. acon. æsc. æth. aga. alli. (alm). anan. aps. ara. art-v. as-o. asr. atp. bi-na. bry. ca-ca. cac. cast. cb-a. chd. chi. cld. clv. cmf. cof. con. cph. crn. crot. cth. cu. dig. dor. drm. dt. eug. eupat. (eupat-p). glo. gn-l. gym. hg. hg-bicl. hg-cl. hg-s. hyo. jat. jnp-s. k-bicr. k-ca. k-na. klm. lac-f. lau-c. lct. li-ca. ly-b. lyc. n-x. na-ba. na-cl. na-sa. ner. ni-ca. nic. p. pb. pet. pnx. ppv. pru-l. pt. rho. rn-b. rs. s. sb-t. sep. spi. spo. str. str-i. thr. thu. trg. trn. vp-t. vr-a. vr-s. vr-v.
  Appearance Bright. (alm). atp. bry. cth. dt. eupat. pb.

Dim. ara. as-o. bry. (cu). dt. hg. k-ca. ppv. sb-t. vr-a.

Glassy. atp. bry. glo. rs.

Staring. atp. cth. (cu). dor. dt. glo. k-ca. lau-c. pru-l. (spo).

Wild. dt.

Color Dark. (as-o). (clv). (cph). (crn). (cu). (dt). (jat). (k-ca). (lyc). (mtr). (ner). (p). (pod). (rs).

Red. acon. atp. bi-na. bry. cld. con. cu. dt. (eupat). (eupat-p). hg. hyo. (k-bicr). (lac-f). na-cl. pnx. ppv. s. (spi). str. str-i. trg.

Yellow. œsc. as-o. chd. chi. con. crn. dig. (eupat). (eupat-p). hg-cl. pb. s. str. vr-a.

Drawing. aga. (chio).

False Sensations. cmf.

Sand. cmf.

Eruptions. (ca-ca). (p). (s).

Styes. (p).

Ulcers. (ca-ca). (s).

Heat. (alm). cb-a. eug. gym. k-bicr. k-na. lct. na-ba. ni-ca. pet. s. sep. thu. trg.

Heaviness. anan. hg-s. k-bicr. (k-o). ppv.

Itching. (grc). hg-bicl. (ly-b). rn-b. s.

Lachrymation. alli. aps. asr. atp. bry. ca-ca. cof. con. crot. cu. drm. (eupat-p). gn-l. k-bicr. k-ca. (lac-f). lct. nic. p. pnx. ppv. pt. s. sb-t. (spi). spo. str. vr-a. vr-s. vr-v.

Hot. (spi).

Motion in. eug.

Rolling. eug.

Movements. (alm). aps. art-v. ca-ca. cit-c. cmf. cth. cu. dig. dt. dt-t. k-o. lyc. (myris). pb. pnx. ppv. s. sep. spi. spo. vr-a.

Convulsions. art-v. cth. cu. dt. pb. ppv.

Squinting. (alm). art-v. dig. dt. (pb). s. spi.

Upwards. aps. cu.

Inwards. (alm). (pb).

Paralysis. (trg).

Pressing. (acon). aga. (chio). cmf. (con). k-ca. klm. (myris). na-ba. (na-cl). sep. (str). thu. vr-a. (zng).

Projecting. æth. atp. cu. pb. (spo). str-i.

Sensitive. (zn).

Shooting. ca-ca. cmf. hg-bicl. k-ca. klm. (lac-f). na-sa. pnx.

Smarting. asr. cast. li-ca. na-ba. trg. trn.

Sunken. as-o. clv. cu. (dt). k-ca. lau-c. p. rs. vp-t. vr-a.

Swelling. (con). dt. (k-ca). (k-i). str-i.

 Feeling of. (aga). cld.

Tearing. (con). na-ba. pul.

Tensive. jnp-s. k-ca. n-x.

Throbbing. (myris). (thr). trg.

Undefined. aps. cth. (spi). thu. (trg).

Same Symptom. dt. hg-bicl. thu.

EYEBALL SUPERIORLY. cac.

Smarting. cac.

EYEBALL ROUND CORNEA. s.

Color Red. s.

SCLEROTIC. con. eupat.

Color Red. con. eupat.

 Yellow. eupat.

CORNEA. ca-ca. con. s.

Eruptions, Ulcers. ca-ca. s.

Opacity. con. s.

IRIS. (alm). arn. art-v. as-o. ast. atp. (br). cic. cmf. cph. dt. glo. morph-a. msc. nic. pb. spi.

 Pupils Contracted. ast. atp. dt. glo.

  Dilated. (alm). art-v. as-o. atp. (br). cic. cmf. cph. dt. morph-a. msc. nic. pb. spi.

  Insensible. arn. as-o. dt.

ORBIT. acon. chio. con. myris. na-cl. trg.

Pressing. acon. chio. na-cl.

Tearing. con.

Undefined. trg.

ORBIT SUPERIORLY. chio. myris.

ORBITAL INTEGUMENTS. art-v. as-o. clv. cph. crn. cu. dt. jat. k-ca. lyc. mtr. ner. p. pod. rs. sep.

Color Dark. art-v. as-o. clv. cph. crn. cu. jat. lyc. mtr. ner. p. rs.

ORBITAL INTEGUMENTS SUPERIORLY. k-ca. sep.

 Movements, Convulsions. sep.

 Swelling. k-ca.

ORBITAL INTEGUMENTS INFERIORLY. dt. pod.

Color Dark. dt. pod.

EYELIDS. aps. bry. cit-c. cmf. con. cop. cro. cu. dt. grc. k-bicr. k-ca. k-o. lyc. myris. p. pnx. ppv. s. sep. spo. trg. vr-a. zn.

Adhesion of. (con). (k-ca).
Color Dark. k-ca.
      Red. con. cu. k-bicr.
Heat. cro.
Itching. grc.
Movements, Closing. aps. (ca-ca). cit-c. cu. dt. k-o.
lyc. pnx. ppv. sep. spo. vr-a.
                Spasmodically. ca-ca. spo.
    Convulsions. cmf. cu.
    Opening Wide. (dt). dt-t.
    Winking. myris.
Paralysis, Opening Difficult. trg.
Swelling. con. cop. cu. k-i.
UPPER EYELID. trg.
Heat. trg.
Smarting. trg.
LOWER EYELID. bry. p.
Swelling. bry.
TARSAL EDGES. s.
Eruptions, Ulcers. s.
Swelling. s.
CANTHI. s.
EXTERNAL CANTHUS. s.
Color Red. s.
FORWARDS. scp. str.
Eyeball, Pressing. sep. str.
BACKWARDS. lac-f.
To HEAD. lac-f.
To FOREHEAD. lac-f.
To TEMPLES. lac-f.
RIGHT. (alm). as-o. chio. cmf. con. k-ca. k-o. lac-f.
ly-b. na-cl. ner. pb. thr. zn.
    Objects Imaginary, **Veil Crooked.** na-cl.
    Photophobia. lac-f.
    Sight Dazzled. na-cl.
    Sight Impaired. na-cl. ner.
    Eyeball, Color Red. as-o. con. lac-f.
           Drawing. as-o.
           Itching. ly-b.
           Lachrymation. con. lac-f.
           Movements, Squinting. (alm). pb.
                   Inwards. (alm). pb.
           Pressing. as-o. cmf. con.

Shooting. lac-f.
Throbbing. thr.
Orbit Superiorly, Drawing. chio.
   Pressing. chio.
Eyelids, Adhesion of. con.
Upper Eyelid, Heaviness. k-o.
   Sensitive. zn.
   Swelling. k-ca.
Backwards. Eyeball, Shooting. lac-f.
To Forehead. Eyeball, Shooting. lac-f.
     Throbbing. lac-f.
To Temple. Eyeball, Shooting. lac-f.
     Throbbing. lac-f.
LEFT. aga. k-ca. myris. spi. zng.
Eyeball, Color Red. spi.
 Lachrymation. spi.
   Hot. spi.
 Pressing. zng.
 Swelling, Feeling of. aga.
 Undefined. spi.
Orbit Superiorly, Pressing. myris.
   Throbbing. myris.
Eyelids, Adhesion of. k-ca.

After ABDOMINAL Symptoms.

cic. grp. k-bicr.
OBJECTS, IMAGINARY. k-bicr.
Veil. k-bicr.
  Yellow. k-bicr.
Yellow. k-bicr.
SIGHT IMPAIRED. k-bicr.
EYEBALL. cic.
To HEAD. cic.
To OCCIPUT. cic.
Eyeball, Shooting. cic.

After URINATION.

eug.
OBJECTS IMAGINARY. eug.
Light. eug.

Before URINARY Symptoms.

(cu).
EYEBALL. (cu).
Movements. (cu).
      Convulsions. (cu).

With URINARY Symptoms.

acon. æsc. (alm). anag. anm. apo. aps. atp. (br). bry.
buf. ca-s. chi. clv. con. cu. dor. dt. eug. eupat. (eupat-p).
grp. hg-cl. hyo. k-ca. k-i. k-o. na-ca. na-cl. pb. s. sep. spo.
str. thu. trg.
OBJECTS, FALSE APPEARANCE of. (alm). atp. pb.
Blue. atp.
Bright. atp.
Grey. atp.
Multiplied. (alm). atp. pb.
Red. atp.
White. atp.
OBJECTS, IMAGINARY. atp.
Bright. atp.
Grey. atp.
Mist. atp.
      Grey. atp.
Spots. atp.
      Bright. atp.
SIGHT IMPAIRED. apo. atp. chi. grp.
EYEBALL. acon. æsc. (alm). anag. anm. aps. atp. buf.
ca-s. clv. con. cu. dor. dt. eug. eupat. hg-cl. hyo. k-ca. k-o.
na-ca. s. str. thu. trg.
Appearance Dim. buf. k-ca.
      Bright. (alm). atp. eupat.
      Glassy. anm. atp.
      Staring. anm. atp. dor. dt. k-o.
      Wild. dt.
Color Dark. (dt). (k-ca).
      Red. atp. buf. (con). cu. dt. (eupat). (eupat-p).
s. str.
      White. (s).
      Yellow. æsc. ca-s. (eupat). hg-cl. pb. str
Heat. eug. na-ca.

Lachrymation. (con). str.
Movements. acon. (alm). aps. atp. buf. cu. dt. (k-o). (pb). (sep). (trg).
        Convulsions.   acon. atp. buf. (cu). dt. (sep). (trg).
                Squinting. (alm). aps. atp. (pb).
                Upwards. aps. buf. cu.
                Inwards. (alm). (pb).
                To Left. buf.
Pressing. anag. (con). (na-cl). thu.
Projecting. anm. atp. hyo. (spo).
Shooting. anag.
Sunken. clv.
Swelling. (bry). (eupat-p). (k-i).
SCLEROTIC. eupat.
Color Red. eupat.
        Yellow. eupat.
CORNEA. s.
Color Red. s.
        White. s.
IRIS. (alm). aps. atp. (br). buf. dt. na-ca. pb.
Pupils Contracted. atp. dt.
        Dilated. (alm). aps. atp. (br). buf. dt. na-ca. pb.
        Insensible. buf.
ORBIT. na-cl.
Pressing. na-cl.
ORBITAL INTEGUMENTS. dt. sep.
ORBITAL INTEGUMENTS SUPERIORLY, sep.
Movements, Convulsions. sep.
ORBITAL INTEGUMENTS INFERIORLY. dt.
Color Dark. dt.
EYELIDS. aps. bry. buf. con. cu. (dt). k-ca. k-i. k-o. sep. trg.
Adhesion of. (con).
Color Dark. k-ca.
Movements, Closing. aps. (buf). cu. k-o. sep.
        Convulsions. cu.
        Opening Wide. (dt).
Swelling. k-i.
LOWER EYELID. bry.
Swelling. bry.
RIGHT. (alm). con. pb.

Eyeball, Color Red. con.
       Lachrymation. con.
       Movements, Squinting. (alm). pb.
           Inwards. (alm). pb.
     Pressing. con.
Eyelids, Adhesion of. con.
LEFT. buf. trg.
Eyeball, Movements, Convulsions. trg.
Eyelids, Movements, Closing. buf.
         Convulsions. trg.

Before MENSES.

atp. hg. lyc. si-x.
OBJECTS, FALSE APPEARANCE of. si-x.
White. si-x.
SIGHT IMPAIRED. atp.
EYEBALL. hg. si-x.
Pressing. hg. si-x.
IRIS. lyc.
Pupils Dilated. lyc.

At Commencement of MENSES.

br.
EYEBALL. br.
Pressing. br.
FORWARDS. br.
Eyeball, Pressing. br.

During MENSES.

br. ca-ca. cast. (chi). grp. hg-s. li-ca. ly-b. lyc. mg-ca. n-x.
ni-ca. p. pnx. pul. sang. sep. si-x. str. zn.
OBJECTS, FALSE APPEARANCE of. li-ca.
Part Visible. li-ca.
SIGHT IMPAIRED. grp. hg-s. li-ca. pul. sep.
EYEBALL. br. ca-ca. cast. (chi). hg-s. mg-ca. n-x. ni-ca.
(str). zn.
Color Red. zn.
Cutting. (hg-s).
Discharge. ca-ca. (mg-ca).

Q

Dryness. mg-ca.
Heat. mg-ca. n-x. ni-ca.
Lachrymation. ca-ca. (chi).
Movements. (chi). (hg-s). (p).
        Convulsions. (chi).
Paralysis. mg-ca.
Projecting. (chi).
Pressing. (br). (hg-s). (sang). (str).
Shooting. ca-ca.
Smarting. cast.
Undefined. ca-ca. mg-ca.
· IRIS. lyc.
Pupils, Contracted. lyc.
ORBIT. hg-s.
ORBIT SUPERIORLY. hg-s.
Cutting. hg-s.
EYELIDS. ca-ca. hg-s. mg-ca. p.
Adhesion of. ca-ca. mg-ca. p.
Movements, Closing. hg-s. p.
        Convulsions. (chi).
UPPER EYELID. hg-s.
Heaviness. hg-s.
CANTHI. mg-ca.
EXTERNAL CANTHUS. mg-ca.
Discharge. mg-ca.
FORWARDS. br. sang. str.
Eyeball, Pressing. br. sang. str.
BACKWARDS. hg-s.
Eyeball, Pressing. hg-s.
·OUTWARDS. hg-s.
Orbit Superiorly, Cutting. hg-s.

After MENSES.

hg-s.
SIGHT IMPAIRED. hg-s.
EYEBALL. hg-s.
Heaviness. hg-s.
Smarting. (hg-s).
Sunken Feeling. hg-s.
Swelling, Feeling of. (hg-s).
ORBIT. hg-s.

ORBIT, SUPERIORLY. hg-s.
Smarting. hg-s.
Swelling, Feeling of. hg-s.

EMISSIONS.

dt.
OBJECTS, IMAGINARY. dt.
Veil. dt.
SIGHT IMPAIRED. dt.

SEXUAL EXCESSES.

p.
SIGHT IMPAIRED. p.

PREGNANCY.

art-v. atp. au. ca-ca. chi. cic. cyc. gel. hyo. k-o. myris.
na-cl. p. pul. s.
OBJECTS, FALSE APPEARANCE of. atp. au. chi.
gel. hyo.
   Confused. chi.
      Outlines. chi.
   Inverted. atp.
   Large. hyo.
   Moving. cic.
   Multiplied. atp. gel.
   Part Visible. au.
      Horizontal. au.
   Red. hyo.
   White. chi.
OBJECTS, IMAGINARY. ca-ca. chi. cyc. k-o. p.
pul. s.
   Bright. cyc.
   Grey. p.
   Halo. chi. s.
      White. chi.
   Mist. ca-ca. k-o. pul.
   Spots. cyc.
      Bright. cyc.
   Veil. p.
      Grey. p.

White. chi.
SIGHT IMPAIRED.   art-v. atp. ca-ca. cyc. gel. k-o.
pul. s.
 EYEBALL.   atp. hyo.
Color Red.   atp. .
Movements.   hyo. (k-o.) (myris). na-cl.
    Convulsions.   (hyo).
    Squinting.   hyo.
EYELIDS.   hyo. k-o. myris. na-cl. str.
Movements, Closing.   k-o. (na-cl).
        Spasmodically.   na-cl.
    Convulsions.   hyo.
    Winking.   myris.
UPPER EYELID.   k-o. str.
Heaviness.   k-o. str.

PARTURITION.

au-cl.
SIGHT IMPAIRED.   au-cl.

With SEXUAL Symptoms.

anag. ara. atp. (br). cap. chi. cmf. cyc. dt. cuphr. gel.
hpm. hyo. k-o. lyc. myris. na-ca. pul. sep. si-x. str. thu.
trg. trn. tss. vr-a.
 OBJECTS, FALSE APPEARANCE of.   atp.
Blue.   atp.
Bright.   atp.
Grey.   atp.
Multiplied.   atp.
Red.   atp.
OBJECTS, IMAGINARY.   atp. cyc.
Grey.   atp.
Mist.   atp. cyc.
    Grey.   atp.
Visions.   atp.
    Horrible.   atp.
SIGHT IMPAIRED.   atp. cap. chi. cyc. gel. hyo. si-x.
(vr-a).
 Hemeralopia.   vr-a.

EYEBALL. anag. ara. atp. cmf. euphr. myris. na-ca. pul. str. thu. trg. trn. tss.
  Appearance Dim. ara.
  Color Dark. (myris).
      Green. (myris).
      Red. atp. euphr. pul. tss.
  Dryness. myris. (thu).
  False Sensations. cmf.
        Sand. cmf.
  Heat. na-ca. (thu).
  Heaviness. (k-o).
  Lachrymation. euphr.
  Movements. (cmf). (hyo). (k-o). (sep).
      Convulsions. (cmf). (hyo). (sep).
  Paralysis. (myris).
  Pressing. anag. cmf. (str).
  Shooting. anag. cmf.
  Smarting. trn.
  Throbbing. trg.
  Undefined. (trg).
LENS. lyc.
  Cataract. lyc.
IRIS. atp. (br). dt.
  Pupils Contracted. atp.
      Dilated. atp. (br). dt.
ORBIT. trg.
  Undefined. trg.
ORBITAL INTEGUMENTS. myris. sep.
  Color Dark. myris.
      Green. myris.
ORBITAL INTEGUMENTS SUPERIORLY. sep.
  Movements, Convulsions. sep.
EYELIDS. cmf. hpm. hyo. k-o. myris. sep. thu.
  Movements, Closing. k-o. sep.
      Convulsions. cmf. hyo.
  Paralysis, Closing Difficult. myris.
UPPER EYELID. k-o.
  Heaviness. k-o.
TARSAL EDGES. hpm. thu.
  Heat. hpm.
LOWER TARSAL EDGE. thu.
  FORWARDS. str.
  Eyeball, Pressing. str.

RIGHT. thu.
Eyeball, Dryness. thu.
Lower Tarsal Edge, Heat. thu.

COUGHING.

acon. art-v. atp. cof. (eupat). grp. k-ca. k-cla. p. par.
ppv. pul. spo. vr-s.
OBJECTS, IMAGINARY. k-ca. k-cla. par.
Bright. k-ca. k-cla. par.
Spots. k-ca. k-cla. par.
      Bright. k-ca. k-cla. par.
EYEBALL. acon. art-v. atp. (eupat). grp. p. ppv. spo.
vr-s.
Color Red. atp.
Lachrymation. acon. art-v. (eupat). grp. p. ppv. vr-s.
Projecting. atp.
Throbbing. spo.

SPEAKING.

p-x.
SIGHT IMPAIRED. p-x.
Myopia. p-x.

Before CHEST Symptoms.

art-v. cu.
EYEBALL. art-v. cu.
Appearance Staring. art-v.
Movements, Convulsions. cu.

With CHEST Symptoms.

acon. æth. ag-na. al-o. alli. (alm). amm-ca. anm. aps.
ara. arn. art-v. as-o. atp. bi-na. br. bry. buf. ca-ca. ca-s.
cac. cast. cb-a. cb-v. chd. chi. cic. cld. clv. cof. cph. crb-x.
cu. cu-ca. dl-s. dor. dph. dro. dt. dt-t. ery. eupat. (eupat-p).
euph. euphr. fe. gel. glo. glp. gym. hg. hpm. hyo. i. k-bicr.
k-ca. k-cla. k-i. klm. kre. lau-c. lct. lyc. mgs. morph-a.
msc. mtr. myris. n-x. na-ba. na-cl. na-sa. os. p. p-x. par.
pb. pnx. pod. pol. ppv. pru-l. pul. qu-sa. rn-b. rs. s. s-x.
sep. smb. sn. spi. spo. spo-f. str. te. thu. trg. trn. urg.
vr-a. vr-s.

OBJECTS, FALSE APPEARANCE of. (alm). amm-ca. atp. cb-v. cic. gel. glo. myris. pb.

Black. amm-ca.

Blue. atp.

Bright. atp.

Far. myris.

Grey. atp.

Inverted. glo.

Moving. amm-ca.

Multiplied. (alm). atp. cic. gel. pb.

Red. atp.

Small. cb-v.

White. atp.

OBJECTS, IMAGINARY. atp. cb-v. (cu). dt. (ery). k-ca. k-cla. par. pru-l. qu-sa. sep. str.

Black. dt. (ery).

Bright. atp. dt. k-ca. k-cla. par. qu-sa. sep.

Figures. (cu). dt.

Grey. atp.

Light. qu-sa.

Mist. atp. (ery).

    Black. (ery).

    Grey. atp.

    Red. (ery).

Red. (ery).

Spirits. (cu).

Spots. atp. dt. k-ca. k-cla. par. qu-sa. sep. str.

    Black. dt.

    Bright. atp. dt. k-ca. k-cla. par. qu-sa. sep. str.

Veil. pru-l.

Vibrations. sep.

    Bright. sep.

Visions. cb-v. str.

    Horrible. cb-v.

PHOTOMANIA. dt.

PHOTOPHOBIA. acon. alli. aps. atp. euph. hg. na-ba.

SIGHT IMPAIRED. amm-ca. as-o. atp. au-cl. bi-na. ca-ca. cof. dt. (ery). gel. klm. myris. pul. s.

EYEBALL. acon. æth. aga. al-o. alli. (alm). anm. aps. ara. arn. art-v. as-o. atp. bi-na. br. bry. buf. ca-ca. ca-s. cac. cast. cb-v. chd. chi. cic. cld. clv. cph. cu. cu-ca. dl-s. dor. dph. dt. (ery). eupat. (eupat-p). euph. euphr. glo. glp. gym. hg. hyo. hyp. i. k-bicr. k-ca. k-i. kre. lau-c. lct. mgs.

morph-a. mtr. myris. na-ba. na-cl. na-sa. p. p-x. pb. pnx. pol. ppv. pru-l. pul. rn-b. rs. s. sep. sn. spi. spo. str. te. thu. trg. trn. urg. vp-t. vr-a. vr-s.

Appearance Bright. acon. (alm). atp. dt. eupat.

Dim. ara. as-o. buf. (cu). dt. k-ca. ppv. sn. vr-a.

Glassy. atp. glo. rs.

Staring. æth. as-o. atp. chi. (cu). dor. dt. glo. hyp. mgs. (spo). urg.

Wild. (alm). cu-ca. dt. hyp. pb.

Color Dark. (art-v). (cph). (cu). (dro). (lyc). (n-x). (p). (p-x). (s). (sn). (spo-f). (trg). (vr-a).

Green. (vr-a).

Red. acon. alli. arn. atp. bi-na. buf. ca-s. cld. clv. cph. cu. cu-ca. dt. (eupat). (eupat-p). euph. euphr. hg. k-bicr. morph-a. mtr. myris. pnx. pol. ppv. pul. .

Yellow. as-o. (eupat). i. (n-x) (spi). vr-a.

Dryness. ca-ca. (mtr). s.

Eruptions. k-bicr.

Blisters. k-bicr.

Hæmorrhage. cb-v. (ery). mtr. str.

Heat. br. lct. mtr. na-ba. (na-cl). pol. sep. thu.

Lachrymation. acon. al-o. alli. aps. art-v. atp. br. bry. ca-ca. ca-s. cb-v. chd. cph. dl-s. dph. (ery). (eupat). euph. euphr. grp. hg. k-ca. kre. lct. mgs. na-cl. (na-sa). pnx. ppv. pul. rs. s. spi. spo. te. trg. urg. vr-a. vr-s.   ·

Hot. bry. euph. euphr. hg. kre. na-cl.

Movements. æth. (alm). anm. aps. art-v. (br). buf. cic. cu. (dph). dt. (dt-t). (glp). hyo. (lau-c). mtr. (na-cl). (pb). (pnx). (pod). ppv. (smb). spi. (spo). (trg). vr-a.

Convulsions. anm. art-v. (br). buf. cic. cu. dt. hyo. lau-c. mtr. vr-a.

Squinting. æth. (alm). aps. art-v. (pb). spi.

Upwards. aps. buf. (cu). ppv. vr-a.

Downwards. æth. (na-cl).

Inwards. (alm). (pb).

To Left. buf.

Paralysis. (cb-a). (trg).

Pressing. atp. gym. na-ba. (na-cl). p. pol. sep.

Projecting. atp. ca-s. cu. dro. hyo. myris. pru-l. spi. (spo).

Sensitive. (na-cl). (spo-f). thu.

Shooting. br. k-ca. pnx. sep.

Smarting. bry. (cac). cast. na-ba. trn.

Sunken. ag-na. as-o. chi. clv. (cu). dl-s. (dt). k-ca. p. p-x. rs. s. sn. vp-t.

Swelling. (bry). (eupat-p). (k-ca). (k-i). (p).

    Feeling of. cld.

Tensive. k-ca. trg.

Tearing. pul. str.

Throbbing. (na-cl). (s-x). spo.

Undefined. k-bicr. k-ca. k-i. rn-b. thu. trg.

Same Symptom. br. gym.

EYEBALL SUPERIORLY. cac.

Smarting. cac.

EYEBALL INTERNALLY. k-bicr.

Eruptions, Blisters. k-bicr.

SCLEROTIC. eupat.

Color Red. eupat.

    Yellow. eupat.

IRIS. acon. æth. (alm). aps. art-v. as-o. atp. (br). buf. ca-ca. cic. crb-x. (cu). dt. glo. hyp. msc. myris. nic. pb. pnx. ppv. pru-l. spi. str. trg.

    Pupils Contracted. atp. crb-x. glo. pnx.

        Dilated. acon. æth. (alm). aps. art-v. as-o. atp. (br). buf. ca-ca. cic. dt. hyp. msc. myris. nic. pb. ppv. pru-l. spi. str. trg.

        Insensible. æth. as-o. buf. crb-x. (cu). dt. myris. ppv.

    Irregular. trg.

ORBIT. na-cl.

ORBIT SUPERIORLY. na-cl.

ORBITAL INTEGUMENTS. art-v. cph. cu. fe. lyc. myris. n-x. p. p-x. rs. s. sn. spi. spo-f. trg. vr-a.

    Color Dark. art-v. cph. cu. lyc. n-x. p. p-x. s. sn. spo-f. trg. vr-a.

        Green. vr-a.

        Yellow. n-x. spi.

Swelling. fe. rs.

ORBITAL INTEGUMENTS INFERIORLY. myris. p.

Color Dark. myris.

Swelling. p.

EYELIDS. aps. atp. br. bry. buf. cb-a. clv. cu. dph. dro. dt. dt-t. (ery). glp. hpm. k-ca. k-i. mtr. na-cl. pnx. pod. ppv. smb. spo. spo-f. trg. trn. vr-a.

Adhesion of. k-ca.
Color Dark. clv. dro. k-ca. ppv.
   Red. cu.
Dryness. mtr.
Hæmorrhage. (ery).
Movements, Closing. aps. atp. (br). cu. dt. glp. pax. pod. ppv. smb. spo.
      Spasmodically. br. spo.
  Convulsions. cu. dph.
  Opening Wide. (cu). dt-t. ppv. (spo).
Paralysis, Opening Difficult. cb-a. trg.
Sensitive. spo-f.
Smarting. trn.
Swelling. clv. cu. k-i.
UPPER EYELID. bry. k-ca. na-cl. vr-a.
Movements, Convulsions. vr-a.
Swelling. bry. k-ca.
LOWER EYELID. bry.
Swelling. bry.
TARSAL EDGES. hpm.
Heat. hpm.
FORWARDS. atp. na-cl. p. pol. trg.
Eyeball, Pressing. atp. p. pol. trg.
RIGHT. (alm). as-o. na-cl. na-sa. pb. s-x.
Eyeball, Color Red. as-o.
   Drawing. as-o.
   Lachrymation. na-cl. na-sa.
   Movements, Squinting. (alm). pb.
      Inwards. (alm) pb.
   Pressing. as-o.
   Throbbing. s-x.
Orbit Superiorly, Heat. na-cl.
   Pressing. na-cl.
   Sensitive. na-cl.
   Throbbing. na-cl.
Upper Eyelid, Heat. na-cl.
   Movements, Hanging down. na-cl.
Forwards. Orbit Superiorly, Pressing. na-cl.
LEFT. buf. trg.
Eyeball, Movements, Convulsions. trg.
Eyelids, Movements, Closing. buf.
   Convulsions. trg.

Before BACK Symptoms.

alm.
SIGHT IMPAIRED. alm.
EYEBALL.
Movements. (alm).
EYELIDS. alm.
Movements, Closing. alm.

With BACK Symptoms.

acon. æsc. (alm). as-o. atp. au. bry. ca-ca. cast. cic. co. con. cro. cu. dig. dor. dt. eupat. (eupat-p). gel. grp. hg-bicl. k-ca. kre. lct. led. lyc. mn-ca. msc. myris. n-x. na-cl. ni-ca. pb. pnx. pru-l. s. sa-l. sc. (spo). thu. trg. trn.
OBJECTS, FALSE APPEARANCE of. (alm). cic. gel. pb.
Multiplied. (alm). cic. gel. pb.
OBJECTS IMAGINARY. cro. myris.
Figures. myris.
Mist. cro.
PHOTOPHOBIA. acon. atp. au. ca-ca. (dt).
SIGHT IMPAIRED. atp. cro. (dt). gel. grp. lyc. msc. na-cl. pru-l.
EYEBALL. acon. æsc. (alm). as-o. atp. au. bry. ca-ca. cast. cic. co. ero. cu. dor. dt. eupat. (eupat-p). hg-bicl. k-ca. lct. led. msc. n-x. ni-ca. pb. s. sa-l. se. (spo). thu. trg. trn.
Appearance, Bright. atp. bry. dt. eupat. trg.
    Dim. bry. k-ca.
    Glassy. bry.
    Staring. atp. cic. dor. msc.
Coldness. (sa-l).
Color Dark. (k-ca).
    Red. acon. atp. (au). bry. (cu). (eupat). (eupat-p). led. s.
    White. (hg-bicl).
    Yellow. æsc. (eupat). s.
Cutting. au.
Discharge. (hg-bicl).
    Pus. (hg-bicl).
Drawing. (se).

Eruptions. (ca-ca). (hg-bicl).
       Ulcers. (ca-ca). (hg-bicl).
Heat. ca-ca. lct. n-x. (na-cl). ni-ca. s. thu.
Itching. ca-ca. s.
Lachrymation. (au). cro. lct. sc.
       Hot. au.
       Appearance of. bry.
       Feeling of. cro.
Movements. as-o. atp. (ca-ca). (hg-bicl). (kre). (na-cl). trg.
       Convulsions. as-o. atp. trg.
       Squinting. atp.
Paralysis. (trg).
Pressing. (na-cl). (se).
Projecting. atp. cu. (spo).
Sensitive. (na-cl).
Shooting. ca-ca. (sa-l). (se).
       Cold. sa-l.
Smarting. cast. cro. trn.
Swelling. (cu). (eupat-p). hg-bicl.
       Feeling of. cro.
Tearing. (con).
Throbbing. (na-cl).
Undefined. bry. co. cro. (s).
Same Symptom. ca-ca. co. (con). (s).
SCLEROTIC: eupat.
Color Red. eupat.
       Yellow. eupat.
CORNEA. au. ca-ca. hg-bicl.
Color Red. au.
       White. hg-bicl.
Eruptions, Ulcers. ca-ca. hg-bicl.
CHAMBERS¯of EYE. hg-bicl.
Discharge, Pus. hg-bicl.
IRIS. (alm). atp. cic. dt. mn-ca. msc. pb. pnx.
Pupils Contracted. mn-ca. msc.
       Dilated. (alm). atp. cic. dt. pb. pnx.
ORBIT. con. na-cl.
Pressing. na-cl.
Tearing. con.
Same Symptom. con.
ORBIT SUPERIORLY. na-cl.

EYELIDS. au. ca-ca. cu. dig. hg-bicl. k-ca. kre. na-cl. trg.

Adhesion of. au. k-ca.
Color Dark. k-ca.
  Red. cu.
Movements, Closing. (ca-ca). (dig). (hg-bicl). kre. (na-cl).
      Spasmodically. ca-ca. hg-bicl.
Paralysis, Opening Difficult. trg.
Swelling. cu.
UPPER EYELID. na-cl.
FORWARDS. na-cl.
RIGHT. (alm). dig. na-cl. pb.
Eyeball, Lachrymation. na-cl.
   Movements, Squinting. (alm). pb.
      Inwards. (alm). pb.
Orbit Superiorly, Heat. na-cl.
     Pressing. na-cl.
     Sensitive. na-cl.
     Throbbing. na-cl.
Eyelids, Movements, Closing. dig. na-cl.
Upper Eyelid, Heat. na-cl.
Forwards. Orbit, Pressing. na-cl.
LEFT. s. se.
Eyeball, Drawing. se.
   Pressing. se.
   Shooting. se.
   Undefined. s.
   Same Symptom. s.

RAISING ARMS.

ba-ca.
OBJECTS, FALSE APPEARANCE of. ba-ca.
Moving. ba-ca.
  Circularly. ba-ca.

Before ARM Symptoms.

na-ca. hyp.
SIGHT IMPAIRED. na-ca.

EYEBALL. hyp.
Appearance Staring. hyp.
        Wild. hyp.
IRIS. hyp.
Pupils, Dilated. hyp.

With ARM Symptoms.

wm. æsc. æth. (alm). anm. apo. atp. buf. euc. cb-v. clv.
ery. (cu). dt. ery. eupat. (eupat-p). grp. hg. hll. hyn. k-ca.
kmn. kre. let. lyc. mgs. mph. msc. myris. na-ba. na-cl. pb.
ppv. pul. s. sep. snb. (spo). str. thr. thu. trg. trn. vr-a.
OBJECTS, FALSE APPEARANCE of   alm. cb-v.
pb. thr.
   Multiplied (alm). pb. thr.
   Small   r.
OBJECTS IMAGINARY. cb-v. thr. trg.
   Black ...
   Bright ...
   Vibrations .. r. trg.
          Black   thr.
          Bright   thr.
   Visions ....
          Horrible. cb-v.
PHOTOPHOBIA. acon. (dt). hg. na-ba. str. thr.
SIGHT IMPAIRED. (alm). apo. atp. (dt). grp. msc.
spo.
EYEBALL. acon. æsc. æth. (alm). anm. atp. buf. clv. cu.
dt. ery. eupat. (eupat-p). hg. hll. hyo. k-ca. klm. let. lyc.
mgs. mph. msc. na-ba. pb. pul. s. (spo). thu. trg. vr-a.
Appearance Bright. (alm). dt. eupat. mgs.
        Dim. (alm). buf. (cu). dt. vr-a.
        Glassy. anm.
        Staring. æth. anm. (cu). dt. ery. msc. (spo).
                Downwards. ery.
        Wild. dt.
Color Dark. (cu). (dt).
        Red. acon. buf. (eupat-p). hg. hyo.
        Yellow. æsc. vr-a.
Heat. let. lyc. mgs. mph. na-ba. thu.
Heaviness ppv.

Itching. (trn).

Lachrymation. dt. (eupat-p). lct. vr-a.

Movements. acon. æth. (alm). atp. buf. con. cu. dt. hll. (kre). (myris). pb. pul. (s). (smb). (trg). (vr-a).

 Convulsions. acon. atp. buf. cu. dt. pul. (trg).

 Squinting. æth. (alm). hll. pb.

 Upwards. buf. con. (cu).

 Downwards. æth.

 Inwards. (alm). (pb).

 To Left. buf.

Pressing. klm. (na-cl). (str).

Projecting. (spo).

Smarting. (cac). (trn).

Sunken. clv. (cu). k-ca.

Swelling. (cop).

Tensive. k-ca.

Undefined. (s).

Same Symptom. acon. dt. lyc. mgs. pul. (s).

EYEBALL, SUPERIORLY. cac.

Smarting. cac.

SCLEROTIC. eupat.

Color Red. eupat.

 Yellow. eupat.

IRIS. æth. (alm). atp. buf. (cu). dt. hll. msc. pb. str.

Pupils Contracted. dt. msc.

 Dilated. æth. (alm). atp. buf. dt. hll. pb. str.

 Insensible. buf. (cu). dt.

ORBIT. na-cl.

Pressing. na-cl.

ORBITAL INTEGUMENTS. (cu). dt.

Color Dark. (cu).

ORBITAL INTEGUMENTS INFERIORLY. dt.

Color Dark. dt.

EYELIDS. (alm). buf. cop. (cu). dt. kre. myris. pb. s. smb. trn. vr-a.

Itching. trn.

Movements, Closing. buf. (cu). dt. kre. s. smb. vr-a.

 Convulsions. trg.

 Opening Wide. (alm). pb.

 Winking. myris.

Smarting. trn.

Swelling. cop.

FORWARDS. str.

Eyeball, Pressing.　str.
RIGHT.　(alm). pb.
Eyeball, Movements, Squinting.　(alm). pb.
　　　　　　　　　　　　Inwards.　(alm). pb.
LEFT.　s. trg.
Eyeball, Movements, Convulsions.　trg.
　　Undefined.　s. trg.
　　Same Symptom.　s.

Before LEG Symptoms.

hyp.
EYEBALL.　hyp.
Appearance, Staring.　hyp.
　　　　Wild.　hyp.
IRIS.　hyp.
Pupils, Dilated.　hyp.

With LEG Symptoms.

　　acon. alm. amb. anm. apo. ast. atp. buf. ca-ca. cast. ccs.
cit-c. cld. clv. cop. cth. (cu). dt. eupat. (eupat-p). hg. hll.
hyo. k-bicr. k-ca. klm. kre. lac-f. lct. mph. mtr. na-ba.
na-cl. pb. ppv. pul. rs. sang. sep. (spo). str. thu. trg. trn.
vr-a.
　OBJECTS, IMAGINARY.　dt. trg.
Figures.　dt.
Vibrations.　trg.
PHOTOPHOBIA.　acon. ca-ca. (dt). hg. (lac-f). na-ba.
SIGHT DAZZLED.　(na-cl).
SIGHT IMPAIRED.　(alm). amb. apo. ast. atp. (dt).
lac-f. na-cl. pb. sep. trn.
　EYEBALL.　acon. (alm). anm. atp. buf. ca-ca. cast.
cit-c. cld. clv. cth. cu. dt. eupat. (eupat-p). hg. hll. hyo.
k-bicr. k-ca. klm. kre. lac-f. lct. mph. mtr. na-ba. ppv.
pul. rho. rs. sang. (spo). str. thu. trg. trn. vr-a.
Appearance Bright.　(alm). atp. dt. eupat. trg.
　　　　Dim.　(alm). buf. (cu). dt. k-ca. vr-a.
　　　　Glassy.　anm. rs.
　　　　Staring.　anm. atp. (cu). dt. (spo).
　　　　Wild.　dt.

Color Dark. (cu). (dt). (k-ca).

Red. acon. atp. buf. (eupat). (eupat-p.) hg. hyo. str.

Yellow. (eupat). str. vr-a.

Discharge. (kre).

Gnawing. kre.

Heat. (alm). (ccs). (cit-c). kre. lct. mph. mtr. na-ba. rho. thu.

Heaviness. ppv.

Itching. (alm). kre. trg.

Lachrymation. dt. (eupat-p). k-bicr. (lac-f). lct. str. vr-a.

Movements. acon. (alm). atp. buf. ca-ca. cu. dt. hll. (pb). (vr-a).

Convulsions. acon. atp. buf. cu. dt.

Squinting. ca-ca. hll.

Upwards. acon. buf.

To Left. buf.

Paralysis. (trg).

Pressing. (cit-c). klm. (na-cl). (str).

Projecting. anm. atp. (spo).

Shooting. (cld).

Smarting. cast. k-bicr. trn.

Sunken. clv. (cu). k-ca. rs.

Swelling. (eupat-p).

Tearing. pul.

Tensive. k-ca.

Undefined. cth. (sang).

Same Symptom. acon. (alm). (ccs). (cld). dt. (sang).

SCLEROTIC. eupat.

Color Red. eupat.

Yellow. eupat.

IRIS. ast. buf. (cu). dt. hll. pul.

Pupils Contracted. ast. dt.

Dilated. buf. dt. hll. pul.

Insensible. buf. (cu). dt.

ORBIT. na-cl.

Pressing. na-cl.

ORBITAL INTEGUMENTS. (cu). dt.

Color Dark. (cu).

ORBITAL INTEGUMENTS INFERIORLY. dt.

Color Dark. dt.

R

EYELIDS. (alm). buf. ccs. cld. cop. cu. dt. k-ca. pb.
trg. vr-a.
>Color Dark. k-ca.
>Heat. ccs.
>Movements, Closing. cu. dt. vr-a.
>>Opening Wide. (alm). pb.
>Paralysis, Opening Difficult. trg.
>Swelling. cop.
>Same Symptom. ccs.
LOWER EYELID. alm. cld.
TARSAL EDGES. alm. cld.
LOWER TARSAL EDGE. alm. cld.
CANTHI. kre.
>Discharge. kre.
RIGHT then LEFT. alm.
>Lower Eyelid, Itching. alm.
FORWARDS. str.
>Eyeball, Pressing. str.
BACKWARDS. lac-f.
To HEAD. lac-f.
To FOREHEAD. lac-f.
To TEMPLE. lac-f.
RIGHT. alm. cld. lac-f.
>Photophobia. lac-f.
>Eyeball, Color Red. lac-f.
>>Lachrymation. lac-f.
>Lower Tarsal Edge, Heat. alm.
>>Itching. alm.
>>Shooting. cld.
>>Same Symptom. alm.
Backwards. Eyeball, Shooting. lac-f.
To Forehead. Eyeball, Shooting. lac-f.
>>>Throbbing. lac-f.
To Temple. Eyeball, Shooting. lac-f.
>>>Throbbing. lac-f.
LEFT. alm. buf. cit-c. cld. na-cl. sang.
>Sight Dazzled. na-cl.
>Sight Impaired. na-cl.
>Eyeball, Heat. cit-c.
>>Pressing. cit-c.
>>Shooting. cld.
>>Undefined. sang.
>>Same Symptom. cld. sang.

Eyelids, Movements, Closing. buf.
Lower Eyelid, Itching. alm.
                    Same Symptom. alm.

On GOING to SLEEP.

cit-c. con. lyc. na-ca.
OBJECTS, IMAGINARY. lyc.
Bright. lyc.
Vibrations. lyc.
            Bright. lyc.
EYEBALL. con.
Pressing. con.
Shooting. (cit-c).
EYELIDS. cit-c.
EYELIDS, INNER SURFACE. cit-c.
LEFT. cit-c.
Eyelids Inner Surface, Shooting. cic-c.

During SLEEP.

anm. atp. bry. chi. cit-c. con. cph. cu. dt. dt-t. fe. hll.
lau-c. lyc. p-x. pod. ppv. pul. rhe. s. sb-t. smb. str-i. vr-a.
OBJECTS, IMAGINARY. lau-c.
Increasing and Decreasing in Size. lau-c.
EYEBALL. anm. bry. chi. con. cu. hll. ppv. pul. vr-a.
Appearance Staring. con.
Discharge. vr-a.
Movements. anm. bry. chi. con. cu. hll. ppv. pul. (rhe).
        Convulsions. anm. bry. chi. con. cu. hll. ppv.
pul. (rhe).
                Upwards. hll. ppv.
EYELIDS. anm. atp. bry. chi. cit-c. con. cph. cu. dt.
dt-t. fe. hll. lyc. p-x. pod. ppv. pul. rhe. s. sb-t. smb. str-i.
vr-a.
Movements, Convulsions. rhe.
            Opening. anm. atp. bry. chi. cit-c. con.
cph. cu. dt. dt-t. fe. hll. lyc. p-x. pod. ppv. pul. s. sb-t.
smb. str-i. vr-a.
RIGHT. (chi). s. (str-i). (vr-a).
Eyelids, Movements, Opening. (chi). s. (str-i).
(vr-a).
LEFT. (chi). (str-i). (vr-a).
Eyelids, Movements, Closing. (chi). (str-i). (vr-a).

WAKING. (After Sleep).

æth. ag-na. aga. al-o. amb. amm-ca. amm-cl. apo. art-v.
atp. bry. ca-a. ca-ca. ca-s. ccs. chd. chi. chio. con. cro. cub.
dig. dl-s. dro. dt. elaps. ery. euph. frm. gel. hll. hydr.
k-bicr. k-ca. k-o. kre. krm. lct. lyc. men. mg-ca. mg-cl.
mgs. mgs-ar. mtr. n-x. na-ca. na-cl. ni-ca. ol-a. p. pb. pul.
rhe. rho. rs. rs-r. rs-v. s. sb-t. sep. smi. so-d. so-t-æg. str.
str-i. te. thr. thu. trg. trn. trx. vr-a. vr-s. woo. zn.

OBJECTS, FALSE APPEARANCE of. dig. gel. p.
   Moving. p.
      Vibrating. p.
   Multiplied. gel.
   White. dig.
OBJECTS, IMAGINARY. amm-ca. ca-s. chio. dt. k-o.
lyc. na-ca. p. so-d. str-i. zn.
   Bright. amm-ca. ca-s. lyc. na-ca.
   Flames. ca-s.
   Flashes Bright. na-ca.
   Mist. chio. k-o. lyc. na-ca. p. str-i. zn.
   Spirits. ca-s. so-d. trg.
   Spots. amm-ca.
      Bright. amm-ca.
   Veil. dt. lyc. str-i.
   Vibrations. lyc.
      Bright. lyc.
SIGHT IMPAIRED. ca-ca. (chd). chio. con. dt. k-o.
lyc. p. pul. str-i. trn. zn.
EYEBALL. ag-na. aga. al-o. amm-ca. amm-cl. art-v.
ca-a. ccs. chd. cub. dl-s. dt. elaps. ery. euph. frm. kre.
krm. lct. lyc. men. mg-ca. mtr. ni-ca. ol-a. p. pb. pul.
rhe. rho. s. sb-t. so-t-æg. thr. trg. trn. trx. vr-s. woo. zn.
   Bruised. (smi).
   Color Red. (ery). (te). woo.
   Contractive. trg.
   Discharge. al-o. amm-cl. art-v. ca-a. (chi). (euph).
krm. mtr. p. rhe. trx.
   Dryness. ag-na. dl-s. elaps. lyc. (mg-cl). (mgs).
(mgs-ar). p. (vr-a).
   False Sensations. ccs. (trn).
      Hair. ccs. (trn).
   Heat. ag-na. al-o. elaps. (k-bicr). krm. ni-ca. ol-a. rho.
(smi). (thr).

Heaviness. (k-bicr). (sep).
Itching. (sep). (te).
Lachrymation. al-o. cub. dt. (ery). (kre). krm. (pb). so-t-æg. zn.
 Hot. kre. pb. zn.
Movements. (amb). (ca-s). (sep). trg.
 As if Taken out, Squeezed, and Put back. trg.
Paralysis. (ag-na). (amm-ca). (ca-s). (cro). (dro). (k-ca). (thu).
Pressing. aga. amm-ca. dl-s. lct. sb-t. vr-s.
Shooting. trn.
Smarting. (te).
Swelling. chd. dt. (n-x). (te). woo.
 Œdematous. (te).
 Red. (te).
 Feeling of. mg-ca. ni-ca.
Tearing. pul.
Tensive. s.
Undefined. frm. (men). (sep).
EYEBALL INTERNALLY. ery. thr.
Heat. thr.
IRIS. mtr.
Pupils, Dilated. mtr.
ORBIT. smi.
ORBIT INFERIORLY. smi.
Bruised. smi.
ORBITAL INTEGUMENTS. n-x.
Swelling. n-x.
EYELIDS. ag-na. amb. amm-ca. ca-s. chd. chi. cro dro. hydr. k-bicr. k-ca. mg-cl. mgs. mgs-ar. rs. sep. smi. te. thu. trn. vr-a. vr-s.
Adhesion of. chd. chi. hydr. k-bicr. rs. smi. trn.
Dryness. mg-cl. mgs. mgs-ar. vr-a.
Movements, Closing. (amb). ca-s. (sep).
 Spasmodically. amb. sep.
Paralysis, Opening Difficult. ag-na. amm-ca. ca-s. cro. dro. k-ca. thu.
Pressing. amm-ca. vr-s.
Undefined. sep.
UPPER. EYELID. k-bicr. sep. te.
Heaviness. k-bicr. sep.
CANTHI. chi. ery. k-bicr. sep.

EXTERNAL CANTHUS. chi.
Discharge. chi.
INTERNAL CANTHUS. ery. k-bicr. sep.
Heat. k-bicr.
Itching. sep.
RIGHT. chd. ery. euph.
Sight Impaired. chd.
Eyeball, Discharge. euph.
      Lachrymation. ery.
Eyeball Internally, Color Red. ery.
Internal Canthus, Color Red. ery.
LEFT. men. rs. te. trn.
Eyeball, False Sensations, Hair. trn.
      Undefined. men.
Eyelids, Adhesion of. rs.
Upper Eyelid, Itching. te.
      Smarting. te.
      Swelling. te.
          Œdematous. te.
          Red. te.

Before SLEEP Symptoms.

jnp-s.
SIGHT IMPAIRED. jnp-s.

With SLEEP Symptoms.

acon. æth. ag-na. aga. al-o. (alm). amm-ca. anm. aps. arn.
art-v. arum-t. as-o. ast. atp. bru. bry. c-bis. cb-a. cb-v. chd.
chi. cic. cl-hx. cof. con. cph. cro. cth. cu. dl-s. dph. dt. dt-t.
ery. eryn. (eupat-p). euphr. fe. fe-a. frm. gel. grc. grt. gui.
gym. hg. hll. hyo. k-ca. kre. lch. led. li-ca. lyc. mg-sa.
mgs-ar. mn-ca. mph. mtr. myris. na-ca. na-cl. ol-a. os. ox-x. p.
p-x. pb. phl. ppv. pru-l. pt. pul. qu-sa. rho. rn-b. rs. s. sb-t. spi.
spo. sr-ca. str-i. thu. trg. trn. trx. vi-o. vi-t. vr-a. vr-s. vrb.
zn. zng.
    OBJECTS, FALSE APPEARANCE of. al-o. (alm).
atp. gel. pb.
    Black. al-o.
    Bright. atp.
    Grey. atp.

Multiplied. (alm). atp. gel. pb.
Red. atp.
White. atp.
Yellow. atp.
OBJECTS IMAGINARY. al-o. atp. cof. cro. dt. hg.
k-ca. led. mtr. myris. na-ca. p. p-x. qu-sa. rs. sb-t. spo. sr-ca.
thu. zn.
   Blue. zn.
   Bright. k-ca. qu-sa. srr.
   Circles. zn.
      Blue. zn.
      Green. zn.
      Yellow. zn.
   Figures. dt. myris.
   Flames. spo.
   Green. zn.
   Grey. atp.
   Light. qu-sa.
   Mist. atp. cro. k-ca.
      Grey. atp.
   Spots. k-ca. qu-sa. sr-ca.
      Bright. k-ca. qu-sa. sr-ca.
   Veil. dt.
   Visions. al-o. atp. cof. dt. hg. led. mtr. na-ca. p. p-x. rs.
sb-t. spo. thu.
PHOTOMANIA. dt.
PHOTOPHOBIA. cb-a. con. hg. k-ca. zng.
SIGHT IMPAIRED. aga. al-o. as-o. ast. atp. cro. dt.
gel. k-ca. mg-sa. ol-a. os. qu-sa.
EYEBALL. ag-na. (alm). aps. art-v. as-o. atp. bru. bry.
chi. con. cph. cro. cth. cu. dph. dt. ery. (eupat-p). euphr.
fe-a. grc. gui. gym. hg. hll. k-bicr. k-ca. krc. lyc. mg-sa.
mn-ca. mph. myris. ox-x. p. pb. ppv. pru-l. pt. rho. rn-b.
rs. s. spi. spo. str-i. trg. trn. vr-a. vr-s. zn.
   Appearance Bright. (alm). atp.
      Dim. bry. cu. mg-sa. spo.
      Glassy. atp.
      Staring. dt. ery. k-ca. pru-l.
   Color Dark. (art-v). (cu).
      Red. (as-o). atp. con. (cu). (eupat-p). hg.
(k-bicr). vr-a. zn.
      Yellow. chi. pb.
   Cutting. s.
   Drawing. (as-o). dph.

Dryness. cph. grc. myris. (pul). spi. zn.
Gnawing. ox-x.
Heat. (cb-v). (cro) gym. kre. mph. pru-l. pt. rho.
Heaviness. (c-bis). (cro). (frm). p.
Itching. rn-b.
Lachrymation. bru. con. cro. (eupat-p). fe-a. k-bicr. k-ca. mph. str-i. vr-s. (zn).
    Hot. zn.
    Feeling of. cro.
Movements. (œth). (alm). (amm-cl). aps. art-v. (c-bis). cu. dt. (dt-t). (ery). hll. (lch). (myris). (pb). ppv. trg.
    Convulsions. art-v. cu. dt. trg.
    Squinting. (alm). art-v. hll. (pb).
    Upwards. aps. ppv.
Paralysis. (cb-v). (hyo). (li-ca).
Pressing. (as-o). (dt). ery. euphr. k-ca. kre. lyc. mn-ca. (myris). (na-cl). p. rn-b. (rs). s.
Projecting. cu.
    Feeling of. gui.
Shooting. k-ca.
Smarting. cro. cth. ox-x. trn.
Strained. dph.
Sunken. ag-na. k-ca.
    Feeling. zn.
Swelling. (con). (cu). (dt). (eupat-p). spo.
    Feeling of. cro. gui.
Tearing. (pb).
Tensive. k-ca. ox-x.
Undefined. cro. zn.
SCLEROTIC. con.
Color Red. con.
CORNEA. con.
Opacity. con.
IRIS. (alm). arn. art-v. as-o. ast. atp. dt. ery. hll. pb.
Pupils Contracted. ast. atp.
    Dilated. (alm). arn. art-v. as-o. atp. dt. ery. hll. pb.
    Insensible. as-o.
ORBIT. k-ca. na-cl. zn.
Pressing. k-ca. na-cl.
ORBIT SUPERIORLY. zn.
Undefined. zn.
ORBITAL INTEGUMENTS. art-v. cu. ox-x. spo.

Color Dark. art-v. cu.
Swelling. spo.
ORBITAL, INTEGUMENTS SUPERIORLY ox-x.
Gnawing. ox-x.
Smarting. ox-x.
Tensive. ox-x.
EYELIDS. æth. amm-cl. aps. c-bis. cb-v. chi. con. cph. cro. cth. cu. dt. dt-t. ery. frm. grt. hyo. k-bicr. k-ca. kre. lch. li-ca. myris. pb. ppv. pul. s. trx. vi-t. vr-s. zn.
Adhesion of. kre.
Color Red. con. cu. k-bicr. zn.
Dryness. cph. pul.
Heat. cb-v. cro.
Heaviness. c-bis. cro. frm.
Movements, Closing. æth. amm-cl. aps. c-bis. chi. cth. cu. ery. grt. lch. myris. ppv. s. trx. vi-t. vr-s.
     Spasmodically. myris.
  Opening Wide. (cu). dt-t.
  Winking. myris.
Paralysis, Opening Difficult. cb-v. hyo. li-ca.
Pressing. dt.
Swelling. con. cu. dt.
  Feeling of. cro.
Tearing. pb.
UPPER EYELID. k-ca.
Swelling. k-ca.
FORWARDS. rs.
Eyeball, Pressing. rs.
BACKWARDS. dph.
Eyeball, Drawing. dph.
RIGHT. (alm). as-o. pb.
Eyeball, Color Red. as-o.
   Drawing. as-o.
   Movements, Squinting. (alm). pb.
     Inwards. (alm). pb.
  Pressing. as-o.

    Before CHILLS.

na-cl.
OBJECTS, IMAGINARY. na-cl.
Bright. na-cl.
Zigzag. na-cl.
  Bright. na-cl.

With CHILLS.

acon. ag-na. alm. anm. aps. as-o. atp. bry. buf. ca-ca. ca-s. cap. cast. cb-a. chi. cic. cit-c. cld. clv. cn-sa. cph. crb-x. cro. cth. cu. cy-hx. dig. dph. dt. ery. eupat. (eupat-p). fe. gel. grp. hg. hyo. jnp-s. k-bicr. k-ca. k-i. kre. lct. led. lyc. mgs-au. msc. mtr. myris. na-ba. na-cl. nic. p. pol. pru-l. pul. qu-sa. rho. s. sep. spi. (spo). srr. str. str-i. thr. trg. trn. vr-a. vr-s.

OBJECTS, FALSE APPEARANCE of. atp. dt. gel. thr.

Blue. atp.

Bright. atp.

Grey. atp.

Large. dt.

Multiplied. atp. gel. thr.

Red. atp.

White. atp.

OBJECTS IMAGINARY. atp. cic. cro. (cu). cy-hx. dt. hyo. jnp-s. k-ca. kre. led. lyc. mtr. pru-l. sep. str. thr. trg. vr-s.

Black. thr.

Bright. atp. hyo. k-ca. led. lyc. mtr. sep. thr.

Figures. (cu). dt.

Flames. atp. hyo.

Grey. atp.

Mist. atp. cro. cy-hx. k-ca. pru-l.

   Grey. atp.

Spirits. (cu).

Spots. k-ca.

   Bright. k-ca.

Veil. kre.

Vibrations. cic. jnp-s. led. lyc. mtr. sep. thr. trg. vr-s.

   Black. thr.

   Bright. led. lyc. mtr. sep. thr.

Visions. dt. str.

PHOTOPHOBIA. acon. aps. as-o. atp. ca-s. (dt). hg. k-ca. kre. lyc. mtr. na-ba. pol. rs. sep. str. thr.

SIGHT DAZZLED. (na-cl).

SIGHT IMPAIRED. alm. atp. ca-ca. chi. cic. cy-hx. dig. (dt). gel. grp. hyo. jnp-s. k-ca. kre. lyc. mgs-au. msc. mtr. na-cl. pru-l. qu-sa. srr. trg. trn.

EYEBALL. acon. ag-na. anm. aps. as-o. atp. bry. buf. ca-ca. cap. cast. cic. cit-c. cld. clv. cth. cu. dig. dph. dt. ery.

eupat. (eupat-p). hg. hyo. k-bicr. k-ca. kre. lct. led. lyc. msc. mtr. na-ba. na-cl. p. pol. pul. rho. rs. s. sep. (spo). str. trg. trn. vr-a.

Appearance Bright. atp. dt. eupat. mtr. sep. trg. trn.

 Dim. as-o. buf. (cu). dt. k-ca. mtr. vr-a.

 Glassy. anm. atp.

 Staring. acon. anm. cic. (cu). k-ca. msc. (spo).

Color Dark. (cu). (k-ca). (myris). p.

 Red. acon. atp. buf. cu. eupat. (eupat-p). hg. kre. na-cl. rs. str.

  Yellow. as-o. eupat. (eupat-p). (spi). str. vr-a.

Dryness. (rs).

Heat. (acon). (aps). (atp.) cro. k-bicr. (kre). lct. mtr. na-ba. pol. rho. (rs). sep.

Itching. (trn).

Lachrymation. ag-na. aps. atp. bry. dph. (enpat-p). k-bicr. k-ca. kre. lct. rs. str. vr-a.

 Hot. bry. kre.

Movements. (acon). buf. (ca-ca). cu. dig. dt. (kre). (mtr). (myris). (rs). (trg). (vr-a).

 Convulsions. cu. dt. (trg).

 Squinting. dig.

 Upwards. buf. (cu).

 To Left. buf.

Pressing. (cit-c). ery. k-ca. kre. lyc. (na-cl). p. rs. s. sep. (str).

Projecting. anm. (spo).

Shooting. acon. aps. cit-c. k-ca. na-ba. rs.

Smarting. bry. cast. k-bicr. trn.

Stiffness. acon. atp. cic. hyo. trg.

Sunken. as-o. clv. (cu). k-ca. p.

Swelling. (aps). (fe). (k-ca). (k-i). (rs).

Tearing. pul.

Tensive. k-ca.

Undefined. acon. aps. atp. ca-ca. cap. cit-c. cld. cth. dph. kre. led. lyc. mtr. na-ba. pol. rho. rs. sep. trg.

SCLEROTIC. eupat.

Color Red. eupat.

 Yellow. eupat.

IRIS. acon. aps. atp. buf. ca-ca. cap. cb-a. cic. cph. crb-x. cro. (cu). dig. dph. dt. hyo. msc. mtr. myris. p. s. sep. si-x. str. str-i. vr-a.

Pupils Contracted. acon. atp. cap. crb-x. dig. dt. msc. mtr. s. sep. si-x. str. vr-a.

    Dilated. aps. atp. buf. ca-ca. cb-a. cic. cph. cro. dph. dt. hyo. mtr. myris. nic. ppv. str-i. trg.

    Insensible. acon. buf. crb-x. (cu). myris. ppv.

    Irregular. trg.

ORBIT. cit-c. na-cl.

Pressing. cit-c. na-cl.

ORBITAL INTEGUMENTS. (cu). myris. p. spi.

Color Dark. (cu). p.

    Yellow. spi.

ORBITAL, INTEGUMENTS INFERIORLY. myris.

Color Dark. myris.

EYELIDS. acon. aps. atp. ca-ca. cro. cu. dig. fe. k-ca. kre. myris. rs. trn. vr-a.

Color Dark. k-ca.

Dryness. rs.

Heat. acon. aps. atp. cro. kre. rs.

Itching. trn.

Movements Closing. (buf). cu. (dig). dt. kre. mtr. vr-a.

    Convulsions. ca-ca. cu. rs.

    Opening Wide. acon.

    Winking. myris.

Smarting. trn.

Swelling. aps. fe. k-i. rs.

UPPER EYELID.. k-ca.

Swelling. k-ca.

FORWARDS. p. s. str.

Eyeball, Pressing. p. s. str.

RIGHT. dig.

Eyelids, Movements, Closing. dig.

LEFT. buf. na-cl. trg.

Sight Dazzled. na-cl.

Sight Impaired. na-cl.

Eyeball, Movements, Convulsions. trg.

Eyelids, Movements, Closing. buf.

    Convulsions. trg.

After CHILLS.

cic. ni-ca. pet.

EYEBALL. ni-ca. pet.

Discharge. ni-ca.
Heat. pet.

Before HEAT.

str.
EYEBALL. str.
Pressing. str.
FORWARDS. str.
Eyeball, Pressing. str.

With HEAT.

acon. alm. aps. art-v. as-o. asr. atp. au. bi-na. buf. ca-ca.
ca-s. cb-a. chi. cic. cit-c. con. cph. cth. (cu). dig. dor. dt.
eupat. (eupat-p). fe. glo. hg. hyo. i. k-ca. k-i. k-o. lch. lct.
led. ly-b. lyc. mn-ca. mtr. myris. na-ba. na-ca. na-cl. p. p-x.
pet. pol. ppv. pul. qu-sa. rho. rs. rut. s. sep. smb. spi. str. trg.
trn. val. vr-a. vr-s.
OBJECTS, FALSE APPEARANCE of. atp. cb-v.
cic. i.
  Blue. atp. i.
  Bright. atp.
  Grey. atp.
  Multiplied. atp. cic.
  Red. atp.
  Small. cb-v.
  White. atp.
OBJECTS IMAGINARY. atp. au. ca-ca. cb-a. cb-v.
chi. dt. hyo. k-ca. ppv. pul. sep.
  Bright. atp. au. cb-a. hyo. k-ca. ppv. sep.
  Figures. dt.
  Flames. atp. ppv.
  Flashes Bright. hyo.
  Green. chi.
  Grey. atp.
  Mist. atp. k-ca. sep.
    Grey. atp.
  Spots. atp. au. cb-a. k-ca. ppv.
    Bright. atp. au. cb-a. k-ca. ppv.
  Vibrations. sep.
    Bright. sep.
  isions. ca-ca. cb-v. (dt). ppv. pul.
    Horrid. cb-v. (dt).

PHOTOPHOBIA. acon. aps. atp. ca-s. con. k-ça. na-ba. s. str.

SIGHT IMPAIRED. atp. bi-na. cb-v. (dt). hg. k-ca. k-o. mtr. na-cl. pul. qu-sa. sep.

EYEBALL. acon. aps. art-v. as-o. asr. atp. bi-na. buf. ca-ca. ca-s. cb-a. cb-v. chi. cic. cit-c. cph. cth. (cu). dig. dor. dt. eupat. (eupat-p). hyo. hyp. k-ca. lch. lct. led. ly-b. lyc. mtr. na-ba. na-ca. na-cl. p. p-x. pet. pol. ppv. pul. rho. rs. rut. s. sep. spi. str. trg. trn. val. vr-a. vr-s.

Appearance Bright. atp. dt. eupat. lch. lyc. mtr. trg. trn.

    Dim. buf. dt.

    Glassy. atp. glo.

    Staring. atp. chi. dor. dt. glo. hyp. lyc.

    Wild. dt. hyp.

Color Dark. (art-v). (dt). (fe).

    Red. acon. atp. bi-na. buf. dt. (eupat-p). hyo. na-cl. (vr-a).

    Yellow. (eupat).

Dryness. spi.

Heat. cb-a. k-ca. lct. na-ba. pet. rho. sep. spi. vr-a.

Itching. (ly-b).

Lachrymation. aps. atp. dt. (eupat-p). k-ca. lct.

Movements. (alm). aps. art-v. buf. (cu). (dt). (lyc). (mtr). (smb). (vr-a).

    Convulsions. art-v. (cu).

    Squinting. aps. art-v.

    Upwards. aps. buf.

    To Left. buf.

Paralysis. na-cl.

Pressing. k-ca. (myris). na-ba. (na-cl). sep.

Projecting. atp. spi.

Shooting. k-ca.

Smarting. asr. na-ba. trn.

Sunken. k-ca.

Swelling. (fe). (k-ca). (k-i).

Tensive. k-ca.

Throbbing. (myris).

Undefined. acon. aps. as-o. atp. ca-ca. ca-s. cb-a. cb-v. cic. cit-c. cph. cth. dig. dt. hyo. led. lyc. na-ba. na-cl. p-x. pol. ppv. pul. rho. rs. rut. s. sep. spi. str. trg. val. vr-a. vr-s.

SCLEROTIC. eupat.

Color Red. eupat.

     Yellow. eupat.

IRIS. acon. aps. art-v. atp. buf. cic. dt. glo. hyp. lyc. mn-ca. mtr. str.

Pupils Contracted. acon. atp. glo. mn-ca. mtr.

     Dilated. aps. art-v. atp. buf. cic. dt. hyp. lyc. str.

     Insensible. buf. dt.

ORBIT. myris. na-cl. val.

Pressing. na-cl.

Undefined. val.

ORBIT SUPERIORLY. myris.

ORBITAL INTEGUMENTS. art-v. dt. fe.

Color Dark. art-v. fe.

Swelling. fe.

ORBITAL INTEGUMENTS INFERIORLY. dt.

Color Dark. dt.

EYELIDS. alm. aps. buf. dt. k-ca. k-i. lyc. smb. vr-a.

Movements, Closing. alm. aps. (buf). dt. lyc. smb. vr-a.

     Opening Wide. (dt). lyc. mtr.

Swelling. k-i.

· UPPER EYELID. k-ca.

Swelling. k-ca.

RIGHT. ly-b. vr-a.

Eyeball, Color Red. vr-a.

     Itching. ly-b.

LEFT. buf. myris.

Orbit Superiorly, Pressing. myris.

     Throbbing. myris.

Eyelids, Movements, Closing. buf.

After HEAT.

au-cl. bry. lyc. spo.

SIGHT. IMPAIRED. au-cl.

EYEBALL. spo.

Shooting. (spo).

Swelling. (bry).

Tearing. (spo).

LENS. lyc.

Cataract. lyc.

EYELIDS. bry.

LOWER EYELID. bry.
Swelling. bry.
LEFT. spo.
Eyeball, Shooting. spo.
          Tearing. spo.

Before SWEAT.

narth.
SIGHT IMPAIRED. narth.

With SWEAT.

acon. ag-na. alm. anm. aps. arn. art-v. as-o. atp. au-cl.
bry. buf. ca-ca. ca-s. cap. cb-v. chi. cl-hx. cld. con. crb-x.
crot. cth. (cu). dl-s. dph. dt. grp. hg. hll. hyo. hyp. k-bicr.
k-ca. k-o. lau-c. led. lyc. mtr. myris. na-ca. na-cl. na-sa.
nic. ox-x. p. p-x. ppv. pul. qu-sa. rho. rs. s. sep. si-x. spi.
(spo). str. thu. vr-a.
OBJECTS, FALSE APPEARANCE **of.** atp. cb-v.
Blue. atp.
Bright. atp.
Grey. atp.
Multiplied. atp.
Red. atp.
Small. cb-v.
White. atp.
OBJECTS, IMAGINARY. as-o. atp. ca-ca. cb-v. (cu).
dl-s. (dt). grp. k-ca. k-o. lyc. mtr. na-cl. pul. sep. spi. str.
Bright. atp. ca-ca. dl-s. grp. k-ca. k-o. lyc. mtr. na-cl.
pul. sep. spi. str.
Figures. (cu).
Flames. atp. k-ca. k-o. na-cl. pul. spi. str.
Grey. atp.
Mist. atp.
     Grey. atp.
Spirits. (cu).
Vibrations. dl-s. grp. k-o. lyc. mtr. sep. str.
     Bright. dl-s. grp. k-o. lyc. mtr. sep. str.
Visions. as-o. cb-v. (dt).
     Horrid. cb-v. (dt).

PHOTOPHOBIA. acon. aps. arn. as-o. atp. bry. ca-ca. ca-s. chi. dt. grp. hg. lyc. mtr. p-x. pul. rs. s. sep. str.

SIGHT IMPAIRED. ag-na. alm. anm. atp. au-cl. ca-ca. ca-s. cb-v. con. crot. dt. hg. hyo. k-o. na-cl. ox-x. p. p-x. qu-sa. s. si-x.

EYEBALL. acon. anm. aps. arn. as-o. atp. bry. buf. ca-ca. ca-s. cld. con. cth. (cu). dt. hg. hll. hyp. k-bicr. k-o. led. lyc. mtr. na-ca. na-sa. p. ppv. pul. rho. rs. s. sep. si-x. spi. (spo). str. thu. vr-a.

Appearance Bright. acon. atp. dt.

> **Dim.** as-o. buf. vr-a.
> **Glassy.** anm. atp.
> **Staring.** anm. as-o. (cu). dt. hyp. (spo).
> **Wild.** dt. hyp.

Color Dark. (cu).

> **Red.** atp. buf. cld. (con). (cu). dt. s.
> **Yellow.** as-o. vr-a.

Eruptions. (ca-ca).

> **Ulcers.** (ca-ca).

Heat. dt.

Heaviness. (crot). ppv.

Lachrymation. aps. bry. (con). k-bicr. (na-sa). vr-a.

> **Hot.** bry.

Movements. acon. buf. (ca-ca). (cu). dt. hll. (myris). (ppv). (vr-a).

> **Convulsions.** buf.
> **Squinting.** hll.
> **Upwards.** acon. buf.
> **To Left.** buf.

Pressing. (con). (na-cl). s.

Projecting. anm. (cu). (spo).

Shooting. ca-ca.

Smarting. bry. k-bicr.

Sunken. as-o. (cu).

Swelling, Feeling of. cld.

Tearing. pul.

Undefined. acon. arn. as-o. atp. bry. ca-ca. ca-s. cth. (cu). hg. k-o. led. lyc. mtr. na-ca. p. pul. rho. rs. s. sep. si-x. spi. str. thu. vr-a.

CORNEA. ca-ca.

Eruptions, Ulcers. ca-ca.

IRIS. anm. art-v. atp. buf. ca-ca. ca-s. cap. cl-hx. crb-x. dph. dt. hll. hyo. hyp. lau-c. mtr. nic. p-x. ppv. pul. s. sep. si-x. spi. thu. vr-a.

s

Pupils Contracted. anm. atp. cap. cl-hx. crb-x. dph. lau-c. mtr. p-x. pul. s. sep. si-x. thu. vr-a.

Dilated. anm. art-v. atp. buf. ca-ca. ca-s. dt. hll. hyo. hyp. nic. ppv. spi.

Insensible. buf. crb-x. dt.

ORBIT. crot. na-cl.

Heaviness. crot.

Pressing. na-cl.

ORBITAL INTEGUMENTS. (cu).

Color Dark. (cu).

EYELIDS. buf. ca-ca. con. crot. myris. ppv. vr-a.

Adhesion of. (con).

Movements, Closing. (buf). (ca-ca). vr-a.

Spasmodically. ca-ca.

Opening Wide. ppv.

Winking. myris.

UPPER EYELID. crot.

Heaviness. crot.

RIGHT. con. na-sa.

Eyeball, Color Red. con.

Lachrymation. con. na-sa.

Pressing. con.

Eyelids, Adhesion of. con.

LEFT. buf.

Eyelids, Movements, Closing. buf.

After SWEAT.

cb-v.

EYEBALL. cb-v.

Heat. cb-v.

Before CONVULSIONS.

hyo. si-x.

OBJECTS, IMAGINARY. hyo.

Bright. hyo.

Spots. hyo.

Bright. hyo.

EYEBALL. si-x.

Lachrymation. si-x.

With CONVULSIONS.

acon. æth. aga. (alm). amm-ca. anm. apo. aps. art-v. as-o. ast. atp. buf. cic. cmf. crb-x. cth. cu. dol. dt. glo. glp. hll. hyo. k-o. lau-c. mtr. phy. ppv. pul. s. si-x. thr. trg. trn. vr-a.

OBJECTS, FALSE APPEARANCE of. amm-ca. cic. dt. hyo.

Black. amm-ca.

Large. dt.

Moving. amm-ca.

Multiplied. cic. hyo.

OBJECTS, IMAGINARY. (dt). hyo. thr.

Bright. hyo.

Flashes Bright. hyo.

Vibrations. thr.

Visions. (dt).

　　Horrid. (dt).

PHOTOPHOBIA. hyo.

SIGHT IMPAIRED. amm-ca. apo. ast. atp. dt. k-o. s.

EYEBALL. acon. æth. (alm). anm. aps. art-v. as-o. atp. buf. cic. cmf. cth. cu. dol. dt. glo. hll. hyo. k-o. lau-c. mtr. phy. ppv. pul. s. si-x. trg. trn.

Appearance Bright. (alm). cmf. cth. dt.

　　Dim. buf. dt. mtr. phy.

　　Glassy. anm.

　　Staring. æth. anm. atp. cic. cth. (cu). dol. dt. k-o. mtr. s. si-x.

　　Wild. dt.

Color Dark. (art-v). (cu). (dt).

　　Red. (aga). buf. cu. dt. hyo. ppv.

Heaviness. ppv.

Itching. (cu).

Movements. acon. æth. (aga). aps. art-v. as-o. atp. buf. cic. cth. cu. dol. dt. glo. glp. hyo. k-o. lau-c. mtr. (ppv). pul. si-x. trg. (vr-a).

　　Convulsions. acon. æth. aps. art-v. as-o. atp. buf. buf. cic. cth. cu. dt. glo. k-o. lau-c. mtr. pul. si-x. trg.

　　Squinting. æth. aps. art-v. atp. hll.

　　Upwards. acon. buf. cic. cu. glo.

　　Downwards. æth.

　　Outwards. glo.

To Left. buf.
Projecting. anm. hyo.
Smarting. trn.
Sunken. (cu). (dt).
Undefined. (cu).
IRIS. æth. anm. aps. art-v. ast. atp. cic. cu. dt. hll.
mtr. phy. ppv.
Pupils Contracted. ast. crb-x.
　　　　Dilated. æth. anm. aps. art-v. atp. cic. dt. hll.
mtr. phy. ppv.
　　　　Insensible. æth. atp. (cu). dt. ppv.
ORBITAL INTEGUMENTS. art-v. (cu). dt.
Color Dark. art-v. (cu).
ORBITAL INTEGUMENTS INFERIORLY. dt.
Color Dark. dt.
EYELIDS. aga. atp. buf. cu. dol. dt. glp. hyo. k-o.
mtr. ppv. pul. vr-a.
Itching. (cu).
Movements, Closing. acon. (buf). cu. dt. glp. k-o.
mtr. ppv. pul. vr-a.
　　　　Convulsions. atp. cu. hyo. mtr.
　　　　Opening Wide. (buf). dol. (dt). ppv.
　　　　Winking. aga.
CANTHI. aga.
INTERNAL CANTHUS. aga.
Color Red. aga.
RIGHT. buf. trg.
Eyelids, Movements, Convulsions. trg.
　　　　　　　Opening Wide. buf. 　　　　　.
LEFT. buf.
Eyelids, Movements, Closing. buf.

After CONVULSIONS.

bru. hyo. s.
EYEBALL. hyo. s.
Lachrymation. s.
Movements. (bru).
Tearing. (hyo).
Throbbing. (hyo).
EYELIDS. bru.
Movements, Closing. bru.

RIGHT. hyo.
Eyeball, Tearing. hyo.
    Throbbing. hyo.

With EMACIATION.

cap. (dt). na-ca.
SIGHT IMPAIRED. cap.
EYEBALL. (dt).
Sunken. (dt).
IRIS. (dt). na-ca.
Pupils Dilated. (dt). na-ca.

With FAINTING.

acon. alm. amb. atp. buf. ca-ca. can. chd. chi. crot. (cu).
dor. dt. fe-a. frm. gel. glo. k-na. ly-b. lyc. mg-cl. morph-a.
myris. na-ba. pb. pet. s-x. str. trg. vr-a. vr-v.
    OBJECTS, FALSE APPEARANCE of. (dt). gel. ly-b.
mg-cl.
    Black. (dt).
    Green. mg-cl.
    Inverted. ly-b.
    Multiplied. gel.
    Red. mg-cl.
    OBJECTS, IMAGINARY. can. (cu). glo. pet. vr-a.
    Black. glo.
    Bright. (vr-a).
    Figures. (cu).
    Mist. can.
    Spirits. (cu).
    Spots. glo. (vr-a).
        Black. glo.
        Bright. (vr-a).
    Veil. pet.
    SIGHT IMPAIRED. alm. amb. ca-ca. can. chd. chi.
dor. dt. fe-a. frm. gel. glo. lyc. myris. pb. pet. s-x. trg. vr-v.
    EYEBALL. atp. buf. crot. k-na. na-ba. str.
    Appearance Staring. atp.
    Color Dark. (myris).
        Red. crot.

Heat. crot. k-na.
Movements. buf.
    Convulsions. buf.
Pressing. na-ba. (str).
Smarting. na-ba.
IRIS. acon. (dt). morph-a.
Pupils Dilated. acon. (dt). morph-a.
    Insensible. (dt).
ORBITAL INTEGUMENTS. myris.
ORBITAL INTEGUMENTS INFERIORLY.   myris.
Color Dark. myris.
FORWARDS. str.
Eyeball, Pressing. str.
LEFT. vr-a.
Objects Imaginary, Bright. vr-a.
    Spots Bright. vr-a.

With HEAVINESS of Body.

aga. myris.
OBJECTS, FALSE APPEARANCE of. myris.
Far. myris.
EYEBALL. aga.
Drawing. aga.
Pressing. aga.

With NUMBNESS of Body.

grp.
SIGHT IMPAIRED. grp.

With SMARTING of Body.

EYEBALL. (eupat-p).
Color Red. (eupat-p).
Swelling. (eupat-p).

With STIFFNESS of Body.

acon. as-o. atp. ppv.
OBJECTS IMAGINARY. atp.
Bright. atp.

Spots. atp.
   Bright. atp.
EYEBALL. acon. as-o. ppv.
Appearance Dim. as-o.
   Staring. acon.
Color Yellow. as-o.
Movements. ppv.
   Convulsions. ppv.
Sunken. as-o.
IRIS. acon.
Pupils Contracted. acon.
   Insensible. acon.
EYELIDS. acon.
Movements, Opening Wide. acon.

With SWELLING of Body.

acon.
EYEBALL. acon.
Projecting. acon.

Before WEAKNESS.

(cu). thr.
OBJECTS, FALSE APPEARANCE of. thr.
Far. thr.
OBJECT IMAGINARY. thr.
Bright. thr.
Veil. thr.
Vibrations. thr.
   Bright. thr.
SIGHT IMPAIRED. thr.
EYEBALL. (cu).
Movements. (cu).
   Convulsions. (cu).

With WEAKNESS.

acon. alm. amm-ca. anm. aps. as-o. atp. cast. cb-v. cic.
cl-hx. clv. cof. cth. cu. dro. dt. ery. eupat-p. euph-a. grp. grt.
hg. hyo. k-ca. k-na. kre. lac-f. mg-cl. myris. na-ba. ni-ca. os.
pb. ppv. qu-sa. rho. rs. s. si-x. smi. so-d. spo. sr-ca. str. thr.
trg. trn. vr-a. vr-s. zn.

OBJECTS, FALSE APPEARANCE of.   (alm).
amm-ca. cic. mg-cl. pb. thr.

Far. thr.

Green. mg-cl.

Moving. amm-ca.

Multiplied. (alm). cic. pb.

Red. mg-cl.

OBJECTS IMAGINARY.   as-o. atp. ery. hyo. k-ca.
smi. sr-ca. thr. trg.

Black. (ery).

Bright. atp. ery. hyo. k-ca. sr-ca. thr.

Flashes Bright. hyo.

Mist. (ery). k-ca. smi.

     Black. (ery).

     Red. (ery).

Red. (ery).

Serpentine Bodies. ery.

     Bright. ery.

Spots. atp. ery. k-ca. sr-ca.

     Bright. atp. k-ca. sr-ca.

     White. ery.

Veil. thr.

Vibrations. thr. trg.

     Bright. thr.

Visions. as-o.

White. ery.

PHOTOPHOBIA. acon. hg. k-na. (lac-f). na-ba.

SIGHT IMPAIRED.   alm. amm-ca. as-o. atp. cb-v.
(ery). euph-c. grp. k-ca. lac-f. os. pb. qu-sa. smi. so-d. thr.
trn. zn.

EYEBALL. acon. (alm). anm. aps. as-o. cast. clv. cof.
cth. cu. dro. dt. ery. eupat-p. hg. hyo. k-ca. k-na. kre. lac-f.
na-ba. ni-ca. pb. ppv. rho. rs. s. si-x. spo. str. trg. trn.
vr-a. zn.

Appearance Bright. (alm). dt.

     Dim. as-o. cu. dt. ery. spo. trg. vr-a.

     Glassy. rs.

     Staring. as-o. dt. eupat-p. k-ca.

Color Dark. (ery).

     Red. acon. (as-o). (cu). hg. hyo. (lac-f) ppv. s.

     Yellow. as-o. pb. s. vr-a.

Drawing. (as-o).

Hæmorrhage. (ery).

Heat. k-na. kre. na-ba. ni-ca. rho. s.

Heaviness. (cro). ppv.

Itching. s.

Lachrymation. cof. dt. k-ca. (lac-f). ppv. spo. (trg). vr-a.

Movements. (alm). anm. aps. (cl-hx). cu. dt. (grt). (myris). (pb). ppv. (spo). trg. (vr-s).

    Convulsions. anm. cu. dt. ppv. trg.

    Squinting. (alm). aps. (pb).

    Inwards. (alm). (pb).

Paralysis. (dro).

Pressing. (as-o). k-ca. (str).

Projecting. (cu).

Shooting. k-ca. (lac-f).

Smarting. cast. trn.

Sunken. as-o. clv. cu. dro. ery. rs.

    Feeling. zn.

Swelling. (k-ca). (spo).

    Feeling of. (cro).

Tensive. si-x.

Throbbing. (lac-f).

Undefined. cth. ery.

IRIS. (alm). anm. aps. as-o. atp. cic. cu. dt. pb.

Pupils Contracted. dt.

    Dilated. (alm). anm. aps. as-o. atp. cic. cu. dt. pb.

    Insensible. as-o. dt.

ORBITAL INTEGUMENTS. ery. spo.

Color Dark. ery.

Swelling. spo.

EYELIDS. (alm). anm. cl-hx. cro. cu. dro. dt. grt. k-ca. myris. pb. spo. trg. vr-s.

Movements, Closing. anm. cl-hx. cu. dt. grt. myris. (spo). vr-s.

                Spasmodically. spo.

    Convulsions. (cu).

    Opening Wide. (alm). dt. pb.

Paralysis, Opening Difficult. dro.

Swelling. spo.

    Feeling of. cro.

UPPER EYELID. cro. k-ca.

Heavy. cro.

Swelling. k-ca.

FORWARDS. str.
Eyeball, Pressing. str.
BACKWARDS. lac-f.
To HEAD. lac-f.
To FOREHEAD. lac-f.
To TEMPLE. lac-f.
RIGHT. (alm). as-o. lac-f. pb.
Photophobia. lac-f.
Eyeball, Color Red. as-o. lac-f.
     Drawing. as-o.
     Lachrymation. lac-f.
     Movements, Squinting. (alm). pb.
        Inwards. (alm). pb.
     Pressing. as-o.
Backwards. **Eyeball, Shooting.** lac-f.
To Forehead. **Eyeball, Shooting.** lac-f.
        Throbbing. lac-f.
To Temple. **Eyeball, Shooting.** lac-f.
        Throbbing. lac-f.
LEFT. trg.
Eyeball, Lachrymation. trg.
     Movements, Convulsions. trg.
Eyelids, Movements, Convulsions. trg.

After WEAKNESS.

as-o. con.
OBJECTS IMAGINARY. con.
Bright. con.
Vibrations. con.
     Bright. con.
PHOTOPHOBIA. as-o.
SIGHT IMPAIRED. con.
EYEBALL. as-o.
Color Red. as-o.
Heat. as-o.
Lachrymation. as-o.

With GLANDULAR Symptoms.

au. ca-ca. con. hg-bicl. rs. s. trn.
OBJECTS, FALSE APPEARANCE of. s.

Multiplied. s.
PHOTOPHOBIA. au. ca-ca. con.
EYEBALL. au. ca-ca. con. s.
Color Red. (au). (con). (s).
    White. (hg-bicl).
Cutting. au.
Eruptions. (ca-ca). (hg-bicl). (rs). (s).
    Pimples. (rs).
    Ulcers. (ca-ca). (hg-bicl). (rs).
    Vesicles. (rs).
Itching. (trn).
Lachrymation. (au) con.
    Hot. au.
Movements. (ca-ca). (hg-bicl).
Shooting. ca-ca.
Smarting. (trn).
Swelling. (con). (hg-bicl). (rs).
Undefined. (s).
Same Symptom. (s).
EYEBALL, ROUND CORNEA. s.
Color Red. s.
SCLEROTIC. con.
Color Red. con.
CORNEA. au. ca-ca. con. hg-bicl. rs. s.
Color Red. au.
    White. hg-bicl.
Eruptions, Pimples. rs.
    Ulcers. ca-ca. hg-bicl. s.
    Vesicles. rs.
Opacity. con. (hg-bicl). s.
CHAMBERS of EYE. hg-bicl.
Discharge, Pus. hg-bicl.
EYELIDS. au. ca-ca. con. hg-bicl. s. trn.
Adhesion of. au.
Color Red. con.
Itching. trn.
Movements, Closing. (ca-ca). (hg-bicl).
                 Spasmodically. ca-ca. hg-bicl.
Smarting. trn.
Swelling. con. hg-bicl.
TARSAL EDGES. s.
Eruptions, Ulcers. s.
Swelling. s.

CANTHI. s.
EXTERNAL CANTHUS. s.
Color Red. s.
LEFT. s.
Eyeball, Undefined. s.
  Same Symptom. s.

With JOINTS Symptoms.

(eupat-p).
EYEBALL. (eupat-p).
Color Red. (eupat-p).
Swelling. (eupat-p).

With SKIN Symptoms.

acon. æsc. (alm). atp. ca-ca. ca-s. cic. clv. cop. cu. dt.
ery. hg. hg-cl. morph-a. pb. s. sa-l. str.
OBJECTS, FALSE APPEARANCE of. (alm). cic.
pb. s.
  Multiplied. (alm). cic. pb. s.
OBJECTS, IMAGINARY. (dt).
Figures. (dt).
PHOTOPHOBIA. ca-ca. hg.
EYEBALL. acon. æsc. (alm). ca-ca. ca-s. clv. cu. dt.
ery. hg. hg-cl. morph-a. pb. s. sa-l. str.
  Appearance Dim. ery.
  Coldness. (sa-l).
  Color Dark. (cu). (ery).
    Red. (cu). dt. hg. morph-a. (s). str.
    Yellow. æsc. ca-s. hg-cl. s. str.
  Eruptions. (s).
    Ulcers. (s).
  Lachrymation. str.
  Movements. (alm). ca-ca. cu. (pb). s.
    Convulsions. cu.
    Squinting. (alm). ca-ca. (pb). s.
  Projecting. acon. cu.
  Shooting. sa-l.
    Cold. sa-l.
  Sunken. clv. (cu). (dt). ery.

Swelling. (cop). (cu). (s).
EYEBALL ROUND CORNEA. s.
Color Red. s.
CORNEA. s.
Eruptions, Ulcers. s.
Opacity. s.
IRIS. (alm). atp. cic. dt. pb.
Pupils Dilated. (alm). atp. cic. dt. pb.
ORBITAL INTEGUMENTS. cu. ery.
Color Dark. cu. ery.
EYELIDS. cop. cu. s.
Color Red. cu.
Movements, Closing. cu.
Swelling. cop. cu.
TARSAL EDGES. s.
Eruptions, Ulcers. s.
Swelling. s.
CANTHI. s.
EXTERNAL CANTHUS. s.
Color Red. s.
RIGHT. (alm). pb.
Eyeball, Movements, Squinting. (alm). pb.
                Inwards. (alm). pb.

ERUPTIONS, Suppressed.

atp. k-o. mg-ca. s. si-x. smi.
SIGHT IMPAIRED. atp. s.
EYEBALL. k-o. smi.
Color Red. k-o. smi.
LENS. mg-ca. s. si-x.
Cataract. mg-ca. s. si-x.

GONORRHŒA, Suppressed.

pul. sb-s.
EYEBALL. pul. sb-s.
Color Red. pul. sb-s.

GOUT.

bry. dig.
EYEBALL. bry. dig.
Color Red. bry. dig.

SCROFULA.

ca-ca. chi. cis. cle. con. dig.
PHOTOPHOBIA.　con.
EYEBALL.　chi. cis. cle. con. dig.
Color Red.　chi. cle. con. dig.
Motion in.　cis.
　　　Passing Round, like something.　cis.
Shooting.　cis.
LENS.　ca-ca.
Cataract.　ca-ca.

SWEAT of FEET, Suppressed.

si-x.
LENS.　si-x.
Cataract.　si-x.

SYPHILIS.

ca-s. n-x.
EYEBALL.　ca-s. n-x.
Color Red.　ca-s. n-x.

LOSS of FLUIDS.

art-v. au-cl. cb-v. chi. dt. p, vr-v.
OBJECTS, IMAGINARY.　dt. vr-v.
Circles.　vr-v.
　　Green.　vr-v.
　　Red.　vr-v.
Green.　vr-v.
Red.　vr-v.
Veil.　dt.
SIGHT IMPAIRED.　art-v. au-cl. cb-v. chi. dt. p.
vr-v.
　EYEBALL.　chi.
Color Red.　chi.
Itching.　chi.

INJURIES.

acon. (alm). con. cro. cyc. euphr. n-x. s.
SIGHT IMPAIRED. con.
EYEBALL. cro. cyc. euphr. n-x.
Color Red. euphr.
Lachrymation. n-x.
    Hot. n-x.
Movements. (cyc).
    Squinting. (cyc).
    Inwards. (cyc).
Shooting. cro.
IRIS. (alm).
Prolapsus. (alm).
LENS. con.
Cataract. con.
RIGHT. con.
Sight Impaired. con.
Lens, Cataract. con.

LEFT. cyc.
Eyeball, Movements, Squinting. cyc.
                  Inwards. cyc.

ALCOHOL.

sb-t. str. zn.
SIGHT IMPAIRED. str.
EYEBALL. sb-t.
Color Red. sb-t.
Eruptions. sb-t.
    Blisters. sb-t.

BEER.

sb-t.
EYEBALL. sb-t.
Color Red. sb-t.
Eruptions. sb-t.
    Blisters. sb-t.

CAMPHOR, Smell of.

k-na.
SIGHT IMPAIRED. k-na.

COFFEE.

alli.
EYEBALL.
Itching. (alli).
EYELIDS. alli.
UPPER EYELID. alli.
LEFT. alli.
Upper Eyelid, Itching. alli.

LEMONADE.

dt.
IRIS. dt.
Pupils Contracted. dt.

MERCURY.

au. ca-s.
PHOTOPHOBIA. au.
EYEBALL. au. ca-s.
Color Red. au. ca-s.
Cutting. au.
Eruptions. (ca-s).
    Ulcers. (ca-s).
Lachrymation. (au).
    Hot. au.
CORNEA. au.
Color Red. au.
Eruptions, Ulcers. au.
EYELIDS. au.
Adhesion of. au.

SILVER, Nitrate of.

na-cl.
EYEBALL. na-cl.
Color Red. na-cl.
Discharge. na-cl.
   Excoriating. na-cl.
   Thin. na-cl.

TOBACCO.

asc. cld.
SIGHT IMPAIRED. asc.
EYEBALL. cld.
Pressing. cld.

VINEGAR.

dt.
OBJECTS, FALSE APPEARANCE **of.** dt.
Small. dt.
SIGHT IMPAIRED. dt.
Myopia. dt.
IRIS. dt.
Pupils Contracted. dt.
   Insensible. dt.

WINE.

zn.

T

II. B. AMELIORATIONS.

BED.

smc.
EYEBALL.
Boring. (smc).
Throbbing. (smc).
ORBIT. smc.
ORBIT SUPERIORLY. smc.
RIGHT. smc.
Orbit Superiorly, Boring. smc.
     Throbbing. smc.

COLD.

ag-na. al-o. alli. amm-ca. asr. k-na. k-o. mg-ca. ni-ca.
ox-x. p. thu.
SIGHT IMPAIRED. al-o. amm-cl. k-o. ni-ca.
EYEBALL. ag-na. al-o. alli. amm-cl. asr. mg-ca. ni-ca.
ox-x. thu.
Color Red. ag-na.
Drawing. (alli).
Gnawing. ox-x.
Heat. al-o. amm-cl. (thu).
Lachrymation. al-o.
    Hot. (al-o).
Pressing. (p).
Smarting. al-o. ox-x.
Swelling, Feeling of. ni-ca.
Tearing. mg-ca.
Tensive. ox-x.
Undefined. ag-na. asr. ni-ca.
ORBITAL INTEGUMENTS. ox-x.
ORBITAL INTEGUMENTS SUPERIORLY. ox-x.
Gnawing. ox-x.
Smarting. ox-x.
Tensive. ox-x,

EYELIDS. mg-ca. p.
Adhesion of. mg-ca.
UPPER EYELID. p.
Pressing. p.
RIGHT. thu.
Eyeball, Heat. thu.
LEFT. al-o. alli.
Eyeball, Drawing. alli.
    Heat. al-o.
      Lachrymation. al-o.
        Hot. al-o.
    Smarting. al-o.

COVERING.

thu.
EYEBALL. thu.
Undefined. thu.

HEAT.

eryn. zn.
EYEBALL. zn.
Heat. zn.
Smarting. zn.
Undefined. zn.

OPEN AIR.

ag-na. alli. amb. cit-c. cl-hx. cof. cro. dig. grc. grt. hæm.
hg. hyo. jcr. jnp-s. k-o. lau-c. lyc. ox-x. p. phy. pol. pt.
pul. rs. sep. smi. trg.
OBJECTS, FALSE APPEARANCE of. grt. hæm.
jnp-s.
Confused. hæm.
Moving. grt. jnp-s.
  Circularly. grt.
  Vibrating. jnp-s.
OBJECTS, IMAGINARY. hæm. jnp-s. trg.
Bright. jnp-s. trg.
Mist. hæm. jnp-s.
Vibrations. jnp-s. trg.
    Bright. jnp-s. trg.

SIGHT IMPAIRED. cof. hæm. hg. jnp-s. k-o.
EYEBALL. ag-na. alli. cit-c. cro. dig. grc. lyc. ox-x.
phy. rs. sep. smi.
    Color Red. ag-na.
    Drawing. (alli).
    False Sensations. smi.
        Sand. smi.
    Gnawing. ox-x.
    Heat. grc.
    Itching. (alli). (grc).
    Lachrymation. cro. (dig). (grc). phy. rs.
            Hot. dig. grc. rs.
    Movements. (sep).
    Pressing. (p). (pol). (rs).
    Shooting. (lau-c). smi.
    Smarting. cit-c. ox-x.
    Swelling, Feeling of. (rs).
    Tearing. lyc.
    Tensive. ox-x.
    Throbbing. (trg).
    Undefined, ag-na. cit-c. (jcr).
ORBIT. jcr. lau-c. pol.
    Pressing. pol.
    Shooting. lau-c.
ORBIT SUPERIORLY. jcr.
    Undefined. jcr.
ORBITAL INTEGUMENTS. ox-x.
ORBITAL INTEGUMENTS SUPERIORLY. ox-x.
    Gnawing. ox-x.
    Smarting. ox-x.
    Tensive. ox-x.
EYELIDS. alli. p. rs. sep.
    Movements, Closing. sep.
UPPER EYELID. alli. p. rs.
    Pressing. p.
CANTHI. grc.
INTERNAL CANTHUS. grc.
    Itching. grc.
RIGHT. jcr. rs. trg.
    Eyeball, Throbbing. trg.
    Orbit Superiorly, Undefined. jcr.
    Upper Eyelid. Pressing. rs.
            Swelling, Feeling of. rs.

LEFT. alli. sep.
Eyeball, Drawing. alli.
Eyelids, Movements, Closing. sep.
Upper Eyelid, Itching. alli.

ROOM, In.

al-o. amm-cl. con. k-o. men. rut. *s.* s-x. zn.
OBJECTS, FALSE APPEARANCE of. k-o.
Large. k-o.
Moving. k-o.
    Circularly. k-o.
SIGHT IMPAIRED al-o. amm-cl. con.
EYEBALL. rut. s. s-x. zn.
False Sensations. (s-x).
    Sand. (s-x).
Heat. s-x. zn.
Lachrymation. rut.
Pressing. s-x.
Smarting. zn.
Tensive. s.
EYEBALL ANTERIORLY. s-x.
Heat. s-x.
Pressing. s-x.
CANTHI. s-x.
EXTERNAL CANTHUS. s-x.
RIGHT. s-x.
External Canthus, False Sensations, Sand. s-x.

WASHING.

al-o. amm-cl. asr. chd. cl-hx. cld. dl-s. frm. k-na. k-o.
mg-ca. na-ca. na-sa. ni-ca. p. pru-l. thu.
OBJECTS IMAGINARY. amm-cl. k-o. na-sa.
Leaf. (na-sa).
    White. (na-sa).
Mist. amm-cl. k-o.
White. (na-sa).
SIGHT IMPAIRED. al-o. amm-cl. chd. k-o. ni-ca.
EYEBALL. al-o. amm-cl. frm. k-na. mg-ca. na-ca. na-sa.
ni-ca. pru-l. thu.
Color Red. ni-ca.

Discharge. (na-sa). pru-l.
> **Pus.** (na-sa).

Heat. al-o. amm-cl. asr. k-na. (thu).
Itching. na-ca.
Lachrymation. al-o. asr. mg-ca.
> **Hot.** (al-o).

Pressing. (p).
Smarting. al-o. na-ca.
Swelling, Feeling of. ni-ca.
Tearing. mg-ca.
Undefined. frm. ni-ca.
EYELIDS. chd. mg-ca. na-sa. p.
Adhesion of. chd. mg-ca. (na-sa).
UPPER EYELID. p.
Pressing. p.
RIGHT. na-ca. na-sa. thu.
Objects Imaginary, Leaf White. na-sa.
> **White.** na-sa.

Eyeball, Heat. thu.
> **Itching.** na-ca.
> **Shooting.** na-ca.

LEFT. al-o. na-sa.
Eyeball, Discharge, Pus. na-sa.
> **Heat.** al-o.
> **Lachrymation.** al-o.
> **Hot.** al-o.
> **Smarting.** al-o.

Eyelids, Adhesion of. na-sa.

LYING.

cb-a. lyc. smc. spo. str.
OBJECTS, FALSE APPEARANCE **of.** cb-a. spo. str.
> **Moving.** cb-a. spo. str.
> **Vertically.** spo. str.
> **Up and Down.** spo. str.

Multiplied. spo.
SIGHT IMPAIRED. spo.
EYEBALL. lyc.

Boring. (smc).
Tearing. lyc.
Throbbing. (smc.)
ORBIT. smc.
ORBIT SUPERIORLY. smc.
RIGHT. smc.
Orbit Superiorly, Boring. smc.
   Throbbing. smc.

REST.

cmc.
EYEBALL. cmc.
Pressing. cmc.
Undefined. cmc.
EYEBALL POSTERIORLY. cmc.
FORWARDS. cmc.
Eyeball, Pressing. cmc.
DOWNWARDS. cmc.
Eyeball, Pressing. cmc.
To HEAD. cmc.
To OCCIPUT. cmc.
Eyeball Posteriorly, Undefined. cmc.

SITTING.

acon. ara-d. arn. asr. led. s.
OBJECTS, FALSE APPEARANCE **of**. acon. arn.
Moving. acon. arn.
  Circularly. acon. arn.
EYEBALL. ara-d. asr. led. s.
Heat. ara-d. asr.
Lachrymation. asr.
Tearing. led.
Tensive. s.

PRESSURE.

al-o. amm-cl. atp. bry. ca-ca. cac. hll. k-o. men. mn-ca.
na-cl. ppv. ptv. pul. trn. vr-a.

EYEBALL. al-o. atp. ca-ca. k-o. men. mn-ca. na-cl. ppv.
ptv. trn. vr-a.
  Bruised. (ptv). vr-a.
  Drawing. mn-ca.
  Dryness. ppv.
  False Sensations. ppv.
      Sand. ppv.
  Heat. atp. (bry).
  Itching. atp.
  Movements. al-o.
     Convulsions. al-o.
  Pressing. (cac). (hll). k-o. (na-cl).
     Like a Nail. (hll).
  Shooting. (trn).
  Tearing. (amm-cl).
  Undefined. (men). na-cl.
EYEBALL EXTERNALLY. vr-a.
  Bruised. vr-a.
ORBIT. amm-cl. cac. hll. mn-ca.
  Drawing. mn-ca.
ORBIT SUPERIORLY. amm-cl. cac. hll.
ORBITAL INTEGUMENTS. bry.
ORBITAL INTEGUMENTS SUPERIORLY. bry.
  Heat. bry.
CANTHI. vr-a.
EXTERNAL CANTHUS. vr-a.
FORWARDS. na-cl.
  Eyeball, Pressing. na-cl.
To HEAD. trn.
To SIDE OF HEAD. trn.
RIGHT. amm-cl. cac. ptv. vr-a.
  Eyeball, Bruised. ptv.
  Orbit Superiorly, Pressing. cac.
             Tearing. amm-cl.
  External Canthus, Bruised. vr-a.
LEFT. al-o. hll. men. trn.
  Eyeball, Movements, Convulsions. al-o.
        Undefined. men.
  Orbit Superiorly, Pressing. hll.
           Like a Nail. hll.
To Side of Head. Eyeball, Shooting. trn.

PRESSURE CONTINUED

amm-cl.
EYEBALL.
Tearing. (amm-cl).
ORBIT. amm-cl.
ORBIT SUPERIORLY. amm-cl.
RIGHT. amm-cl.
Orbit Superiorly, Tearing. amm-cl.

PRESSURE UPWARDS.

atp.
EYEBALL. atp.
Heat. atp.
Itching. atp.

RUBBING.

aga. al-o. alli. amm-ca. amm-cl. aps. art-v. atp. bar. ca-a.
ca-ca. ca-o. cap. cb-a. ccs. chd. co. cro. cth. dl-s. dt. eupat-p.
euph. f-hx. grc. grt. gym. hyo. ind. jat. jnc. k-bicr. k-i. k-o.
kre. krm. lam. lct. ly-b. mg-ca. mg-cl. mll. mrl. msc. na-ba.
na-ca. na-cl. na-sa. ol-a. os. p. p-x. pb. phl. phy. ppv. pru-l.
pt. pul. rn-b. rs. s. s-x. se. smr. sn. spi. spo. sr-ca. str. thu.
trg. trn. tx-b. urt. vi-t. vtx. zn. zng.
OBJECTS, FALSE APPEARANCE of. cro.
White. cro.
OBJECTS IMAGINARY. al-o. art-v. cro. kre. krm.
(ly-b). p. pb. pul. trg.
Feathers. al-o. kre.
Mist. al-o. art-v. cro. (ly-b). (p). pb. pul. trg.
Spots. krm.
White. krm.
Threads. al-o.
White. krm.
SIGHT IMPAIRED. al-o. art-v. cap. cro. (k-o). (ly-b).
mll. na-ca. p. p-x. pb. pul. trg.
EYEBALL. aga. amm-ca. amm-cl. ca-o. cb-a. ccs. chd.
co. cro. dt. eupat-p. k-i. k-o. mg-ca. mg-cl. msc. na-ba. na-cl.
na-sa. ol-a. p. phl. ppv. pru-l. pt. rn-b. sn. spi. sr-ca. str. trn.
tx-b. vtx. zng.

Crampy. (msc).

Creeping. atp. (na-sa). (pt).

Discharge. aga.

Drawing. tx-b.

Dryness. ppv.

False Sensations. atp. ca-o. (cb-a). ccs. (co). (dt). (k-o). mg-cl. na-ba. p. ppv. rn-b. (trn). zng.

 Hair. ccs. (trn).

 Pellicle. (k-o).

 Sand. atp. (cb-a). (co). (dt). mg-cl. na-ba. p. ppv. rn-b. zng.

 Splinter. ca-o.

Heat. cro. ol-a. (phl). (spi). (tx-b).

Itching. aga. (alli). amm-ca. (art-v). (atp). (bar). (ca-a). cb-a. (chd). (dl-s). (dt). (euph). (f-hx). (grt). (hyo). (jat). (jnc). k-o. (lam). (mg-ca). (mg-cl). msc. na-cl. ol-a. (os). p. phl. (phy). pru-l. pt. (rs). (se). (sn). (spi). (spo). str. tx-b. (vi-t).

Lachrymation. eupat-p. (na-sa).

Movements. amm-cl. (hyo).

 Convulsions. amm-cl.

Paralysis. (mrl).

Pressing. atp. (chd). cro. mg-cl. na-sa. (ol-a).

Shooting. (atp). (ca-a). (cb-a). (grt). (ind). (ol-a). phl. (spo). (vi-t).

Smarting. amm-ca. (cb-a). (grc). (hyo). (ind). (jat). (k-i). (k-o). (lct). (mg-ca). (phl). (rs). (s-x). smr. (sr-ca) (vtx). (zn).

Tearing. (hyo).

Tensive. (k-o).

Throbbing. (chd).

Tingling. (art-v).

EYEBALL SUPERIORLY. co.

False Sensations, Sand. co.

ORBITAL INTEGUMENTS. f-hx. na-cl. ol-a. pru-l. spi. spo. vi-t.

ORBITAL INTEGUMENTS SUPERIORLY. f-hx. na-cl. ol-a. pru-l. spi. vi-t.

 Itching. f-hx. na-cl. pru-l.

 Shooting. ol-a.

ORBITAL INTEGUMENTS INFERIORLY. spo.

EYELIDS. alli. art-v. chd. dl-s. euph. grt. jat. jnc. lam. mrl. ol-a. phl. pru-l. rs. s-x. se. tx-b.

Heat. tx-b.
Itching. grt. tx-b.
Tingling. art-v.
UPPER EYELID. alli. chd. dl-s. mrl. pru-l. rs.
Itching. pru-l.
Paralysis, Opening Difficult. mrl.
LOWER EYELID. euph. lam. ol-a. phl. s-x.
Itching. euph. lam. ol-a.
Smarting. s-x.
TARSAL EDGES. dl-s. jat. jnc. grt. se.
Itching. jat.
Smarting. dl-s.
UPPER TARSAL EDGE. dl-s.
Itching. dl-s.
CANTHI. art-v. atp. bar. ca-a. cb-a. dl-s. euph. grc. grt. hyo. ind. k-o. lam. lct. mg-ca. mg-cl. msc. os. phl. phy. pru-l. pt. zn.
Crampy. msc.
Creeping. pt.
Itching. art-v. hyo. k-o. lam.
Movements, Convulsions. hyo.
Smarting. hyo. lct.
EXTERNAL CANTHUS. ca-a. euph. grc. ol-a.
Shooting. ca-a.
Smarting. grc.
INTERNAL CANTHUS. atp. bar. ca-a. cb-a. dl-s. grt. ind. mg-ca. mg-cl. os. phl. phy. pru-l. zn.
Heat. phl.
Itching. atp. bar. ca-a. dl-s. grt. mg-ca. phl. pru-l.
Shooting. atp. ca-a. grt. ind. phl.
Smarting. cb-a. ind. zn.
RIGHT. chd. dt. k-i. k-o. mg-ca. mg-cl. na-sa. ol-a. rs. sr-ca. spi. vtx.
Sight Impaired. k-o.
Eyeball, False Sensations, Pellicle. k-o.
Sand. dt.
Itching. chd. dt. ol-a.
Lachrymation. na-sa.
Smarting. k-i. mg-ca. sr-ca. vtx.
Tensive. k-o.
Orbital Integuments Superiorly, Heat. spi.
Itching. spi.
Pressing. ol-a.

Upper Eyelid, Itching. rs.

        Smarting. rs.

External Canthus, Heat. ol-a.

        Throbbing. chd.

Internal Canthus, Itching. mg-cl.

        Smarting. mg-ca.

LEFT. alli. cb-a. chd. euph. lct. ly-b. mg-ca. na-sa. ol-a. os. p. pru-l. sn. spi. spo. trn. vi-t. zng.

Objects Imaginary, Mist. ly-b.

Sight Impaired. ly-b.

Eyeball, Creeping. na-sa.

        False Sensations, Hair. trn.

            Sand. cb-a. p. zng.

        Itching. mg-ca. ol-a. sn. spi.

        Shooting. ol-a.

        Smarting. mg-ca. zu.

Orbital Integuments Superiorly, Itching. pru-l. vi-t.

        Shooting. vi-t.

Orbital Integuments Inferiorly, Itching. spo.

        Shooting. spo.

Upper Eyelid, Itching. alli. chd.

Lower Eyelid, Smarting. phl.

Canthus, Smarting. lct.

External Canthus, Itching. euph.

Internal Canthus, Itching. os.

        Smarting. cb-a.

TOUCH.

gui. hyo. k-o. men. spo. thu.

EYEBALL.

Gnawing. (hyo).

Heat. (men).

Pressing. (hyo).

Shooting. (spo).

Smarting. (thu).

Tearing. (thu).

Tensive. (men). (spo).

ORBITAL INTEGUMENTS. gui. hyo. thu.

ORBITAL INTEGUMENTS SUPERIORLY. hyo. thu.

Gnawing. hyo.
Pressing. hyo.
Smarting. thu.
EYELIDS. men.
UPPER EYELID. men.
CANTHI. spo.
EXTERNAL CANTHUS. spo.
LEFT. men. spo. thu.
Orbital Integuments Superiorly, Tearing. thu.
Upper Eyelid, Heat. men.
　　　　Tensive. men.
External Canthus, Shooting. spo.
　　　　Tensive. spo.

RISING. (Generally).

atp. au. cb-v. glo. ol-a. p. rn-b. rs. str.
OBJECTS, FALSE APPEARANCE of. au.
Moving. au.
　　Circularly. au.
EYEBALL. glo. ol-a. rs.
Heat. ol-a. rs.
Pressing. glo. rs.

RISING from LYING.

atp. cb-v. glo. ol-a. p. rn-b. rs. str.
EYEBALL. glo. ol-a. rs.
Heat. ol-a. rs.
Pressing. glo. rs.

RISING from STOOPING.

au.
OBJECTS, FALSE APPEARANCE of. au.
Moving. au.
　　Circularly. au.

STOOPING.

acon. arn. ba-ca.
OBJECTS, FALSE APPEARANCE of. arn.

Moving. arn.
   Circularly. arn.
EYEBALL.   acon.
Bursting.   (acon).
Pressing.   (ba-ca).
Undefined.   (acon).
EYEBALL SUPERIORLY.   acon.
Bursting.   acon.
Undefined.   acon.
ORBIT.   ba-ca.
Pressing.   ba-ca.

WALKING.

acon. amb. bry. grc. hyo. na-cl. ol-a. ox-x. pul. trg.
OBJECTS, FALSE APPEARANCE **of**.   acon. bry.
Moving.   acon. bry.
   Circularly.   acon. bry.
OBJECTS IMAGINARY.   trg.
Bright.   trg.
Vibrations.   trg.
   Bright.   trg.
SIGHT IMPAIRED.   na-cl.
EYEBALL.   grc. ol-a. ox-x.
Gnawing.   ox-x.
Heat.   grc. ol-a.
Smarting.   ox-x.
ORBITAL INTEGUMENTS.   ox-x.
ORBITAL INTEGUMENTS SUPERIORLY.   ox-x.
Gnawing.   ox-x.
Smarting.   ox-x.
Tensive.   ox-x.

EFFORT of WILL.

atp. gel.
OBJECTS, FALSE APPEARANCE **of**.   atp. gel.
Moving.   atp.
   Undulating.   atp.
Multiplied.   atp. gel.
SIGHT IMPAIRED.   atp.

MENTAL EXERTION.

p.
EYEBALL.
Pressing. (p).
EYELIDS. p.
UPPER EYELID. p.
Pressing. p.

MOVING HEAD BACKWARDS.

atp. pol.
OBJECTS, FALSE APPEARANCE **of.** pol.
Multiplied. pol.
SIGHT IMPAIRED. atp.

MOVING HEAD ROUND to RIGHT.

ca-ca.
SIGHT IMPAIRED. ca-ca.

DARKNESS.

atp. dt. k-i. myris. p. s. si-x.
SIGHT IMPAIRED. (atp). dt. myris. p. s. si-x.
LEFT. atp.
Sight Impaired. atp.

LIGHT, **Artificial.**

ag-na. amm-cl. (atp).
SIGHT IMPAIRED. ag-na. (atp).
EYEBALL. amm-cl.
Heat. amm-cl.
LEFT. atp.
Sight Impaired. atp.

LIGHT, **Natural.**

(dt). srr.
SIGHT IMPAIRED. (dt). srr.

When FIRST LOOKING.

con.
OBJECTS, FALSE APPEARANCE of. con.
Multiplied. con.

LOOKING FIXEDLY. (Long).

al-o. bap. cb-v. con. drm. dt. eug. lac-c. lct. li-ca. p-x.
pet. smc.
OBJECTS, FALSE APPEARANCE of. eug. li-ca. smc.
Moving. smc.
   Vibrating. smc.
Multiplied. eug.
Part Visible. li-ca.
OBJECTS, IMAGINARY. dt. lac-c.
Figures. lac-c.
   Side of Visual Ray, at. lac-c.
Side of Visual Ray, at. lac-c.
Vibrations. dt.
SIGHT IMPAIRED. bap. con. drm. dt. eug. lct. p-x.
Presbyopia. dt.

LOOKING through a DOUBLE CONVEX LENS.

atp.
SIGHT IMPAIRED. atp.
Presbyopia. atp.

LOOKING through a PIN-HOLE.

atp.
SIGHT IMPAIRED. atp.
Presbyopia. atp.

LOOKING UP.

cast.
OBJECTS, IMAGINARY. cast.
Veil. cast.

LOOKING DOWN.

ba-a. vr-s.
EYEBALL. ba-a. vr-s.
Pressing. ba-a. vr-s.

LOOKING SIDEWAYS.

ca-ca. mg-cl. qu-sa. s.
OBJECTS IMAGINARY. mg-cl.
High up. mg-cl.
Mist. mg-cl.
Rocks. mg-cl.
    High up. mg-cl.
SIGHT IMPAIRED. ca-ca. qu-sa. s.

LOOKING STRAIGHT.

gel. pol.
OBJECTS, FALSE APPEARANCE of. gel.
Multiplied. gel.
OBJECTS, IMAGINARY. pol.
Bright. pol.
Spots. pol.
    Bright. pol.

LOOKING at DISTANT **Objects.**

dt.
OBJECTS, IMAGINARY. (dt).
Figures. (dt).
SIGHT IMPAIRED. dt.
Presbyopia. dt.

LOOKING at SMALL **Objects.**

ca-ca. ca-s. cof. dt. mgs-au.
OBJECTS, FALSE APPEARANCE of. dt.
Oblique. dt.
SIGHT IMPAIRED. ca-ca. cof. mgs-au.

LOOKING AWAY for a MOMENT.

p-x.
SIGHT IMPAIRED. p-x.
Presbyopia. p-x.

HOLDING FINGER VERTICALLY before NOSE.

gel.
SIGHT IMPAIRED. gel.

LACHRYMATION.

ca-ca. p-x. snp. spi.
OBJECTS, IMAGINARY. ca-ca. spi.
Bright. spi.
Feathers. ca-ca.
Flames. spi.
Veil. ca-ca.
SIGHT IMPAIRED. ca-ca. p-x. spi.
EYEBALL. snp.
Shooting. (snp).
LEFT. snp.
Eyeball, Shooting. snp.

MOVING EYES.

cit-c. n-x. p.
OBJECTS, IMAGINARY. cit-c. n-x. p.
Bright. cit-c.
Circle. p.
    Variegated. p.
Cobweb. n-x.
Spots. cit-c.
    Bright. cit-c.
Variegated. p.

MOVING EYELIDS.

sn.
EYEBALL. sn.
Scraping. sn.

OPENING EYELIDS.

ag-na. asr. si-x. spo.
OBJECTS, FALSE APPEARANCE of. si-x.
Moving. si-x.
    Circularly. si-x.
OBJECTS, IMAGINARY. spo.
Bright. spo.
Flames. spo.
SIGHT IMPAIRED. ag-na.
EYEBALL.
Movements. (asr).
    Convulsions. (asr).
EYELIDS. asr.
UPPER. EYELID. asr.
LEFT. asr.
Upper Eyelid, Movements, Convulsions. asr.

CLOSING EYELIDS.

al-o. anan. asr. au. ba-a. chd. cic. cmc. cro. cth. dt. gel.
grt. hpm. k-o. lyc. myris. n-x. narth. p-x. pol. pt. sep.
snp-n. spi. str.
OBJECTS, FALSE APPEARANCE of. pol. str.
Moving. str.
    Vertically. str.
        Up and Down. str.
Multiplied. pol.
OBJECTS, IMAGINARY. n-x.
Cobweb. n-x.
PHOTOPHOBIA. k-o.
SIGHT IMPAIRED. anan. asr. cro. grt.
EYEBALL. au. ba-a. chd. dt. gel. hpm. k-o. p-x. pt.
snp-n. spi.
Dryness. spi.
False Sensations. chd. (dt).
        Sand. chd. (dt).
Heat. pt. spi.
Movements. gel.
    Convulsions. gel.
Paralysis. (myris).
Pressing. ba-a. (cic). k-o. snp-n.

Shooting. (p-x).
Tensive. au.
Undefined. chd. snp-n.
EYEBALL SUPERIORLY. p-x.
Shooting. p-x.
EYEBALL EXTERNALLY. dt.
EYELIDS. myris.
CANTHI. cic. p-x. snp-n.
INTERNAL CANTHUS. cic. p-x. snp-n.
Heat. p-x.
Pressing. snp-n.
DOWNWARDS. snp-n.
Internal Canthus, Pressing. snp-n.
RIGHT. cic. myris.
Eyelids, Paralysis, Opening Difficult. myris.
Internal Canthus, Pressing. cic.
RIGHT. dt.
Eyeball Externally, False Sensations, Sand. dt.

CLOSING ONE EYE.

ca-ca. gel. p. pol.
OBJECTS, FALSE APPEARANCE of. ca-ca. pol.
Multiplied. ca-ca. pol.
SIGHT IMPAIRED. gel.

CLOSING LEFT EYE.

pol.
OBJECTS, FALSE APPEARANCE of. pol.
Multiplied. pol.

BLOWING NOSE.

(au).
EYEBALL. (au).
Undefined. (au).

DISCHARGE from NOSE.

k-i. mgs.
SIGHT IMPAIRED. k-i.
EYEBALL. k-i.
Dryness. (mgs).

Smarting. k-i.
EYELIDS. mgs.
Dryness. mgs.

HÆMORRHAGE. from NOSE.

br.
EYEBALL. br.
Undefined. br.

SNEEZING.

mgs.
EYEBALL.
Dryness. (mgs).
EYELIDS. mgs.
Dryness. mgs.

EATING.

chi. fe-mgs. li-ca. men. smc. snp-s.
OBJECTS, IMAGINARY. fe-mgs.
Blue. fe-mgs.
Bright. fe-mgs.
Circles. fe-mgs.
　　Blue. fe-mgs.
　　Bright. fe-mgs.
　　Red. fe-mgs.
　　Zigzags. fe-mgs.
Red. fe-mgs.
Zigzags. fe-mgs.
SIGHT IMPAIRED. fe-mgs.
EYEBALL. men. snp-s.
Boring. (smc).
Movements. (men).
　　Convulsions. (men).
Pressing. men. snp-n.
Throbbing. (smc).
Undefined. snp-n.
ORBIT. chi. li-ca. smc.
Undefined. li-ca.
ORBIT SUPERIORLY. chi. smc.
Undefined. chi.

EYELIDS. men.
Movements, Convulsions. men.
DOWNWARDS. snp-n.
Eyeball, Pressing. snp-n.
RIGHT. smc.
Orbit Superiorly, Boring. smc.
         Throbbing. smc.
LEFT. li-ca.
Orbit, Undefined. li-ca.

FLATUS, Emission of.

ca-a.
OBJECTS, FALSE APPEARANCE of. ca-a.
Strange. ca-a.
PHOTOMANIA. ca-a.

VOMITING.

rph.
SIGHT IMPAIRED. rph.

URINATING.

gel.
SIGHT IMPAIRED. gel.

SPEAKING.

lac-d.
EYEBALL. lac-d.
Undefined. lac-d.

On GOING to SLEEP.

smc.
EYEBALL.
Boring. (smc).
Throbbing. (smc).
ORBIT. smc.
ORBIT SUPERIORLY. smc.
RIGHT. smc.
  bit Superiorly, Boring. smc.
        Throbbing. smc.

WAKING.

ca-ca. chi. cro.
SIGHT IMPAIRED. chi.

SWEAT.

rho.
EYEBALL. rho.
Heat.. rho.

TOUCHING the OBJECT.

pru-l.
OBJECTS, FALSE APPEARANCE **of.** pru-l.
Large. pru-l.

COFFEE.

trg.
EYEBALL. trg.
Itching. trg.
Pressing. trg.

TOBACCO.

ara-d.
EYEBALL. ara-d.
Heat. ara-d.

WINE.

aga.
EYEBALL. aga.
Contractive. (aga).
Lachrymation. (aga).
Movements. (aga).
    Convulsions. (aga).
Smarting. (aga).
CHANGING CHARACTER **or** PLACE. aga.

Eyeball, Contractive then Lachrymation. (aga).

             „   **then Smarting.** (aga).

       Lachrymation then Movements, Convul-sions. (aga).

       Smarting then   „   (aga).

RIGHT then LEFT. aga.

Eyeball, Movements, Convulsions. aga.

Right Eyeball Contractive, then Left Eyeball Movements, Convulsions. aga.

          Lachrymation, then   „   aga.

          Smarting, then   „   aga.

RIGHT. aga.

Eyeball, Contractive. aga.

       Lachrymation. aga.

       Movements, Convulsions. aga.

       Smarting. aga.

Changing. Eyeball Contractive then Lachry-mation. aga.

       „   „   **then Smarting.** aga.

LEFT. aga.

Eyeball, Movements, Convulsions. aga.

APPENDIX.

In the Rubric **Changing Character or Place**, at page 62, the collectives of the varieties of Change, either of Character or Place, were omitted. As they are rather numerous, to give them as **addenda** would confuse; I have therefore here reprinted the entire Rubric in its complete form. A strict arrangement would also require a similar change to be made in the Rubric **Alternating in Character or Place** at page 65, but as the symptoms in this Rubric are very few, I have not thought it necessary to make any alteration.

CHANGING CHARACTER or PLACE in EYES.

aga. amb. atp. ba-ca. ber. bru. ca-a. ca-ca. ca-s. can. cb-a. ccs. chd. chio. cic. cl-hx. con. cot. cro. crot. cu. cy-hx. dl-s. dt. (ery). eryn. f-hx. gn-l. grp. jnp-s. k-bicra. k-ca. k-o. kre. lam. lau-c. men. mg-ca. mgs. mgs-ar. msc. n-x. na-ba. na-cl. na-sa. ner. p. p-x. pb. phy. pnx. pol. pru-l. pul. qu-sa. s. sb-t. sep. si-x. smb. smc. smi. sn. spi. spo. sr-ca. str-i. thu. trg. trn. trx. u-na.

OBJECTS, FALSE APPEARANCE of. **Blue then Grey.** atp.

    Blue then White. atp.

    Bright then Red. atp.

    Red then Blue. atp.

OBJECTS IMAGINARY. **Bright then White.** p-x.

Bright then Red. f-hx.

Mist then Bright. (na-sa).

   ,, then **Green.** (na-sa).

   ,, then **Stars.** (na-sa).

   ,, then ,, **Bright Green Yellow Near Eye.** (na-sa).

   ,, then **Yellow.** (na-sa).

Plain White then Bright. p-x.

Spots Bright then White. p-x.

Vibrations then Flames. f-hx.

   ,, **Bright Red then** ,, **Red.** f-hx.

White then Bright. p-x.

SIGHT IMPAIRED. **Presbyopia then Myopia.** dt. phy.

EYEBALL. **Coldness then False Sensations, Sand.** f-hx.

   ,,   **then Shooting.** mgs-ar.

Color Red then Discharge, Pus. (eryn).

   ,,   **then Itching.** (bru).

   ,,   **then Lachrymation.** grp.

Contractive then Lachrymation. (aga).

   ,,   **then Smarting.** (aga).

Drawing then Lachrymation. grp.

   ,,   **then Pressing.** (rho).

Eruptions, Blisters then Granulations. sb-t.

False Sensations, Hairs then Pressing. (ccs).

            Pellicle then Shooting. (k-o).

            Wind (cold) then Sand. f-hx.

Gnawing then Discharge. (kre).

Heat then Coldness. chd.

   ,,   **then Color Red.** sr-ca.

   ,,   **then Discharge.** (kre).

   ,,   **then Pressing.** (atp).

   ,,   **then Shooting.** sr-ca.

Itching then Color Red. kre.

   ,,   **then Discharge.** (kre).

   ,,   **then False Sensations, Sand.** kre.

   ,,   **then Heat.** cb-a. k-bicra. kre.

   ,,   **then Lachrymation.** cb-a. k-o.

   ,,   **then Pressing.** ca-ca. cb-a. kre. (pru-l). trg.

   ,,   **then Smarting.** kre.

   ,,   **then Undefined.** k-bicra.

Lachrymation then Dryness. s.

      ,,   **then Movements, Convulsions.** (aga).

Motion in then Sensitive. (cb-a).

Movements, Convulsions then Itching.

Pressing then Color Red. kre.

   ,,   **then Discharge, Pus.** (eryn).

   ,,   **then Lachrymation.** ca-s. grp. kre.

   ,,   **Hot.** grp. kre.

   ,,   **then Shooting.** k-ca.

Sensitive then Drawing. (ber).

   ,,   **then Pressing.** (na-sa).

   ,,   **then Shooting.** (gn-l).

   ,,   **then Throbbing.** (ber).

Shooting then **Color Red.** n-x.
     „   then **Drawing.** (mgs).
     „   then **Heat.** (p-x).
     „   then **Lachrymation.** (snp).
              Feeling of. (ba-ca).
     „   then **Numbness.** (s).
     „   then **Pressing.** (ba-ca). (na-sa). spo.
Smarting then **Dryness.** (s).
     „   then **Lachrymation.** s.
     „   then **Movements, Convulsions.** (aga).
Softness, Feeling of, then **Pressing.** (na-sa).
Swelling then **Color Red.** (chio).
     „   then **Discharge, Pus.** (eryn).
     „   then **Eruptions, Pustules.** (chio).
     „   then **Itching.** (chio).
     „   then **Wrinkled.** (chio).
Tearing then **Lachrymation.** mg-ca.
     „   then **Shooting.** (thu).
Tensive then **Shooting.** (k-o).
Throbbing then **Pressing.** (amb).
     „   then **Sensitive.** (thu).
Tingling then **Drawing.** (ber).
     „   then **Pressing.** (amb).
     „   then **Throbbing.** (ber).
Undefined then **Color Red.** crot.
     „   then **Shooting.** (gn-l).
IRIS. **Pupils Contracted** then **Dilated.** aga-p.
atp. can. cic. cl-hx. cu. dl-s. jnp-s. k-o. lam. lau-c. men.
pb. pnx. pol. pul. smb. smc. sn. trx.
        Dilated then **Contracted.** aga. atp. ca-a.
cy-hx. ner. p-x. qu-sa.
ORBIT. **Shooting** then **Pressing.** ba-ca.
·TARSAL EDGES. **Sensitive** then **Drawing.** ber.
                       then **Throbbing.** ber.
Tingling then **Drawing.** ber.
     „   then **Throbbing.** ber.
EYELIDS, INNER SURFACE. **Smarting then
Dryness.** s.
CANTHI. **Color Red** then **Itching.** bru.
OBJECTS, IMAGINARY then SIGHT IMPAIRED.
p.
OBJECTS, IMAGINARY then EYEBALL. (ery).
na-sa. spi.

Flames Red then Lachrymation. spi.
Mist Red then Lachrymation. (ery).
Red then Lachrymation. (ery). spi.
OBJECTS, IMAGINARY then IRIS. spi.
Flames Red then Pupils Dilated. spi.
Red then Pupils Dilated. spi.
SIGHT IMPAIRED then OBJECTS IMAGINARY.
na-sa.
SIGHT IMPAIRED then SIGHT DAZZLED. na-cl.
SIGHT IMPAIRED then EYEBALL. ca-ca. dt. kre.
p-x. spi.

„	then **Appearance Dim**. dt.	
„	then **Color Red**. kre.	
„	then **Lachrymation**. ca-ca. dt. kre.	

p-x. spi.

Hot. kre.

„	then **Pressing**. dt.	
„	then **Smarting**. dt.	

SIGHT IMPAIRED then IRIS. spi.

„   then **Pupils Dilated**. spi.
EYEBALL then OBJECTS IMAGINARY. k-ca. spi.
Heat, then Flames Red. spi.
„   then **Red**. spi.
Shooting then Mist. k-ca.
EYEBALL, then SIGHT IMPAIRED. cic. con. cro.
k-ca. msc. sep. spi.

Appearance Staring, then	„	cic. msc.
Heat, then	„	spi.
Lachrymation, then	„	cro.
Pressing, then	„	cro. (sep).
Shooting, then	„	k-ca.
Undefined, then	„	con. cro.

EYEBALL, then CORNEA. phy.
Color Red, then Opacity. phy.
EYEBALL, then IRIS. msc.
Appearance Staring, then Pupils Contracted. msc.
EYEBALL, then LENS. atp. n-x.
Color Red, then Cataract. atp. n-x.
EYEBALL, then ORBIT. cb-a.
EYEBALL, then EYELIDS. eryn. gn-l. k-bicra. u-na.
Itching, then Adhesion of. k-bicra.
EYEBALL, then UPPER EYELID. gn-l.

Sensitive, then **Shooting.** gn-l.
Undefined, then ,, gn-l.
EYEBALL, then CANTHI. cot. kre.
Gnawing, then Discharge. kre.
Heat, then ,, kre.
Itching, then ,, kre.
EYEBALL, then EXTERNAL CANTHUS. cot.
ORBIT, then EYEBALL. ba-ca.
Shooting, then Lachrymation, Feeling of. ba-ca.
ORBIT, then ORBIT SUPERIORLY. chio.
Pressing, then Downwards Pressing. chio.
ORBIT, then EYELIDS. ba-ca.
EYELIDS, then OBJECTS IMAGINARY. spi.
Movements, Closing, then Flames Red. spi.
          ,,   **then Red.** spi.
EYELIDS, then SIGHT IMPAIRED. spi.
Movements, Closing then ,, spi.
EYELIDS, then EYEBALL. f-hx. lau-c. smi. str-i.
Adhesion, then Lachrymation. smi, str-i.
Movements, Closing, then Appearance Staring.
lau-c.
          ,,   **then** ,, **Upward**
Looking. lau-c.
          ,,   **Opening Spasmodically, then False**
Sensations, Sand. f-hx.
EYELIDS, then ORBIT. cb-a. na-ba.
UPPER EYELID, then ORBIT. cb-a.
CANTHI, then EYELIDS. k-bicra. pul.
EXTERNAL CANTHUS, then EYELIDS. pul.
Pressing, then Adhesion. pul.
INTERNAL CANTHUS, then LOWER EYELID.
k-bicra.
Heat, then Heat. k-bicra.
EYEBALL to JAW, then EYEBALL to ABDOMEN.
mgs.
          ,,   **then** ,, **to CHEST.** mgs.
          ,,   **then** ,, **to BACK.** mgs.
          ,,   **then** ,, **to LEGS.** mgs.

ERRATA.

All through the volume make the following corrections :—

  For ara. *read* ara-d.

    „ hg-bi. „ hg-bini.

    „ k-bicr. „ k-bicra.

    „ lac-ac. „ lac-cg.

    „ pru. „ pru-sp.

    „ so-t. „ so-t-æg.

Page 9, line I2, *for* clf. *read* clv.

Page 16, line 4 from bottom, *for* (pb). *read* (pul).

Page 21, line 5, *for* (Al-o). *read* (al-o).

Page 60, line 9, *for* fc-mgs. *read* fe-mgs.

Page 75, lines 11 to 13, *for*   **Black.** ⎱ *read* **Black.**

                        Moving. ⎰   **Moving.**

                    Moving.   **Moving.**

      lines 13 and 14 from bottom, *for* **Near Eye.**

                                    Yellow.

                    read—**Near Eye.**

                                    Yellow.

Page 120, line 4 from bottom, *for* na-sa. *read* (na-sa).

Page 130, *Heading, for* POSTURE, *read* SITUATION.

Page 269, line 2 from bottom, *for* isions *read* **Visions.**

INDEX.

—o—

SYMPTOMS PP. 1-99.

OPINIONS OF THE PRESS, &c.

"Carefully arranged."——"A valuable Repertory."—(*Hahnemannian Monthly,* 1869, p. 344).

"This work is rapidly making its way into favor as its character and scope become more developed. We have received numerous letters from our subscribers, who are delighted with it, and who are looking forward to the publication of 'The Head Chapter.' "—(*Hahnemannian Monthly,* 1869, p. 479.)

"Those who have made use of it pronounce it the most perfect and useful Repertory for the Head and Eye thus far published. It makes a book of 220 pages, which will often be consulted by those who are desirous to make exact prescriptions for affections of the eyes and head."—(*Hahnemannian Monthly,* 1871, p. 230.)

"*It is the only complete one we have; it is the clearest and best arranged;* and it will enable us to do twice as much as formerly in diseases of the eyes."——"Those who do not like to be fed by what others have chewed for them, will be glad to have it."—(*Constantine Hering, M.D.,* 1869.)

"Whenever I have used your Repertory, I have found it very complete."—
(*A. Lippe, M.D.,* 1870.)

"Your work is practical, and a safe guide into that vast labyrinth of our Materia Medica"——"I am well aware that the getting up of such a work requires a peculiar tact and considerable lexicographical talent, which you (to me) seem to possess."—(*B. Finck?, M.D.,* 1870.)

"I am glad your complete Repertory is about to be published. Through your kindness I have used a MS. copy of it for some time, and have found it most useful in the elucidation of the Eye cases that have come under my care. I have been repeatedly directed to medicines which would never have suggested themselves, but for the aid supplied by the Repertory. For completeness and fulness of symptoms it seems to me unique,—and the arrangement both of symptoms and conditions is as nearly perfect as the present state of our knowledge admits. I believe it will become indispensible to every medical man who desires to practice with scientific accuracy and precision, and I hope it will encourage others to take up other regions of the body to make Repertories of them with equal earnestness and perseverance."—
(*R. M. Theobald, M.A., M.R.C.S.,* 1873.)

BY THE SAME AUTHOR,

THE PATHOGENETIC RECORD;

AN ARRANGEMENT OF THE PHYSIOLOGICAL AND TOXICOLOGICAL
EFFECTS OF DRUGS, COLLECTED FROM MEDICAL AND
GENERAL LITERATURE.

*Now being published as an Appendix to the British Journal
of Homœopathy.*

In course of Preparation (arranged like the present Volume),

DISEASES OF THE HEAD AND MIND.

DISEASES OF THE EARS.

DISEASES OF THE ABDOMEN.

DISEASES OF THE CHEST.

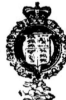

Milton Keynes UK
Ingram Content Group UK Ltd.
UKHW020654220923
429186UK00006B/409